Medical Dosage Calculations

Eighth Edition

June Looby Olsen, RN, MS
Professor of Nursing (Emeritus)
The College of Staten Island
Staten Island, New York

Anthony Patrick Giangrasso, PhD
Professor of Mathematics
La Guardia Community College
Long Island City, New York

Dolores M. Shrimpton, RN, MA
Associate Professor
Chairperson, Department of Nursing
Kingsborough Community College
Brooklyn, New York

PEARSON
Prentice Hall

Upper Saddle River, New Jersey, 07458

Library of Congress Cataloging-in-Publication Data

Olsen, June Looby.
    Medical dosage calculations / June Looby Olsen, Anthony Patrick Giangrasso, Dolores
M. Shrimpton.—8th ed.
        p. ; cm.
    Includes index.
    ISBN 0-13-113479-5
    1. Pharmaceutical arithmetic.   2. Pharmaceutical arithmetic—Problems, exercises, etc. I.
Giangrasso, Anthony Patrick. II. Shrimpton, Dolores M. III. Title.
    [DNLM: 1. Pharmaceutical Preparations—administration & dosage—Nurses' Instruction.
2. Mathematics—Nurses' Instruction. QV 748 O52m 2004]
RS57.M425 2004
615'.14—dc21

2003042866

Publisher: Julie Levin Alexander
Executive Assistant and Supervisor: Regina Bruno
Editor-in-Chief: Maura Connor
Senior Acquisitions Editor: Nancy Anselment
Editorial Assistant: Malgorzata Jaros-White
Director of Production and Manufacturing: Bruce Johnson
Managing Editor: Patrick Walsh
Production Liaison: Julie Li
Production Editor: Lisa Garboski, bookworks
Manufacturing Buyer: Pat Brown
Design Director: Cheryl Asherman
Senior Design Coordinator: Maria Guglielmo Walsh
Cover Designer: Mary Siener
Interior Designer: Mary Siener
Senior Marketing Manager: Nicole Benson
Channel Marketing Manager: Rachele Strober
Marketing Coordinator: Janet Ryerson
Supplements Editor: Yesenia Kopperman
Media Editor: John Jordan
Media Production Manager: Amy Peltier
Media Project Manager: Stephen Hartner
Compositor: Preparé
Printer/Binder: Banta Menasha
Cover/Printer: Phoenix Color Corporation

Pearson Education Ltd.
Pearson Education Singapore Pte. Ltd.
Pearson Education Canada, Ltd.
Pearson Education—Japan
Pearson Education Australia Pty. Limited

Pearson Education North Asia Ltd.
Pearson Educación de Mexico, S.A. de C.V.
Pearson Education Malaysia Pte. Ltd.

10 9 8 7 6 5 4 3 2
ISBN 0-13-113479-5

DEDICATION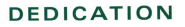

To my husband, Bill, my children, Keith and Michelle, and to my granddaughter, Taylor, who has brought so much joy to our family.

June Looby Olsen

To my darling wife, Susan, and to my children, Anthony, Michael, and Jennifer.

Anthony Patrick Giangrasso

To my son, Shawn, daughter-in-law, Kim, and grandaughter, Brooke Elizabeth for all the love and happiness they have brought into my life.

Dolores M. Shrimpton

PREFACE

In a growing range of health-care settings, nursing and allied health professionals are assuming increasing responsibilities in every aspect of drug administration. The first step in assuming this responsibility is learning to calculate drug dosages accurately. Dosage calculation is not just about math skills, it is an introduction to the **professional context** of drug administration. Calculation skills and the reason for their application—this is what *Medical Dosage Calculations* has taught thousands of students with unmatched success through seven editions.

Medical Dosage Calculations is a combined text and workbook designed for the student of dosage calculations. Its consistent focus on safety, accuracy, and professionalism make it a valuable part of a dosage calculation course for nursing or allied health-care programs. It is also highly effective for independent study and may be used as a refresher to dosage calculation skills or as a professional reference.

Topics introduced and developed in *Medical Dosage Calculations* include:

- basic arithmetic skills
- systems of measurement
- dosage calculations for all common forms of drug preparations
- IV and specialized calculations

In addition to these topics, this edition includes substantially more information about basic drug administration. Readers will learn how to interpret actual drug labels, package inserts, and various forms of medication orders, as well as how to recognize a wide variety of syringes.

Key Features of *Medical Dosage Calculations*

We have built on the strengths of the previous editions by continuing to provide the thoroughness of a textbook with the practicality and convenience of a workbook. Here are the important features that have made *Medical Dosage Calculations* an effective and popular book through seven editions.

- *Dimensional Analysis Calculation Method.* Dimensional analysis is a technique in which the units on the drug package are systematically converted to the units on the drug order. Conversion factors have traditionally been used to simplify complex calculations in physics and chemistry. However, before the first edition of this textbook in 1972, these methods had not been applied to drug calculations. Dosage calculation methods were limited to either the *ratio-and-proportion* method or the use of *memorized formulas*. Our innovation in dosage calculation has come to be imitated in many textbooks and accepted by an ever-increasing number of medical professionals over the three decades since we coined the phrase *Dimensional Analysis*.

- *Learn by Example.* Each chapter unfolds basic concepts and skills through the use of examples like the following:

  How many scored tablets would you give a patient, if the order is for 30 milligrams of codeine sulfate and each tablet contains 20 milligrams?

  In this problem you want to convert the order, 30 milligrams, to tablets.

  $$30 \, mg = ? \, tablets$$

  You want to cancel the milligrams and determine the equivalent amount in tablets.

  $$30 \, mg \times \frac{? \, tab}{? \, mg} = ? \, tab$$

  Since 1 tab = 20 mg, the fraction is $\dfrac{1 \, tab}{20 \, mg}$

  $$30 \, \cancel{mg} \times \frac{1 \, tab}{20 \, \cancel{mg}} = \frac{30 \, tab}{20} = 1\frac{1}{2} \, tab$$

  So, 30 milligrams is equivalent to $1\frac{1}{2}$ tablets, and you should give the patient $1\frac{1}{2}$ tablets of codeine sulfate.

- *Case Studies.* Realistic case scenarios allow the student to apply concepts and techniques presented in the text to a clinical setting.

- *Problem Sets.* This text/workbook offers learners more than 1000 practice opportunities. Answers to all but the Additional Exercises can be found in the book. Answers to the Additional Exercises are in the Instructor's Guide, and on the companion Website. Each chapter's practice opportunities are grouped into four problem sets:

  - Try These for Practice
  - Exercises
  - Additional Exercises
  - Cumulative Review Exercises

- *Comprehensive Self-Tests.* Upon completion of this text/workbook, these Self-Tests quiz the students' comprehensive knowledge. Answers to the Self-Tests can be found in the book.

Organization. The skills mastered in *Medical Dosage Calculations* are arranged into four basic learning units:

- **Unit 1: Basic Calculation and Administration Skills**

  After a review of basic number skills, this section introduces the essentials of drug administration. A separate chapter introduces dimensional analysis using a friendly, commonsense approach.

- **Unit 2: Systems of Measurement for Dosage Calculations**

  This section covers the three systems of measurement that nurses and other allied health professionals must understand to interpret medication orders and calculate dosages. Readers learn to convert measurements between and within measurement systems.

- **Unit 3: Common Medication Preparations**

  The chapters in this unit prepare readers to calculate oral and parenteral medication dosages and introduce the preparation of solutions.

- **Unit 4: Specialized Medication Preparations**

  This important final section provides a solid base for calculating IV and enteral flow rates, intravenous piggyback infusions and duration of infusions, as well as pediatric dosages.

Benefits of Using *Medical Dosage Calculations*

- Constant skill reinforcement through frequent practice opportunities.
- More than 1000 problems for students to solve.
- Commonly used medications featured.
- Actual drug labels, syringes, drug package inserts, and medication orders are illustrated throughout the text.
- Ample work space on every page for note-taking and problem-solving.
- Answers to the problem sets are found in Appendix A at the end of the text.

Supplemental Materials

Instructor's Manual

This combined *Instructor's Manual with Test Bank* provides extra test questions, answers to test questions, answers to Additional Exercises, a list of Key Terms, possible teaching approaches relevant to each chapter, an overview of chapter objectives, and seven comprehensive examinations with answers. In addition we have included six self-tests with answers. This guide helps instructors prepare lectures and examinations quickly.

Companion Website: www.prenhall.com/olsen   This on-line Study Guide includes objectives, multiple-choice questions, fill-in-the-blank, matching exercises, case studies, know-your-label exercises, comprehensive tests, and Web links.

Instructor's Resource CD-ROM   This resource includes Instructor's Manual, Test Bank, and PowerPoint Slides.

REVIEWERS FOR THE EIGHTH EDITION

Lisa M. Fiorentino, PhD, RN, CRNP
Assistant Professor of Nursing and Chair, Department of Nursing
University of Pittsburgh at Bradford
Bradford, Pennsylvania

Julie Garrison, Pharm.D
Clinical Instructor/Clinical Pharmacist
University of Washington School of Pharmacy
Seattle, Washington

Rebecca Crews Gruener, RN, MS
Associate Professor of Nursing
Louisiana State University at Alexandria
Alexandria, Louisiana

Peggy L. Hawkins, RN, PhD
Associate Professor of Nursing
College of Saint Mary
Omaha, Nebraska

Connie S. Heflin, MSN, RN
Professor
Paducah Community College
Paducah, Kentucky

Patricia K. Leary, MS
Allied Health Instructor
MOISD and FSU
Big Rapids, Michigan

Shirley F. Lishman, RN, MSN
Associate Professor
Texarkana College
Texarkana, Texas

Hope M. Moon, RN, MSN, CNS
Program Director, Associate Degree Nursing Program
Lorain County Community College
Elyria, Ohio

Scott Thigpen, RN, MSN, CCRN, CEN
Assistant Professor of Nursing
South Georgia College
Douglas, Georgia

Penelope S. Wright, PhD, RN
Associate Professor
University of Alabama School of Nursing
Birmingham, Alabama

Jan Clifton, MS, ATCL, CSCS
Professor
Danville Area Community College
Danville, IL

Kelly Dempsey, MSN, RN
Professor
Indiana University East
Richmond, IN

Janice Hausauer, MS, RN
Adjunct Assistant Professor
Montana State University College of Nursing
Bozeman, MT

Reviewers for the Seventh Edition

Jeannette May Anderson, RN, MSN
Tarrant County Junior College, Fort Worth, Texas
M&M Nurse Review Centre, Arlington, Texas

Deborah Dalrymple, RN, MSN, CRNI
Montgomery County Community College
Blue Bell, Pennsylvania

Patricia Graham, RN, BSN
Georgia School of Nursing
Augusta, Georgia

ACKNOWLEDGMENTS

Our special thanks to the faculty of the Department of Nursing at the College of Staten Island and La Guardia Community College, especially Eugenia Borgia Murray, who have participated with support and suggestions for the past 28 years. Also, a thank you to our editor, Nancy Anselment, media editor John Jordan, and the production and marketing teams at Prentice Hall.

My loving thanks and warmest regards to my daughter, Michelle Olsen Keefe.

Special thanks also to our former coauthor, Leon J. Ablon, for his contributions to previous editions. To our friend and former coauthor, the late Helen Siner Weisman, we remember you. You honored our writing group by your professional attitude and knowledge. We miss you.

CONTENTS

UNIT ONE

Basic Calculation and Administration Skills

CHAPTER ONE

Review of Arithmetic for Medical Dosage Calculations

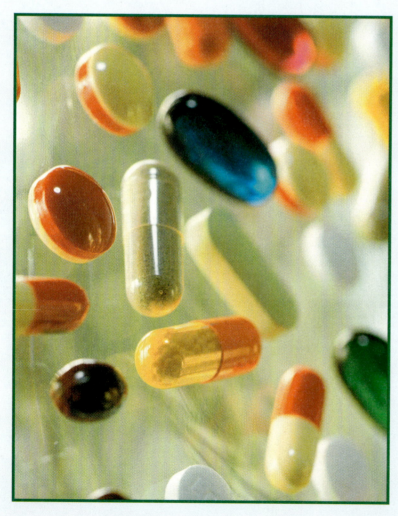

Objectives

After completing this chapter, you will be able to

- Convert decimal numbers to fractions.
- Convert fractions to decimal numbers.
- Round decimal numbers to a desired number of places.
- Multiply and divide decimal numbers.
- Multiply and divide fractions.
- Simplify complex fractions.
- Write percentages as decimal numbers.
- Write percentages as fractions.

Medical dosage calculations can involve whole numbers, fractions, decimal numbers, and percentages. Your results on the *Diagnostic Test of Arithmetic*, found on the next page, will identify your areas of strength and weakness. You can use Chapter 1 to improve your math skills or simply to review the kinds of calculations you will encounter in this text.

Name: _____   Date: _____

Class: _____   Instructor: _____

Diagnostic Test of Arithmetic

The following Diagnostic Test illustrates all the arithmetic skills needed to do the computations in this text. Take the test and compare your answers with the answers found in Appendix A. If you discover areas of weakness, carefully review the relevant review materials in Chapter 1 so that you will be mathematically prepared for the rest of the test.

1. Write 0.625 as a fraction. _____

2. Write $\dfrac{2750}{1000}$ as a decimal number. _____

3. Round 4.781 to the nearest tenth. _____

4. Write $\dfrac{2}{3}$ as a decimal number rounded to the nearest hundredth. _____

5. $\dfrac{8.4}{0.21} =$ _____

6. $3.267 \times 100 =$ _____

7. $42.51 \div 10 =$ _____

8. $65 \div 0.05 =$ _____

9. $\dfrac{10}{21} \times 7 \times \dfrac{3}{5}$ _____

10. $4\dfrac{2}{3} \div 21 =$ _____

11. $\dfrac{3}{4} \div \dfrac{9}{16} =$ _____

12. $\dfrac{\frac{3}{4}}{12} =$ _____

13. Write 35% as a fraction. _____

14. Write 2.5% as a decimal number without using the % symbol.

_____

15. Write $4\dfrac{3}{5}$ as an improper fraction. _____

Answers can be found in Appendix A.

Changing Decimal Numbers and Whole Numbers to Fractions

A decimal number represents a fraction with a denominator of 10, 100, 1000, and so on. Each decimal number has three parts: the whole-number part, the decimal point, and the fraction part. Table 1.1 shows the names of the decimal positions.

Reading a decimal number will help you to write it as a fraction.

Decimal Number	$\longrightarrow$	Read	$\longrightarrow$	Fraction
4.1	$\longrightarrow$	four and one tenth	$\longrightarrow$	$4\dfrac{1}{10}$
0.3	$\longrightarrow$	three tenths	$\longrightarrow$	$\dfrac{3}{10}$
0.07	$\longrightarrow$	seven hundredths	$\longrightarrow$	$\dfrac{7}{100}$
0.231	$\longrightarrow$	two hundred thirty-one thousandths	$\longrightarrow$	$\dfrac{231}{1000}$
0.0025	$\longrightarrow$	twenty-five ten thousandths	$\longrightarrow$	$\dfrac{25}{10,000}$

A number can be written in many different forms. For example, the decimal number 3.5 is read as *three and five tenths*. In fraction form, it is $3\dfrac{5}{10}$ or $3\dfrac{1}{2}$. You can also write $3\dfrac{1}{2}$ as an **improper fraction**, as follows:

$$3\frac{1}{2} = \frac{3 \times 2 + 1}{2} = \frac{7}{2}$$

Table 1.1

Names of Decimal Positions

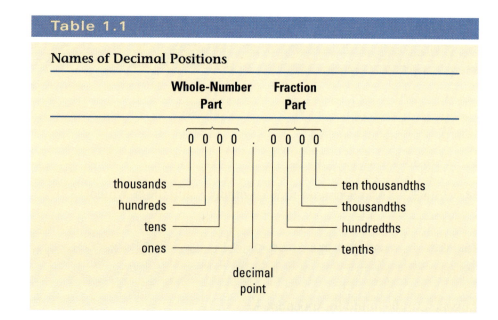

Example  1.1

Write 2.25 as an improper fraction.

The number 2.25 is read *two and twenty-five hundredths* and written $2\frac{25}{100}$.

You can simplify:

$$2\frac{25}{100} = 2\frac{\overset{1}{\cancel{25}}}{\underset{4}{\cancel{100}}} = 2\frac{1}{4} = \frac{2 \times 4 + 1}{4} = \frac{9}{4}$$

> **NOTE**
>
> Simplify $\frac{25}{100}$ to $\frac{1}{4}$ by dividing both numerator and denominator by the same number, 25. This is called **canceling**.

Changing Fractions to Decimal Numbers

To change a fraction to a decimal, think of the fraction as a division problem. For example:

$$\frac{2}{5} \quad \text{means} \quad 2 \div 5 \quad \text{or} \quad 5\overline{)2}$$

Here are the steps for this division.

Step 1   Replace 2 with 2.0 and then place a decimal point directly above the decimal point in 2.0

$$5\overline{)2.0}^{\,\cdot}$$

Step 2   Perform the division.

$$\begin{array}{r} 0.4 \\ 5\overline{)2.0} \\ \underline{2\ 0} \\ 0 \end{array}$$

So,

$$\frac{2}{5} = 0.4$$

Example 1.2

Write $\frac{5}{2}$ as a decimal number.

$$\frac{5}{2} \quad \text{means} \quad 2\overline{)5}$$

Step 1 $2\overline{)5.0}^{\,\cdot}$

Step 2

$$
\begin{array}{r}
2.5 \\
2\overline{)5.0} \\
4 \\
\hline
1\,0 \\
1\,0 \\
\hline
\end{array}
$$

So,

$$
\frac{5}{2} = 2.5
$$

Example 1.3

Write $\dfrac{193}{10}$ as a decimal number.

$$
\frac{193}{10} \quad \text{means} \quad 10\overline{)193}
$$

Step 1

$$
10\overline{)193.0}^{\,\cdot}
$$

Step 2

$$
\begin{array}{r}
19.3 \\
10\overline{)193.0} \\
10 \\
\hline
93 \\
90 \\
\hline
30 \\
30 \\
\hline
0 \\
\end{array}
$$

So,

$$
\frac{193}{10} = 19.3
$$

There is a quicker way to do this problem. To divide any decimal number by 10, you move the decimal point in the number one place to the left. Notice that there is one zero in 10.

$$
\frac{193}{10} = \frac{193.}{10} = 19\underset{\smile}{3.} = 19.3
$$

To divide a number by 100, move the decimal point in the number two places to the left, because there are two zeros in 100. So, the quick way to divide by 10, 100, 1000, and so on, is to count the zeros and then move the decimal point to the left the same number of places. The answer should always be a smaller number than the original. Check your answer to be sure.

Example 1.4

Write $\dfrac{9.25}{100}$ as a decimal number.

There are two zeros in 100, so move the decimal point in 9.25 two places to the left, and fill the empty position with a zero.

$$\frac{9.25}{100} = \;\;\underset{\frown\frown}{}9.25 = 0.0925$$

Rounding Decimal Numbers

Sometimes it's convenient to round answers—that is, to find an approximate answer rather than an exact one. To round 0.257 to the nearest tenth—that is, to round the answer to one decimal place—you do the following:

Look at the hundredths (second) decimal place digit. Because this digit is 5 or more, round 0.257 by adding 1 to the tenths (first) decimal place digit. Finally, drop all the digits after the tenths place. So 0.257 becomes 0.3 when rounded to the nearest tenth.

To round 6.4345 to the nearest hundredth—that is, to round the answer to two decimal places—you do the following:

Look at the thousandths (third) place digit. Since this digit is less than 5, round 6.4345 by leaving the hundredths digit alone. Finally, drop all the digits after the hundredths place. So 6.4345 becomes 6.43 when rounded to the nearest hundredth.

Example 1.5

Round 4.8075 to the nearest hundredth, tenth, and whole number.

4.8075 rounded to the nearest: hundredth = 4.81

tenth = 4.8

whole number = 5

Multiplying and Dividing Decimal Numbers

To multiply two decimal numbers, first multiply, ignoring the decimal points. Then count the total number of decimal places in the original two numbers. That sum equals the number of decimal places in the answer.

Example 1.6

$304.2 \times 0.16 = ?$

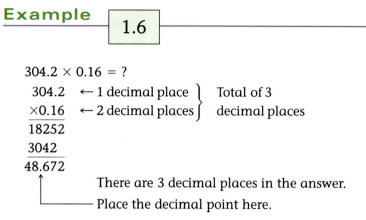

So,

$$304.2 \times 0.16 = 48.672$$

Example 1.7

$304.25 \times 10 = ?$

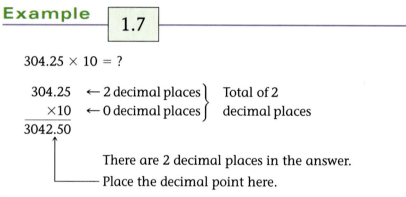

So,

$$304.25 \times 10 = 3042.50 \quad \text{or} \quad 3042.5$$

There is a quicker way to do this problem. To multiply any decimal number by 10, move the decimal point in the number being multiplied one place to the right. Notice that there is one zero in 10.

$$304.25 \times 10 = 304.2\underset{\frown}{\,}5 \text{ or } 3042.5$$

To multiply a number by 100, move the decimal point in the number two places to the right, because there are two zeros in 100. So, the quick way to multiply by 10, 100, 1000, and so on, is to count the zeros and then move the decimal point to the right the same number of places. The answer should always be a larger number than the original. Check your answer to be sure.

Example 1.8

$23.597 \times 1000 = ?$

There are three zeros in 1000, so move the decimal point in 23.597 three places to the right.

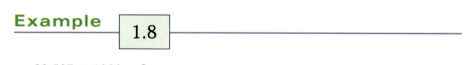

So,

$$23.597 \times 1000 = 23{,}597$$

Example 1.9

Write $\dfrac{106.8}{15}$ as a decimal number to the nearest tenth; that is, round the answer to one decimal place.

$\dfrac{106.8}{15}$ means $15\overline{)106.8}$

Step 1 $15\overline{)106.8}$ with decimal point above

Step 2 Because you want the answer to the nearest tenth (one decimal place), do the division to two decimal places and then round the answer. Since the second place digit in the answer is *less than 5*, leave the first decimal place digit alone. Finally, drop the digit in the second (hundredths) decimal place.

$$
\begin{array}{r}
7.12 \\
15\overline{)106.80} \\
\underline{105} \\
18 \\
\underline{15} \\
30 \\
\underline{30} \\
0
\end{array}
$$

So, $\dfrac{106.8}{15}$ is 7.1 to the nearest tenth.

Example 1.10

$\dfrac{48}{0.002} = ?$

Note that there are three decimal places in 0.002, so move the decimal points in both numbers three places to the right.

$\dfrac{48}{0.002}$ means $0.002\overline{)48.}$ or $0.002\overline{)48.000}$

$$
\begin{array}{r}
24000. \\
2\overline{)48000.} \\
\underline{4} \\
8 \\
\underline{8} \\
0
\end{array}
$$

So,

$$\frac{48}{0.002} = 24{,}000$$

Multiplying and Dividing Fractions

To *multiply* fractions, multiply the numerators to get the new numerator and multiply the denominators to get the new denominator.

Example 1.11

$$\frac{3}{5} \times 6 \times \frac{1}{5} = ?$$

A whole number can be written as a fraction with 1 in the denominator. In this example, write 6 as $\frac{6}{1}$.

$$\frac{3}{5} \times \frac{6}{1} \times \frac{1}{5} = \frac{3 \times 6 \times 1}{5 \times 1 \times 5} = \frac{18}{25}$$

Example 1.12

$$\frac{4}{5} \times \frac{3}{10} \times \frac{20}{7} = ?$$

It is often convenient to cancel before you multiply.

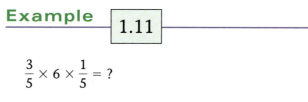

To *divide* fractions, change the division problem to an equivalent multiplication problem by inverting the second fraction.

Example 1.13

$$1\frac{2}{5} \div \frac{7}{9} = ?$$

Write $1\frac{2}{5}$ as the fraction $\frac{7}{5}$. Division $\left(\frac{7}{5} \div \frac{7}{9}\right)$ becomes the multiplication $\left(\frac{7}{5} \times \frac{9}{7}\right)$.

Sometimes you must deal with whole numbers, fractions, and decimal numbers in the same multiplication and division problems.

Example 1.14

$$\frac{1}{300} \times 60 \times \frac{1}{0.4} = ?$$

$$\frac{1}{\cancel{300}\,\underset{5}{}} \times \frac{\overset{1}{\cancel{60}}}{1} \times \frac{1}{0.4} = \frac{1}{5 \times 0.4} = \frac{1}{2}$$

NOTE

Avoid canceling decimal numbers. It is a possible source of error.

Sometimes you will need to simplify a fraction that contains decimal numbers.

Example 1.15

$$0.35 \times \frac{1}{60} = ?$$

$$\frac{0.35}{1} \times \frac{1}{60} = \frac{0.35}{60}$$

The numerator of this fraction is 0.35, a decimal number. You can write an equivalent form of the fraction by multiplying the numerator and denominator by 100.

$$\frac{0.35}{60} \times \frac{100}{100} = \frac{0.3\,5}{60.0\,0} = \frac{35}{6000} = \frac{7}{1200}$$

Example 1.16

Give the answer to the following problem in a fractional form containing no decimal numbers.

$$0.88 \times \frac{1}{2.2} = ?$$

$$\frac{0.88}{1} \times \frac{1}{2.2} = \frac{0.88}{2.2}$$

Multiply the numerator and the denominator of this fraction by 100 to eliminate both decimal numbers.

$$\frac{0.88}{2.2} \times \frac{100}{100} = \frac{0.8\,8}{2.2} = \frac{88}{220} = \frac{2}{5}$$

You can do this problem a different way by dividing 0.88 by 2.2.

$$\begin{array}{r} 0.4 \\ 2.2\overline{)0.88} \end{array} \quad \text{and} \quad 0.4 = \frac{2}{5}$$

Complex Fractions

Fractions that have numerators or denominators that are fractions are called **complex fractions**. The longer fraction line separates the numerator from the denominator and indicates division.

$$\dfrac{1}{\dfrac{2}{5}} \quad \text{means} \quad 1 \div \frac{2}{5} \quad \text{or} \quad 1 \times \frac{5}{2} \quad \text{which is} \quad \frac{5}{2}$$

$$\dfrac{\dfrac{1}{2}}{5} \quad \text{means} \quad \frac{1}{2} \div 5 \quad \text{or} \quad \frac{1}{2} \times \frac{1}{5} \quad \text{which is} \quad \frac{1}{10}$$

$$\dfrac{\dfrac{3}{5}}{\dfrac{2}{5}} \quad \text{means} \quad \frac{3}{5} \div \frac{2}{5} \quad \text{or} \quad \frac{3}{\cancel{5}_{1}} \times \frac{\cancel{5}^{1}}{2} \quad \text{which is} \quad \frac{3}{2}$$

Example | 1.17

$$\dfrac{\dfrac{1}{25} \times 500}{\dfrac{1}{4}} = ?$$

Convert to a simpler form.

$$\left(\frac{1}{25} \times \frac{500}{1}\right) \div \frac{1}{4} = ?$$

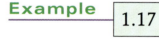

$$\left(\frac{1}{\cancel{25}_{1}} \times \frac{\overset{20}{\cancel{500}}}{1}\right) \div \frac{1}{4} =$$

$$\frac{20}{1} \div \frac{1}{4} =$$

$$\frac{20}{1} \times \frac{4}{1} = 80$$

Example | 1.18

$$\dfrac{\dfrac{2}{3} \times \dfrac{1}{3}}{4} = ?$$

Convert to a simpler form.

$$\frac{2 \times 1}{\frac{3}{1} \times \frac{3}{4}} = ?$$

$$\frac{2}{\frac{9}{4}} =$$

$$\frac{2}{1} \div \frac{9}{4} = \frac{2}{1} \times \frac{4}{9} = \frac{8}{9}$$

This problem could be done another way:

$$\frac{2}{3} \times \frac{1}{\frac{3}{4}} = ?$$

$$\frac{2}{3} \times \left(1 \div \frac{3}{4} \right) =$$

$$\frac{2}{3} \times \left(\frac{1}{1} \times \frac{4}{3} \right) =$$

$$\frac{2}{3} \times \frac{4}{3} = \frac{8}{9}$$

Percentages

Percent (%) means *parts per 100* or *divided by 100*. In calculations dealing with a percentage, you drop the % symbol, divide the number by 100, and write it as a fraction or a decimal number.

13%   means $\frac{13}{100}$ or   0.13

100%   means $\frac{100}{100}$ or   1

12.3%   means $\frac{12.3}{100}$ or   0.123

$6\frac{1}{2}\%$ means   6.5%   or $\frac{6.5}{100}$ or   0.065

Example   1.19

Write 0.5% as a fraction.

$$0.5\% = \frac{0.5}{100} = \frac{5}{1000} = \frac{1}{200}$$

There is another way to get the answer. You know that $0.5 = \frac{1}{2}$ so,

$$0.5\% = \frac{1}{2}\% = \frac{1}{2} \div 100 = \frac{1}{2} \times \frac{1}{100} = \frac{1}{200}$$

PRACTICE SETS

You will find the answers to *Try These for Practice* and the answers to *Exercises* in Appendix A at the back of the book. The answers to the *Additional Exercises* can be found on the companion Website or ask your instructor.

Try These for Practice

Test your comprehension after reading the chapter.

1. Write $\dfrac{3}{5}$ as a decimal number. _____

2. $\left(\dfrac{2}{5} \times \dfrac{18}{20}\right) \times \dfrac{5}{9} =$ _____

3. $\dfrac{7.37 \times 1.5}{0.5} =$ _____

4. $\dfrac{\dfrac{3}{14}}{\dfrac{6}{28}} =$ _____

5. Write 4.5% as a decimal number. _____

Exercises

Reinforce your understanding in class or at home. *Check your answers in Appendix A at the back of the book.*

Convert the decimals to fractions.

1. 0.62 = _____

2. 5.75 = _____

Convert the fractions to decimals.

3. $\dfrac{3}{8} =$ _____

4. $\dfrac{7}{25} =$ _____

5. $\dfrac{1}{5} =$ _____

6. $\dfrac{1}{300} =$ _____

7. $\dfrac{1}{150} =$ _____
(nearest thousandth)

8. $\dfrac{9200}{100} =$ _____

9. $\dfrac{3.75}{1000} =$ _____

10. $\dfrac{193.4}{7} =$ _____
(nearest tenth)

Convert to decimals.

11. $\dfrac{0.36}{0.4} =$ _____

12. $\dfrac{0.036}{0.04} =$ _____

Multiply the decimals.

13. $278.2 \times 100 = $ _____

14. $10.175 \times 10.3 = $ _____

15. $64.73 \times 1000 = $ _____

Divide the decimals.

16. $95 \div 0.05 = $ _____

17. $9.5 \div 0.05 = $ _____

Write the answers to Problems 18 through 22 in fractional form.

18. $\dfrac{7}{15} \times 20 \times \dfrac{1}{2} = $ _____

19. $3\dfrac{1}{2} \div 6 = $ _____

20. $13 \div 2\dfrac{1}{3} = $ _____

21. $6.35 \times \dfrac{1}{5} = $ _____

22. $\dfrac{1}{500} \times 175 \times \dfrac{1}{0.5} = $ _____

Write the answers to Problems 23 through 26 in fractional form and in decimal form to the nearest tenth.

23. $7.75 \times \dfrac{1}{0.5} = $ _____

24. $\dfrac{7}{\frac{3}{8}} = $ _____

25. $\dfrac{\frac{1}{5}}{4} \times 9 = $ _____

26. $\dfrac{\frac{2}{3} \times 170}{\frac{3}{8}} = $ _____

Write the percentages as decimals.

27. $24\dfrac{3}{5}\% = $ _____

28. $63\% = $ _____

Write the percentages as fractions.

29. $2.75\% = $ _____

30. $7.5\% = $ _____

Additional Exercises

Now, on your own, test yourself! The answers to the *Additional Exercises* can be found on the companion Website or ask your instructor.

Convert the decimals to fractions.

1. $0.24 = $ _____

2. $3.24 = $ _____

Convert the fractions to decimals.

3. $\dfrac{5}{8} = $ _____

4. $\dfrac{4}{25} = $ _____

5. $\dfrac{1}{10} = $ _____

6. $\dfrac{1}{200} = $ _____

7. $\dfrac{1}{300} =$ _____
(nearest thousandth)

8. $\dfrac{4500}{100} =$ _____

9. $\dfrac{6.25}{1000} =$ _____

10. $\dfrac{142.6}{7} =$ _____
(nearest tenth)

Convert to decimals.

11. $\dfrac{7.2}{0.06} =$ _____

12. $\dfrac{72}{0.006} =$ _____

Multiply the decimals.

13. $123.4 \times 100 =$ _____

14. $5.125 \times 1.3 =$ _____

15. $36.42 \times 1000 =$ _____

Divide the decimals.

16. $85 \times 0.05 =$ _____

17. $8.5 \times 0.5 =$ _____

Write the answers to Problems 18 through 22 in fractional form.

18. $\dfrac{4}{15} \times 30 \times \dfrac{1}{2} =$ _____

19. $6\dfrac{1}{2} \div 3 =$ _____

20. $26 \div 3\dfrac{1}{4} =$ _____

21. $4.25 \times \dfrac{1}{5} =$ _____

22. $\dfrac{1}{250} \times 125 \times \dfrac{1}{0.5} =$ _____

Write the answers to Problems 23 through 26 in fractional form and in decimal form to the nearest tenth.

23. $4.75 \times \dfrac{1}{1.5} =$ _____

24. $\dfrac{3}{\frac{5}{10}} =$ _____

25. $\dfrac{\frac{1}{4}}{6} \times 8 =$ _____

26. $\dfrac{\frac{1}{4} \times 160}{\frac{5}{8}} =$ _____

Write the percentages as decimals.

27. $38\dfrac{2}{5}\% =$ _____

28. $35\% =$ _____

Write the percentages as fractions.

29. $6.75\% =$ _____

30. $1.5\% =$ _____

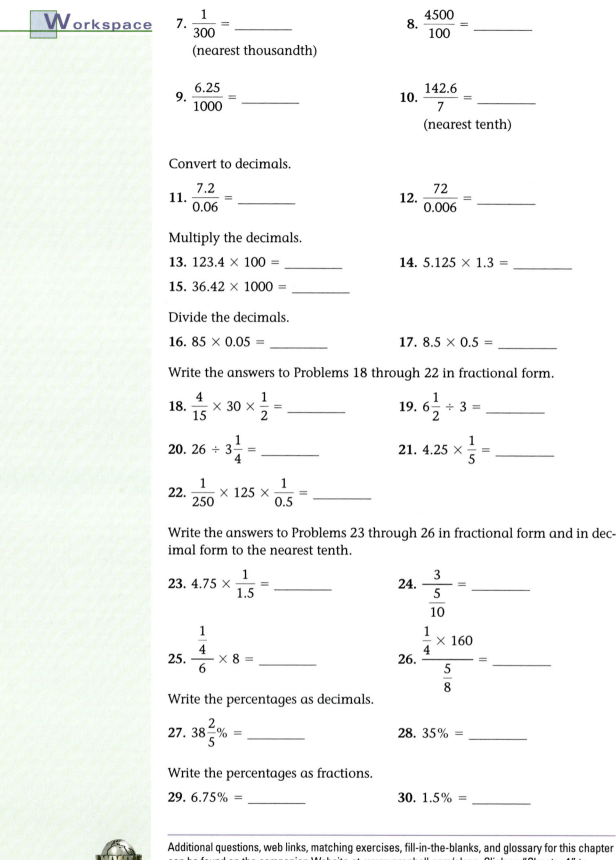

Additional questions, web links, matching exercises, fill-in-the-blanks, and glossary for this chapter can be found on the companion Website at www.prenhall.com/olsen. Click on "Chapter 1" to select the activities for this chapter.

CHAPTER TWO

Drug Administration

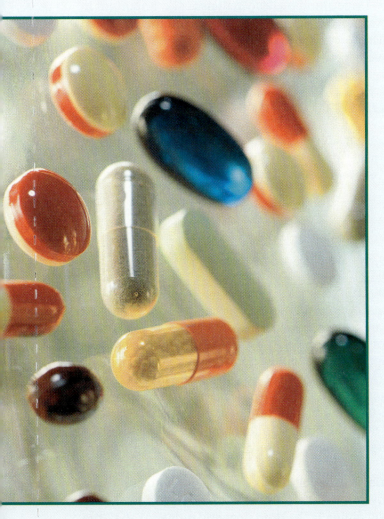

Objectives

After completing this chapter,
you will be able to

- Identify the parts of a medication order.
- Describe the information listed on a physician's order sheet and a medication administration record.
- Identify the routes of drug administration.
- Describe the forms in which medication is supplied.
- Interpret information found on medication labels and package inserts.
- Explain the "five rights" concerning medication administration.
- Identify the trade name and the generic name of a drug.
- Explain the legal implications involved in the administration of drugs.

This chapter presents the components of the **drug order**, **drug label**, **drug package insert**, **physician's order sheet**, and **medication administration record**. Each is discussed in the context of their use in an institutional health care setting, such as a hospital or extended-care facility.

Who Administers Drugs?

To a patient, drugs can be life saving, therapeutic, or life threatening. Physicians and dentists can legally prescribe medications. In many states, physician's assistants and nurse practitioners can also prescribe a range of medications related to their areas of practice.

The registered professional nurse (RN), licensed practical nurse (LPN), and the vocational nurse (VN) are responsible for administering drugs ordered by the prescriber. Physicians, dentists, physician's assistants, and nurse practitioners can also administer drugs to patients.

In most cases, however, drug administration is a process involving a chain of health care professionals. The **prescriber writes** the drug order, the **pharmacist fills** the order, and the **nurse administers** the drug to the patient. Everyone involved is equally responsible for the accuracy of the order and the safety of the patient.

In order to ensure patients' safety, health care professionals who administer medications must understand how drugs act. This knowledge helps them determine when a drug should not be administered or when it should be used cautiously. Understanding drug actions is also important in determining whether a prescribed drug will interact with another drug that the patient is receiving. Drug actions are discussed in pharmacology textbooks and drug handbooks.

The Drug Administration Process

As someone who will be responsible for administering drugs to clients, you must know how to administer them safely. In particular, you must know the classic **Five "Rights" of Medication Administration**:

- right drug
- right dose
- right route
- right time
- right patient

The Right Drug

A drug is a substance that acts therapeutically on the physiologic processes of the human body. For example, the drug insulin is given to patients whose bodies do not manufacture sufficient insulin for the metabolism of food. Some drugs have more than one therapeutic property. Aspirin, for example, is an antipyretic (fever-reducing), analgesic (pain-relieving), and anti-inflammatory drug and has anticoagulant properties (decreases the viscosity of blood). A drug may be taken for any one, or all, of its therapeutic properties.

A drug can be prescribed using either its **generic name** or its **trade name**. For example, many companies manufacture the anti-anginal drug nifedipine (Figure 2.1). Nifedipine is the drug's generic name. As the drug label in the figure shows, the manufacturer calls this drug Procardia. So, in this case, Procardia is the drug's trade name. A drug has only one generic

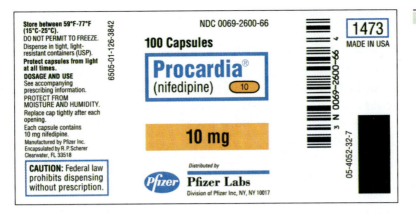

Figure 2.1 Drug Label for Procardia. A drug's trade name and generic name. The trade name (Procardia) can be identified by the raised ® to the right of the name. The drug's generic name (nifedipine) usually appears in lowercase letters. The manufacturer (Pfizer) chose the name Procardia for its version of this anti-anginal drug.

(Registered Trademark of Pfizer Inc. Reproduced with permission.)

name but can have many trade names. Each trade name is patented by the particular manufacturer of the drug.

The drug's trade name usually has the symbol™ or ® printed to the right of the name (for example, Procardia®). This is the drug's trademark or registration symbol. In addition, the trade name usually begins with an uppercase letter, whereas the generic name is printed in lowercase letters (see Figure 2.1). If the prescriber writes an order for Procardia, then the brand Procardia **must** be used, and no substitutions are allowed. But if the order uses the drug's generic name (for example, nifedipine) or if the order indicates a trade name but states "substitution permitted," then nifedipine made by any manufacturer may be administered. Each drug has a unique identification number which is assigned by the Drug Enforcement Agency (DEA). This number is called the **National Drug Code (NDC) number**. The NDC number for Procardia (0069260066) is printed in two places on the label and is also encoded in the bar code.

WARNING

Read drug names carefully! Many drugs have similar looking names. For example, digoxin is *not* digitoxin, and cefotetan is *not* cefoxitin.

Here is a list of some of the drugs whose names could be confused:

amiodarone hydrochloride (Cordarone)	amrinone lactate (Inocor)
cefepine hydrochloride (Maxipime)	cefixime (Suprax)
ceftazidime (Tazidime)	ceftizoxime sodium (Cefizox)
Celexa (citalopram hydrobromide)	Celebrex (celacoxib)
Ceftin (cefuroxime axetil)	Cefzil (cefprozil)
cephalexin hydrochloride (Keftab)	cephalexin monohydrate (Keflex)
fluconazole (Diflucan)	fluorouracil (Adrucil)
fludarabine phosphate (Fludara)	vinorelbine (Navelbine)
glipizide (Glucotrol)	glyburide (Micronase)
hydralazine hydrochloride (Apresoline)	hydroxyzine embonate (Atarax)

Inderal (propanolol hydrochloride)	Inderide (propanolol hydrochlorothiazide)
metolazone (Zaroxolyn)	miconazole (Monistat)
nizatidine (Axid)	nifedipine (Procardia)
pentamidine isethionate (Pentam)	pentazocine hydrochloride (Talwin)
Protapam Chloride (pralidoxime chloride)	protamine sulfate
triazolam (Halcion)	trazodone hydrochloride (Desyrel)

The Right Dose

There are many drug references available. They indicate the correct dose for a specific drug. These resources include pharmacology texts and drug handbooks, the *United States Pharmacopeia,* the *Physicians' Desk Reference,* and manufacturers' package inserts. Those prescribing and administering medications must learn the correct dose. It is their **legal responsibility** to know this information.

The right dose can be affected by the patient's weight or body surface area (BSA). Many drug doses administered to children or for cancer therapy are calculated based on BSA.

Body surface area is an estimate of the total skin area of a person measured in meters squared (m^2). Body surface area is determined by formulas or by the use of a BSA nomogram. You can measure the BSA of a child or an adult if you know his or her height and weight.

The Right Route

Medications must be administered in the form and via the route specified by the prescriber. Medications are manufactured in a variety of forms: liquids, vapors, and solids. Each drug can be administered by one or more routes: by injections (parenteral), by absorption through the skin or mucous membranes (cutaneous), or by mouth (oral).

Parenteral medications are those that are injected into the body by various routes. See Table 2.1. The most common parenteral drug administration sites are listed in Table 2.1. Learn these abbreviations for the major routes of drug administration.

Table 2.1

Major Parenteral Drug Administration Routes

Route	Abbreviation	Meaning
Intramuscular	IM	into the muscle
Subcutaneous	SC	into the subcutaneous tissue
Intravenous	IV	into the vein
Intracardiac	IC	into the cardiac muscle
Intradermal	ID	beneath the skin

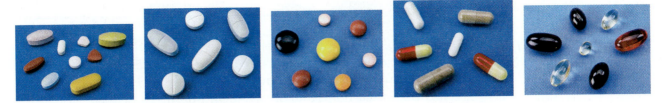

Figure 2.2 (Photos by Al Dodge.)

Medications can also be administered **cutaneously**—that is, through the skin or mucous membrane. This route includes topical administration on the skin surface; transdermal through the skin; inhalation through the nose or mouth; and application of solutions and ointments to the mucosa of the eyes, nose, ears, and mouth. A nitroglycerin patch and the now-familiar nicotine patch, which are applied to the skin, are examples of cutaneously administered drugs. Suppositories containing medications are inserted into the appropriate orifice (vagina, rectum, or urethra).

Oral drugs are administered **by mouth** (po). Oral drugs are supplied in both solid and liquid form. The most common forms are **tablets**, **capsules**, and **caplets** (Figure 2.2). Some tablets and capsules are manufactured in **sustained-release** (SR) or **extended-release** (XL) form. These slowly release a controlled amount of medication over a period of time (usually 24 hours). There are also tablets for **buccal administration** (absorbed by the mucosa of the oral cavity) and tablets for **sublingual administration** (absorbed under the tongue). Oral drugs also come in liquid form: **oral suspensions** and **elixirs**.

> **NOTE**
>
> The prescriber specifies the drug's route of administration. You cannot substitute one route of administration for another.

The Right Time

The prescriber will indicate when and how often a medication should be administered. For example, po medications can be given either before or after meals, depending on the action of the drug. A drug's frequency of administration may be stated specifically; for example, once a day (qd), twice a day (bid), three times a day (tid), and four times a day (qid). Also, medications can be ordered at varying times in a 24-hour day; for example, q4h (every four hours), q6h, q8h, or q12h.

The Right Patient

In a hospital setting, the identification bracelet identifies the patient. The patient's response to the question, "What is your name?" must match the name on the drug order form and the name on the patient's identification bracelet. Some patients are allergic to certain drugs or have an idiosyncratic (unusual) reaction to a drug. Therefore, the person administering the drug must question the patient concerning allergies and record this information on the appropriate form.

WARNING

Anticipate side effects! A side effect is an undesired physiologic response to a drug. For example, codeine relieves pain. But its side effects include constipation, nausea, drowsiness, and itching. Record any side effects noted and discuss them with the prescriber.

Drug Orders

A drug order (prescription) includes the patient's name, name of the drug, the dose, route of administration, and frequency of administration. This order must be written by a health professional licensed by the state to practice as a physician, dentist, advanced nurse practitioner, or a physician's assistant. This book uses the title "prescriber" to designate anyone with the authority to write a prescription. The pharmacist who fills the order by providing the medication ordered by the prescriber is also licensed by the state. A pharmacist cannot write an order or administer medications to patients.

A drug order can take various forms. Figure 2.3 is an example of a *physician's order sheet*. The essential components of a correctly written physician's order include the following information:

Date order written:	1/12/03
Time order written:	9:30 A.M.
Name of drug:	dexamethasone
Dose:	2 mg (milligram)
Route of administration:	po (by mouth)
Frequency of administration:	qhs (at hour of sleep)
Name of prescriber:	J. Olsen, MD

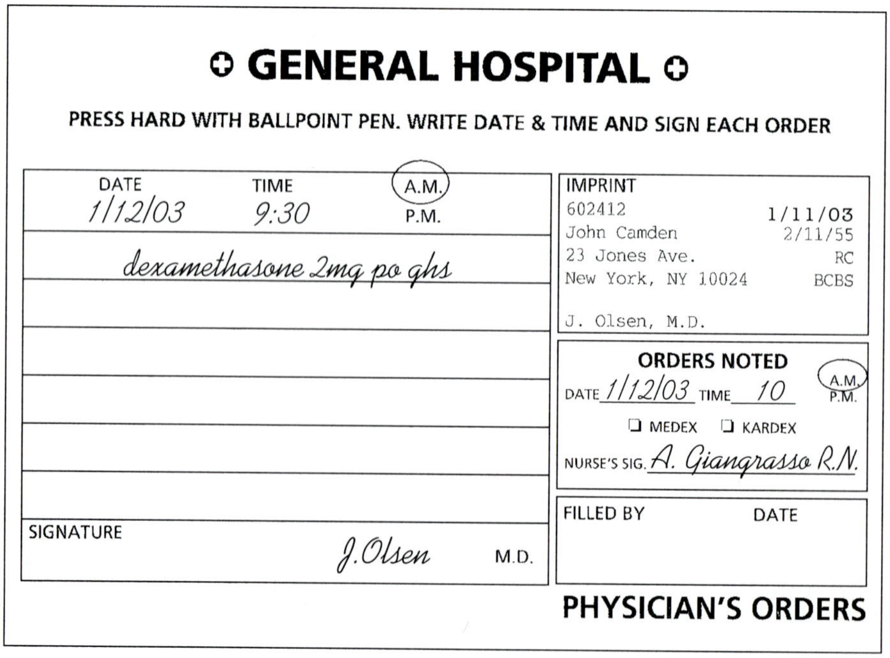
⊕ GENERAL HOSPITAL ⊕

PRESS HARD WITH BALLPOINT PEN. WRITE DATE & TIME AND SIGN EACH ORDER

DATE 1/12/03 TIME 9:30 A.M. P.M.

dexamethasone 2mg po qhs

SIGNATURE J.Olsen M.D.

IMPRINT
602412 1/11/03
John Camden 2/11/55
23 Jones Ave. RC
New York, NY 10024 BCBS
J. Olsen, M.D.

ORDERS NOTED
DATE 1/12/03 TIME 10 A.M. P.M.
❑ MEDEX ❑ KARDEX
NURSE'S SIG. A. Giangrasso R.N.

FILLED BY DATE

PHYSICIAN'S ORDERS

Figure 2.3 Physician's order sheet.

In addition, the physician's order sheet provides basic patient information:

Name of patient:	John Camden
Patient's registration number:	602412
Address:	23 Jones Ave., New York, NY 10024
Physician:	J. Olsen
Birthdate:	2/11/55
Date of admission:	1/11/03
Religion:	Roman Catholic
Insurance:	Blue Cross, Blue Shield

You will find a list of the most common abbreviations that might appear on a drug order in Appendix B. Now, try interpreting the physician's order sheet in Figure 2.4. Record the following information:

Date order written: _____

Time order written: _____

Name of drug: _____

Dose: _____

Route of administration: _____

Frequency of administration: _____

Name of prescriber: _____

Name of patient: _____

Patient's registration number: _____

Address: _____

Physician: _____

Birthdate: _____

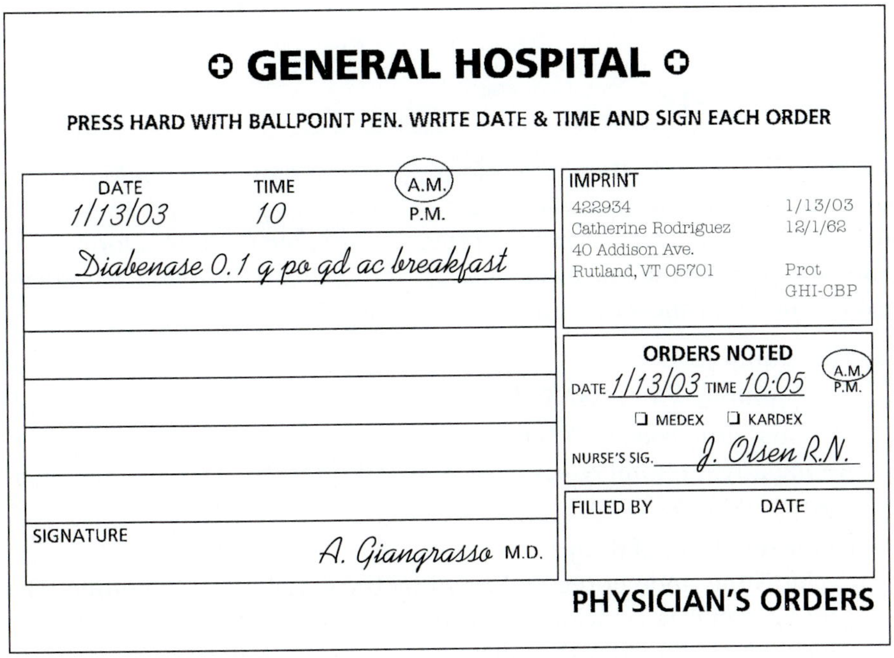

⊕ GENERAL HOSPITAL ⊕

PRESS HARD WITH BALLPOINT PEN. WRITE DATE & TIME AND SIGN EACH ORDER

DATE 1/13/03	TIME 10	(A.M.) P.M.

Diabenase 0.1 g po qd ac breakfast

IMPRINT
422934   1/13/03
Catherine Rodriguez   12/1/62
40 Addison Ave.
Rutland, VT 05701   Prot
                         GHI-CBP

ORDERS NOTED
DATE 1/13/03 TIME 10:05 (A.M.) P.M.
❏ MEDEX ❏ KARDEX
NURSE'S SIG. J. Olsen R.N.

FILLED BY   DATE

SIGNATURE   A. Giangrasso M.D.

PHYSICIAN'S ORDERS

Figure 2.4 Physician's order sheet.

Date of admission: _____

Religion: _____

Insurance: _____

Here is what you should have found:

Date order written: <u>1/13/03</u> _____

Time order written: <u>10 A.M.</u> _____

Name of drug: <u>Diabenase</u> _____

Dose: <u>0.1 g</u> _____

Route of administration: <u>po (by mouth)</u> _____

Frequency of administration: <u>qd ac breakfast (every day before breakfast)</u>

Name of prescriber: <u>A. Giangrasso M.D.</u> _____

Name of patient: <u>Catherine Rodriguez</u> _____

Patient's registration number: <u>422934</u> _____

Address: <u>40 Addison Ave, Rutland, VT 05701</u> _____

Physician: <u>A. Giangrasso</u> _____

Birthdate: <u>12/1/62</u> _____

Date of admission: <u>1/13/03</u> _____

Religion: <u>Protestant</u> _____

Insurance: <u>GHI-CBP</u> _____

Note that just under the patient "imprint" there is a small section entitled "Orders Noted." This section indicates the date and time that the order was transcribed to the medication administration record (discussed later in this chapter). The signature belongs to the nurse who transcribed this order from the physician's order sheet to the medication administration record.

Drug Labels

You will need to understand the information found on drug labels in order to calculate drug dosages and to ensure that a drug is prepared and administered safely. Every drug label provides the same kinds of information. Study the parts of the label in Figure 2.5 for Ceclor, a drug that has bacteriostatic action. Follow the numbers on the label.

1. The manufacturer:
   The company that produced the drug is Lilly.

2. National drug code (NDC) number:
   An identifying number assigned to this drug by the Drug Enforcement Agency: 0002-5130-87.

3. Name and form of drug:
   Ceclor is the trade name, indicated by the ® following the name. The generic name is cefaclor. The drug is in the form of a dry powder, which, when diluted with water, will become an oral suspension.

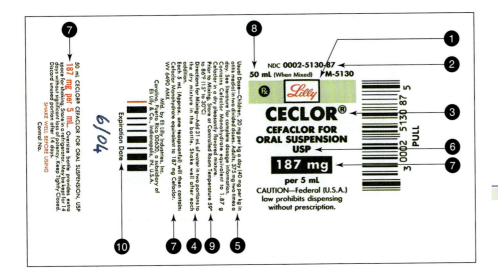

Figure 2.5 Drug label for Ceclor; see text for explanation. (Courtesy of Eli Lilly Company.)

4. Directions for mixing:
   Add 31 mL of water in two portions to the dry mixture in the bottle. Shake well after each addition.

5. Dosage recommendations:
   Children, 20 mg per kg per day (40 mg per kg in otitis media) in two divided doses. Adults, 375 mg two times a day. See package insert for complete dosage information.

6. USP:
   This means that the drug is prepared according to the standards set by the *United States Pharmacopeia,* which specifies the accepted formulations of drugs available in the United States.

7. Amount of drug per dose (shown in three places):
   Each dose contains 187 milligrams per 5 milliliters.

8. Volume of the reconstituted drug:
   When the drug is mixed according to the directions, there will be 50 mL of the oral suspension.

9. Storage directions:
   Some drugs have to be stored under controlled conditions if they are to retain their effectiveness. This drug should be stored at 59°F to 86°F (15°C to 30°C).

10. Expiration date:
    The expiration date specifies when the drug should be discarded. For example, 6/04 indicates that after June 30, 2004, the drug cannot be dispensed and should be discarded.

11. After mixing Ceclor, store in refrigerator.

> **WARNING**
>
> Always read the expiration date! After the expiration date, the drug may lose its potency or act differently in the patient's body. Discard expired drugs. *Never* give expired drugs to patients!

Study the major kinds of information provided in Figure 2.6 for Dolophine Hydrochloride (methadone hydrochloride).

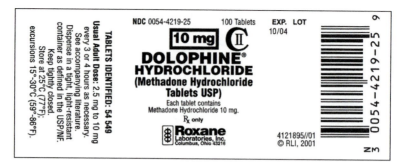

Figure 2.6 Drug label for Dolophine Hydrochloride: 1. Trade name: Dolophine Hydrochloride. 2. Generic name: methadone hydrochloride. 3. Drug form: 10 mg tablets. 4. Manufacturer: Roxane. 5. Expiration date: October 2004. 6. Storage temperature: Store at 25°C (77°F). 7. Dose: 2.5 mg to 10 mg every 3 or 4 hours as necessary.

(Used with permission of Roxane Laboratories, Inc.)

Study the kinds of information provided by the label for the antibiotic Vibramycin in Figure 2.7.

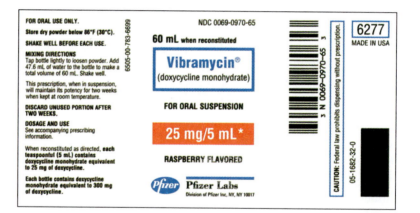

Figure 2.7 Drug label for Vibramycin; see text for information.

(Registered Trademark of Pfizer Inc. Reproduced with permission.)

1. Trade name and generic name:
   The trade name is Vibramycin, and the generic name is doxycycline monohydrate.

2. Storage:
   Store dry powder below 86°F (30°C).

3. Mixing directions:
   Tap bottle lightly to loosen powder. Add 47.6 mL of water to the bottle to make a total volume of 60 mL. Shake well.

4. Strength of drug after mixing:
   Five milliliters of the prepared solution will contain 25 milligrams of Vibramycin.

5. When should the unused portion of the reconstituted drug be discarded?
   Discard unused portion after two weeks.

You will learn more about preparing drug solutions in Chapter 8.

Example 2.1

Examine the label shown in Figure 2.8 and record the following information:

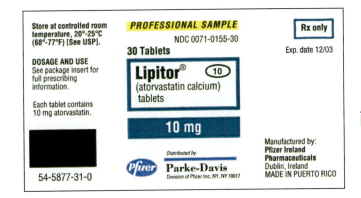

Figure 2.8 Drug label for Lipitor.
(Registered Trademark of Pfizer Inc. Reproduced with permission.)

Trade name: _____

Generic name: _____

Form: _____

Dosage or strength: _____

Amount of drug in container: _____

Usual dosage: _____

Expiration date: _____

Storage temperature: _____

Here is what you should have found:

Trade name: <u>Lipitor</u>

Generic name: <u>atorvastatin calcium</u>

Form: <u>tablets</u>

Dosage or strength: <u>10 mg per tablet</u>

Amount of drug in container: <u>30 tablets</u>

Usual dosage: <u>See package insert</u>

Expiration date: <u>December 2003</u>

Storage temperature: <u>20°–25°C (68°–77°F)</u>

Example 2.2

Examine the label shown in Figure 2.9 and record the information below:

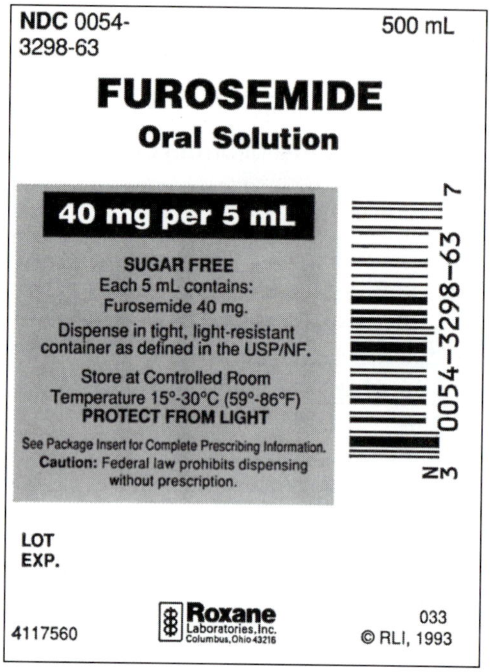

Figure 2.9 Drug label for FUROSEMIDE.

(Used with permission of Roxane Laboratories, Inc.)

Trade name: _____

Generic name: _____

Form: _____

Strength: _____

Amount in the bottle: _____

Usual dosage: _____

Caution: _____

Here is what you should have found:

Trade name: _none_

Generic name: _furosemide_

Form: _oral solution_

Strength: _40 mg per 5 mL_

Amount in the bottle: _500 mL_

Usual dosage: _See package insert._

Caution: _Federal law prohibits dispensing without prescription._

Drug Package Inserts

Sometimes information you need to safely prepare, administer, and store medications is not located on the drug label. In such cases, you may need to read the **package insert**. The pharmaceutical manufacturer includes a package insert with each container of a prescription drug.

The information on a drug package insert is intended for the physician, pharmacist, or the person who administers the drug to patients. It contains complex descriptions of a drug's chemistry and how it acts in the body. Figure 2.10a, b, and c shows an example of two pages from a drug package insert for Diazepam.

ROXANE LABORATORIES, INC.

DIAZEPAM ORAL SOLUTION
5 mg per 5 mL
DIAZEPAM *INTENSOL*™ Ⓒ IV
Oral Solution (Concentrate)
5 mg per mL

R_x only

DESCRIPTION

Each 5 mL of Oral Solution contains:
Diazepam .... 5 mg
Each mL of *Intensol*™ Oral Solution (Concentrate) contains:
Diazepam .... 5 mg
Alcohol 19%

Inactive Ingredients:
The wintergreen-spice flavored 5 mg/5 mL Oral Solution contains citric acid, D&C Yellow No. 10, FD&C Red No. 40, flavoring, polyethylene glycol, propylene glycol, sodium citrate, sorbitol, and water.
The 5 mg/mL *Intensol*™ Oral Solution (Concentrate) contains alcohol, D&C Yellow No. 10, polyethylene glycol, propylene glycol, succinic acid, and water.
Diazepam is a benzodiazepine derivative. Chemically, diazepam is 7-chloro-1,3-dihydro-1-methyl-5-phenyl-2H-1,4-benzodiazepin-2-one. It is a colorless crystalline compound, insoluble in water and has a molecular weight of 284.74. Its structural formula is as follows:

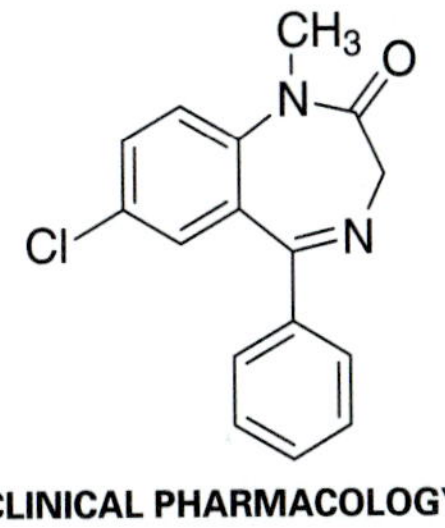

CLINICAL PHARMACOLOGY

In animals diazepam appears to act on parts of the limbic system, the thalamus and hypothalamus, and induces calming effects. Diazepam, unlike chlorpromazine and reserpine, has no demonstrable peripheral autonomic blocking action, nor does it produce extrapyramidal side effects; however, animals treated with diazepam do have a transient ataxia at higher doses. Diazepam was found to have transient cardiovascular depressor effects in dogs. Long-term experiments in rats revealed no disturbances of endocrine function.
Oral LD_{50} of diazepam is 720 mg/kg in mice and 1240 mg/kg in rats. Intraperitoneal administration of 400 mg/kg to a monkey resulted in death on the sixth day.
Reproduction Studies: A series of rat reproduction studies was performed with diazepam in oral doses of 1, 10, 80 and 100 mg/kg. At 100 mg/kg there was a decrease in the number of pregnancies and surviving offspring in these rats. Neonatal survival of rats at doses lower than 100 mg/kg was within normal limits. Several neonates in these rat reproduction studies showed skeletal or other defects. Further studies in rats at doses up to and including 80 mg/kg/day did not reveal teratological effects on the offspring.
In humans, measurable blood levels of diazepam were obtained in maternal and cord blood, indicating placental transfer of the drug.

INDICATIONS AND USAGE

Diazepam is indicated for the management of anxiety disorders or for the short-term relief of the symptoms of anxiety. Anxiety or tension associated with the stress of everyday life usually does not require treatment with an anxiolytic.
In acute alcohol withdrawal, diazepam may be useful in the symptomatic relief of acute agitation, tremor, impending or acute delirium tremens and hallucinosis.
Diazepam is a useful adjunct for the relief of skeletal muscle spasm due to reflex spasm to local pathology (such as inflammation of the muscles or joints, or secondary to trauma); spasticity caused by upper motor neuron disorders (such as cerebral palsy and paraplegia); athetosis; and stiff-man syndrome.
Oral diazepam may be used adjunctively in convulsive disorders, although it has not proved useful as the sole therapy.
The effectiveness of diazepam in long-term use, that is, more than 4 months, has not been assessed by systematic clinical studies. The physician should periodically reassess the usefulness of the drug for the individual patient.

Figure 2.10a Drug package insert for Diazepam.
(Used with permission of Roxane Laboratories, Inc.)

CONTRAINDICATIONS

Diazepam is contraindicated in patients with a known hypersensitivity to this drug and, because of lack of sufficient clinical experience, in children under 6 months of age. It may be used in patients with open angle glaucoma who are receiving appropriate therapy, but is contraindicated in acute narrow angle glaucoma.

WARNINGS

Diazepam is not of value in the treatment of psychotic patients and should not be employed in lieu of appropriate treatment. As is true of most preparations containing CNS-acting drugs, patients receiving diazepam should be cautioned against engaging in hazardous occupations requiring complete mental alertness such as operating machinery or driving a motor vehicle.

As with other agents which have anticonvulsant activity, when diazepam is used as an adjunct in treating convulsive disorders, the possibility of an increase in the frequency and/or severity of grand mal seizures may require an increase in the dosage of standard anticonvulsant medication. Abrupt withdrawal of diazepam in such cases may also be associated with a temporary increase in the frequency and/or severity of seizures.

Since diazepam has a central nervous system depressant effect, patients should be advised against the simultaneous ingestion of alcohol and other CNS-depressant drugs during diazepam therapy.

Usage in Pregnancy: An increased risk of congenital malformations associated with the use of minor tranquilizers (diazepam, meprobamate and chlordiazepoxide) during the first trimester of pregnancy has been suggested in several studies. Because use of these drugs is rarely a matter of urgency, their use during this period should almost always be avoided. The possibility that a woman of childbearing potential may be pregnant at the time of institution of therapy should be considered. Patients should be advised that if they become pregnant during therapy, or intend to become pregnant, they should communicate with their physicians about the desirability of discontinuing the drug.

Management of Overdosage: Manifestations of diazepam overdosage include somnolence, confusion, coma and diminished reflexes. Respiration, pulse and blood pressure should be monitored, as in all cases of drug overdosage, although, in general, these effects have been minimal following overdosage. General supportive measures should be employed, along with immediate gastric lavage. Intravenous fluids should be administered and an adequate airway maintained. Hypotension may be combated by the use of norepinephrine or metaraminol. Dialysis is of limited value. As with the management of intentional overdosage with any drug, it should be borne in mind that multiple agents may have been ingested.

Flumazenil, a specific benzodiazepine receptor antagonist, is indicated for the complete or partial reversal of the sedative effects of benzodiazepines and may be used in situations when an overdose with a benzodiazepine is known or suspected. Prior to the administration of flumazenil, necessary measures should be instituted to secure airway, ventilation, and intravenous access. Flumazenil is intended as an adjunct to, not as a substitute for, proper management of benzodiazepine overdose. Patients treated with flumazenil should be monitored for re-sedation, respiratory depression, and other residual benzodiazepine effects for an appropriate period after treatment. **The prescriber should be aware of a risk of seizure in association with flumazenil treatment, particularly in long-term benzodiazepine users and in cyclic antidepressant overdose.** The complete flumazenil package insert including **CONTRAINDICATIONS, WARNINGS,** and **PRECAUTIONS** should be consulted prior to use.

Withdrawal symptoms of the barbiturate type have occurred after the discontinuation of benzodiazepines (see DRUG ABUSE AND DEPENDENCE section).

[Oral Solution (Concentrate)] are classified by the Drug Enforcement Administration as a Schedule IV con

PRECAUTIONS

It diazepam is to be combined with other psychotropic agents or anticonvulsant drugs, careful consideration should be given to the pharmacology of the agents to be employed–particularly with known compounds which may potentiate the action of diazepam such as phenothiazines, narcotics, barbiturates, MAO inhibitors and other antidepressants. The usual precautions are indicated for severely depressed patients or those in whom there is any evidence of latent depression: particularly the recognition that suicidal tendencies may be present and protective measures may be necessary. The usual precautions in treating patients with impaired renal or hepatic function should be observed.

In elderly and debilitated patients, it is recommended that the dosage be limited to the smallest effective amount to preclude the development of ataxia or oversedation (2 mg to 2 1/2 mg once or twice daily, initially, to be increased gradually as needed and tolerated).

The clearance of diazepam and certain other benzodiazepines can be delayed in association with Tagamet (cimetidine) administration. The clinical significance of this is unclear.

Information for Patients: To assure the safe and effective use of benzodiazepines, patients should be informed that, since benzodiazepines may produce psychological and physical dependence, it is advisable that they consult with their physician before either increasing the dose or abruptly discontinuing this drug.

ADVERSE REACTIONS

Side effects most commonly reported were drowsiness, fatigue and ataxia. Infrequently encountered were confusion, constipation, depression, diplopia, dysarthria, headache, hypotension, incontinence, jaundice, changes in libido, nausea, changes in salivation, skin rash, slurred speech, tremor, urinary retention, vertigo and blurred vision. Paradoxical reactions such as acute hyperexcited states, anxiety, hallucinations, increased muscle spasticity, insomnia, rage, sleep disturbances and stimulation have been reported; should these occur, use of the drug should be discontinued.

Because of isolated reports of neutropenia and jaundice, periodic blood counts and liver function tests are advisable during long-term therapy. Minor changes in EEG patterns, usually low-voltage fast activity, have been observed in patients during and after diazepam therapy and are of no known significance.

DRUG ABUSE AND DEPENDENCE

Diazepam Oral Solution and *Intensol™* trolled substance.

Figure 2.10b

Withdrawal symptoms, similar in character to those noted with barbiturates and alcohol (e.g., convulsions, tremor, abdominal and muscle cramps, vomiting and sweating), have occurred following abrupt discontinuance of diazepam. The more severe withdrawal symptoms have usually been limited to those patients who received excessive doses over an extended period of time. Generally milder withdrawal symptoms (e.g., dysphoria and insomnia) have been reported following abrupt discontinuance of benzodiazepines taken continuously at therapeutic levels for several months. Consequently, after extended therapy, abrupt discontinuance should generally be avoided and a gradual dosage tapering schedule followed. Addiction-prone individuals (such as drug addicts or alcoholics) should be under careful surveillance when receiving diazepam or other psychotropic agents because of the predisposition of such patients to habituation and dependence.

DOSAGE AND ADMINISTRATION

Dosage should be individualized for maximum beneficial effect. While the usual daily dosages given below will meet the needs of most patients, there will be some who may require higher doses. In such cases dosage should be increased cautiously to avoid adverse effects.

Adults:	*Usual Daily Dosage*
Management of Anxiety Disorders and Relief of Symptoms of Anxiety.	Depending upon severity of symptoms - 2 mg to 10 mg, 2 to 4 times daily.
Symptomatic Relief in Acute Alcohol Withdrawal.	10 mg, 3 or 4 times during the first 24 hours, reducing to 5 mg, 3 or 4 times daily as needed.
Adjunctively for Relief of Skeletal Muscle Spasm.	2 mg to 10 mg, 3 or 4 times daily.
Adjunctively in Convulsive Disorders.	2 mg to 10 mg, 2 to 4 times daily.
Geriatric Patients or in the presence of debilitating disease.	2 mg to 2 1/2 mg, 1 or 2 times daily initially; increase gradually as needed and tolerated.

Children:
Because of varied responses to CNS-acting drugs, initiate therapy with lowest dose and increase as required. Not for use in children under 6 months. | 1 mg to 2 1/2 mg, 3 or 4 times daily initially; increase gradually as needed and tolerated.

Proper Use of an Intensol™:

An Intensol is a concentrated oral solution as compared to standard oral liquid medications. It is recommended that an Intensol be mixed with liquid or semi-solid food such as water, juices, soda or soda-like beverages, applesauce and puddings.

Use only the calibrated dropper provided with this product. Draw into the dropper the amount prescribed for a single dose. Then squeeze the dropper contents into a liquid or semi-solid food. Stir the liquid or food gently for a few seconds. The Intensol formulation blends quickly and completely. The entire amount of the mixture, of drug and liquid or drug and food, should be consumed immediately. Do not store for future use.

HOW SUPPLIED

5 mg per 5 mL Oral Solution (Orange-colored, wintergreen-spice flavored solution)

NDC 0054-8207-16: Unit dose Patient Cup™ filled to deliver 5 mL (Diazepam 5 mg), ten 5 mL Patient Cups™ per shelf pack, 4 shelf packs per shipper.

NDC 0054-8208-16: Unit dose Patient Cup™ filled to deliver 10 mL (Diazepam 10 mg), ten 10 mL Patient Cups™ per shelf pack, 4 shelf packs per shipper.
NDC 0054-3188-63: Bottle of 500 mL.

5 mg per mL *Intensol*™
Oral Solution (Concentrate)
NDC 0054-3185-44: Bottles of 30 mL with calibrated dropper [graduations of 0.2 mL (1 mg), 0.4 mL (2 mg), 0.6 mL (3 mg), 0.8 mL (4 mg), and 1 mL (5 mg) on the dropper].

Store at Controlled Room Temperature
15°-30°C (59°-86°F).

PROTECT FROM MOISTURE.

4048501
088

Revised August 1998
© RLI, 1998

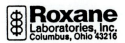

Figure 2.10c

Always consult the package insert when you need detailed information about

- mixing and storing a drug
- preparing a drug dose
- when the drug should *not* be used
- side effects and adverse reactions

The categories of information usually listed on a package insert are described in Table 2.2.

Table 2.2

Types of Information on Drug Package Inserts

Information	Comments
Name of pharmaceutical company	
Name of the drug (trade/generic)	
Strength of drug and clinical formulation	
Clinical pharmacology	How the drug acts in the body.
Indications for using the drug	The conditions the drug is approved to treat.
Contraindications	Conditions under which the drug must *not* be given.
Warning information	Relative to the safety of the patient. For example, a potent diuretic drug that can deplete the body of electrolytes and fluid can cause a state of dehydration. Therefore, *close* medical supervision would be required for the patient.
Precautions	Indicate the assessments that must be done by a nurse to identify untoward results that could occur when a patient is given a medication. Serum diagnostic tests also identify changes in the patient's overall condition.
Adverse reactions	Drug reactions that could affect patient comfort and safety but that don't necessarily deter the prescriber from prescribing the drug.
Dosage	Indicates the amount of drug that can be administered to the patient.

Example 2.3

Read the excerpts provided from the package inserts in Figures 2.11 through 2.14, and fill in the requested information.

1. What is the name of the concentrated form of the drug (Figure 2.11)?

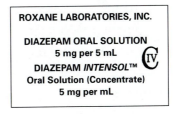

ROXANE LABORATORIES, INC.

DIAZEPAM ORAL SOLUTION
5 mg per 5 mL
DIAZEPAM *INTENSOL™*
Oral Solution (Concentrate)
5 mg per mL

Figure 2.11 Drug names from the Diazepam package insert.
(Used with permission of Roxane Laboratories, Inc.)

2. What are the most commonly reported side effects of this drug (Figure 2.12)?

ADVERSE REACTIONS

Side effects most commonly reported were drowsiness, fatigue and ataxia. Infrequently encountered were confusion, constipation, depression, diplopia, dysarthria, headache, hypotension, incontinence, jaundice, changes in libido, nausea, changes in salivation, skin rash, slurred speech, tremor, urinary retention, vertigo and blurred vision. Paradoxical reactions such as acute hyperexcited states, anxiety, hallucinations, increased muscle spasticity, insomnia, rage, sleep disturbances and stimulation have been reported; should these occur, use of the drug should be discontinued.

Because of isolated reports of neutropenia and jaundice, periodic blood counts and liver function tests are advisable during long-term therapy. Minor changes in EEG patterns, usually low-voltage fast activity, have been observed in patients during and after diazepam therapy and are of no known significance.

Figure 2.12 Adverse reactions to Diazepam.
(Used with permission of Roxane Laboratories, Inc.)

3. According to the information in Figure 2.13, how is Intensol supplied?

HOW SUPPLIED

5 mg per 5 mL Oral Solution (Orange-colored, wintergreen-spice flavored solution)
NDC 0054-8207-16: Unit dose Patient Cup™ filled to deliver 5 mL (Diazepam 5 mg), ten 5 mL Patient Cups™ per shelf pack, 4 shelf packs per shipper.

NDC 0054-8208-16: Unit dose Patient Cup™ filled to deliver 10 mL (Diazepam 10 mg), ten 10 mL Patient Cups™ per shelf pack, 4 shelf packs per shipper.

NDC 0054-3188-63: Bottle of 500 mL.

5 mg per mL *Intensol™*
Oral Solution (Concentrate)
NDC 0054-3185-44: Bottles of 30 mL with calibrated dropper [graduations of 0.2 mL (1 mg), 0.4 mL (2 mg), 0.6 mL (3 mg), 0.8 mL (4 mg), and 1 mL (5 mg) on the dropper].

Figure 2.13 How Diazepam Intensol is supplied.
(Used with permission of Roxane Laboratories, Inc.)

4. According to Figure 2.14, would this drug be ordered for an infant who is 5 months of age?

CONTRAINDICATIONS

Diazepam is contraindicated in patients with a known hypersensitivity to this drug and, because of lack of sufficient clinical experience, in children under 6 months of age. It may be used in patients with open angle glaucoma who are receiving appropriate therapy, but is contraindicated in acute narrow angle glaucoma.

Figure 2.14 Contraindications for Diazepam.
(Used with permission of Roxane Laboratories, Inc.)

5. According to Figure 2.15, what is an appropriate dose for convulsive disorders?

DOSAGE AND ADMINISTRATION

Dosage should be individualized for maximum beneficial effect. While the usual daily dosages given below will meet the needs of most patients, there will be some who may require higher doses. In such cases dosage should be increased cautiously to avoid adverse effects.

Adults:	**Usual Daily Dosage**
Management of Anxiety Disorders and Relief of Symptoms of Anxiety.	Depending upon severity of symptoms –2 mg to 10 mg, 2 to 4 times daily.
Symptomatic Relief in Acute Alcohol Withdrawal.	10 mg, 3 or 4 times during the first 24 hours, reducing to 5 mg, 3 or 4 times daily as needed.
Adjunctively for Relief of Skeletal Muscle Spasm.	2 mg to 10 mg, 3 or 4 times daily.
Adjunctively in Convulsive Disorders.	2 mg to 10 mg, 2 to 4 times daily.

Figure 2.15 Dosage of Diazepam.
(Used with permission of Roxane Laboratories, Inc.)

Here is what you should have found:

1. Diazepam Intensol.
2. Drowsiness, fatigue, and ataxia.
3. 5 mg per mL
4. No.
5. 2 mg to 10 mg, 2 to 4 times daily.

Medication Administration Records

Medication administration records (MARs) are used to record information about the drugs a patient receives under a prescriber's orders. The following list indicates the kinds of information recorded on a MAR.

- Person receiving the medications:
  Name
  Date of birth
  Patient registration number
  Allergies
- Medication:
  Name
  Dosage
  Time of administration
  Route of administration
  Date started
  Date discontinued
- Staff member administering medications:
  Initials of those administering medications
  Signatures of staff members administering medications

Although the type of information appearing on a MAR is fairly standard, the appearance of these records varies from one health care provider to another. For example, some MARs record the time of drug administration using the military clock. This system of recording time does not use A.M. or P.M. after the hour designation. Instead, the hours past 12 noon are designated by higher numbers. For example, 2:00 P.M. according to the standard clock is written as 1400 (pronounced "fourteen hundred hours"). Figure 2.16 compares military and standard clock hours.

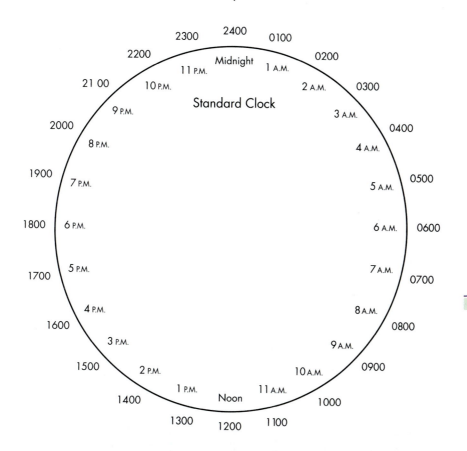

Figure 2.16 A comparison of the military (outer) and standard (inner) clock. 10 P.M. on a standard clock is 2200 (twenty-two hundred hours) on a military clock.

In some health care facilities, the MAR is computerized. Hard copy of a MAR can be readily printed from the computerized patient data base. Each time a medication is administered to a patient, the MAR is updated at a computer terminal by the staff member who administered the drug.

Let's look at a MAR in detail (Figure 2.17). This MAR reveals the following information:

Drug administered at 6 A.M. (0600) on 9/12/04: Amoxicillin 1250 mg
Drugs administered between 12 noon and 11 P.M. (1200–2300) on 9/15/04: Lotensin 20 mg, Ticlid 250 mg, Xanax 0.5 mg, and Amoxicillin 1500 mg
Did Ms. Kim receive Amoxicillin 1250 mg on 9/12/04, at 6 A.M. (0600)? Yes.
When did Ms. Kim receive the last dose of Xanax?
9 P.M. (2100) on 9/15/04.

UNIVERSITY HOSPITAL

DAILY MEDICATION ADMINISTRATION RECORD

789652
Wendy Kim
44 Chester Ave.
N.Y., N.Y. 10003

Dr. Leon Ablon

7/12/01
8/24/54
Christian
Aetna

PATIENT NAME *Wendy Kim*

ROOM # *422*

IF ANOTHER RECORD IS IN USE ☐

ALLERGIC TO (RECORD IN RED): *tomatoes, codeine*

DATES GIVEN ↓ DATE DISCHARGED:

RED CHECK INITIAL	ORDER DATE	INITIAL	EXP DATE	MEDICATION, DOSAGE, FREQUENCY AND ROUTE	HOURS	12	13	14	15	16	17
	9/12	JO	9/17	Amoxicillin 1250 mg	0600	LA	LA	LA			
				po q 12 h	1800	MS	SG	SG			
	9/12	JO	9/17	Digoxin 0.125 mg qd po	0900	JO	JO	JO	LA		
	9/12	JO	9/17	Lotensin 20 mg po bid	0900	JO	JO	JO	LA		
					1900	JO	JO	JO	JO		
	9/12	JO	9/17	Ticlid 250 mg po qd	1900	JO	JO	SG	SG		
	9/12	JO	9/17	Xanax 0.5 mg hs po	2100	MS	MS	SG	SG		
	9/15	JO	9/17	Amoxicillin 1550 mg	X	X	X	X	LA		
				q 12 h po	0600				LA		
					1800				SG		

INT.	NURSES' FULL SIGNATURE AND TITLE	INT.	NURSES' FULL SIGNATURE AND TITLE
MS	Mary Smith R.N.		
SG	Susan Green R.N.		
LA	Louise Alvarez R.N.		
JO	Jane Olsen L.P.N.		

39171 (10/91)

Figure 2.17 Medication administration record.

Example 2.4

Study the MAR in Figure 2.18; then fill in the following chart and answer the questions.

Name of Drug	Dose	Route of Administration	Time of Administration

1. Which drugs were administered at 9 A.M. on 7/15? _____
2. Identify the drug administered IV at 6 P.M. on 7/14. _____
3. Which drug was administered subcutaneously on 7/16? _____
4. Who administered the folic acid on 7/16? _____
5. When was the thioguanine given on 7/15? _____

Here is what you should have found:

Name of Drug	Dose	Route of Administration	Time of Administration
Centrum	1 tablet	po	0900 (9 A.M.)
folic acid	5 mg	po	0900 (9 A.M.)
cytarabine	150 mg	IV	0600 (6 A.M.) 1800 (6 P.M.)
thioguanine	150 mg	po	0900 (9 A.M.) 1700 (5 P.M.)
erythropoietin	3000 units	sc	0900 (9 A.M.) tiw (Monday, Wednesday, Friday only)

1. Centrum 1 tablet, folic acid 5 mg, thioguanine 150 mg
2. cytarabine 150 mg
3. erythropoietin 3000 units
4. Leon Ablon
5. 9:00 A.M. and 5:00 P.M.

UNIVERSITY HOSPITAL

DAILY MEDICATION ADMINISTRATION RECORD

12481632
David Samuels
378-12 Horida Ave.
Stocie, Il. 63642

Dr. June Olsen

7/3/01
12/20/60
RC
Medicaid

PATIENT NAME *David Samuels*

ROOM # *5421*

IF ANOTHER RECORD IS IN USE ☐

ALLERGIC TO (RECORD IN RED): *penicillin*

DATES GIVEN ↓

DATE DISCHARGED:

RED CHECK INITIAL	ORDER DATE	INITIAL	EXP DATE	MEDICATION, DOSAGE, FREQUENCY AND ROUTE	HOURS	14	15	16
	7/14	Jo	7/19	Centrum 1 Tab qd po	0900	LA	LA	LA
				—				
	7/14	Jo	7/19	Folic acid 5 mg qd po	0900	LA	LA	LA
				—				
	7/14	Jo	7/18	Cytarabine 150 mg IV	0600	AG	AG	AG
				q 12 h in 250 ml 5% D/W	1800	SG	SG	SG
				for 5 days				
				—				
	7/12	Jo	7/21	thioguanine 150 mg po				
				bid for 5 days	0900	LA	LA	LA
					1700	SG	SG	SG
	7/14	Jo	7/20	Erythropoietin 3000 units s/c	0900	X	X	LA
				TIW (MWF) only				

INT.	NURSES' FULL SIGNATURE AND TITLE	INT.	NURSES' FULL SIGNATURE AND TITLE
LA	Leon Ablon R.N.		
AG	Anthony Giangrasso R.N.		
SG	Suson Green R.N.		

39171 (10/91)

Figure 2.18 Medication administration record.

PRACTICE SETS

You will find the answers to *Try These for Practice* and the answers to *Exercises* in Appendix A at the back of the book. The answers to the *Additional Exercises* can be found on the companion Website or ask your instructor.

Try These for Practice

Test your comprehension after reading the chapter. Study the drug labels in Figure 2.19, and supply the following information.

1. What is the route of administration for Zyprexa?

   _____

2. How many capsules are in the container of Geodon?

   _____

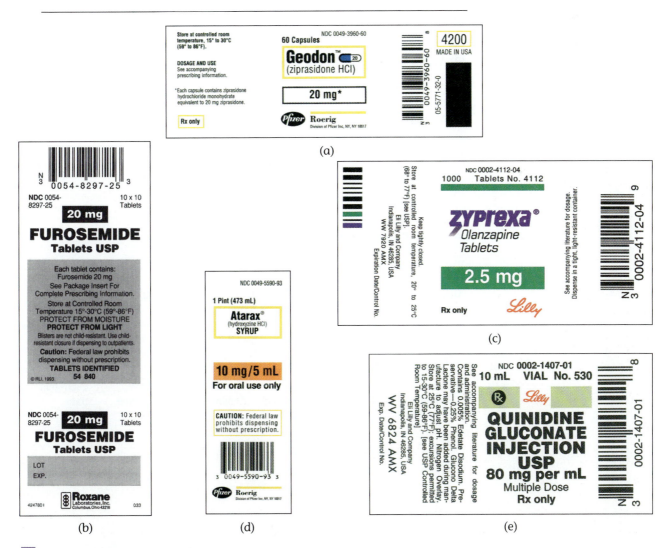

Figure 2.19 Drug labels.

((a, d) Registered Trademark of Pfizer Inc. Reproduced with permission. (b) Used with permission of Roxane Laboratories, Inc. (c, e) Courtesy of Eli Lilly and Company.)

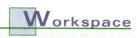

3. What is the quantity of drug in each milliliter of quinidine gluconate?

_____

4. Write the trade name for the drug hydroxyzine HCl.

_____

5. What is the quantity of drug in each tablet of furosemide?

_____

Exercises

Reinforce your understanding in class or at home. Study the drug labels shown in Figure 2.19, and supply the following information. *Check your answers in Appendix A at the back of the book.*

1. Write the generic name for Zyprexa.

_____

2. Write the trade name for ziprasidone HCl.

_____

3. Which drug can be administered by injection?

_____

4. What is the route of administration for furosemide?

_____

5. Write a trade name for the drug whose NDC number is 0049-5590-93.

_____

6. Study the MAR in Figure 2.20. Fill in the following chart and answer the questions.

Name of Drug	Dose	Route of Administration	Time of Administration	Date Started	Expiration Date
Celebrex					
Flomax					
Ditropan					
Zoloft					
Seraquel					
Valium					
Fluconazole					

MEDICATION RECORD

Jane Ellington
2335 15ª Ave
Queens, NY
10221

12/20/20
Protestant
BCBS *

DIAGNOSIS	urinary tract infection
	cronic depression
	osteoarthritis

Dr. A. Giangrasso MD
#324689

12/07/03

ALLERGIES (LIST IN RED)

KNOWN ALLERGIES   Yes ☐   No ☒   WEIGHT ___104 lb___

ORDER DATE	EXP. DATE	MEDICATION, DOSAGE, FREQUENCY & ROUTE	HOURS	2003 DATES GIVEN															DO NOT WRITE IN THIS COLUMN
				7	8	9	10	11	12	13	14	15	16	17	18	19	20	
12/7	12/18	Celebrex 100 mg po	8AM	RG	RG	RG	RG	RG	MD	MD								
		bid q 12h	8PM	TK	TK	TK	TK	TK	JO	JO								
12/7	12/13	Flomax 0.4 mg po 30 min AC dinner	5PM	RD	RD	RD	RD	RD	JO	JO								
12/7	12/13	Ditropan 0.005 g po qd	8AM	RG	RG	RG	RG	RG	MD	MD								
12/8	12/14	Zoloft 0.1 g po q AM	8AM	X	RG	RG	RG	RG	MD	MD								
12/7	12/13	Seraquel 100 mg po hs	9PM	RD	RD	RD	RD	RD	JO	JO								
12/9	12/16	Valium 10 mg po prn q hs	9PM	X	X	RD	X	RD	JO	JO								
12/8	12/15/03	100 ml D5/NS with	8AM	X	X	RG	RG	RG	MD	MD								
		Fluconazole 400 mg	8PM	X	RD	RD	RD	RD	JO	JO								
		IV q 12 hours																

INIT.	NURSES' FULL SIGNATURE & TITLE	INIT.	NURSES' FULL SIGNATURE & TITLE	INIT.	NURSES' FULL SIGNATURE & TITLE
RG	Robert Graham	JO	Joan Olsen		
MD	Martha Daly				
TK	Taylore Keife				
RD	Rachel Dugas				

Figure 2.20 Medication record.

a. Which drugs were administered at 8 P.M. on 12/7/03?

_____

b. How many doses of Valium did the patient receive in seven days?

_____

c. What is the name of the drug administered IV?

_____

d. How many medications were administered at 5 P.M.? Name the medication(s).

_____

e. Designate the time of day the patient received Ditropan.

_____

f. Identify the nurse who administered the medication on 12/7/03 at 8 A.M.

_____

g. Identify the medication(s) administered at 9 P.M. on 12/08/03.

_____

h. What is the name of the patient's physician?

_____

7. Study the physician's order sheet in Figure 2.21; then answer the following questions.

		PHYSICIAN'S ORDERS	CHART COPY

FORM 01 109

ORDER DATE	DATE DISC.		
4/20/03	4/27/03	Cefaclor 250 mg q 8 h po for 7 days	
4/20/03	4/27/03	Nitroglycerine transdermal 10 cm² qd. remove from 10 PM - 7 AM daily	
4/20/03	4/27/03	Diabenase 0.1 g daily po AC breakfast	
4/22/03	4/29/03	Vioxx 25 mg po daily oral suspension with breakfast	
4/22/03	4/29/03	Forosemide 80 mg po bid	
4/23/03	4/30/03	Monopril 20 mg po daily	

PATIENT CERTIFICATION

2/28/52 Episcopal Aetna

4/20/03

Jane Myers 23 College Ave Salt Lake City Utah 46082

Dr. D. Looby #212332

PLEASE INDICATE BEEPER # → *222*

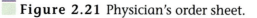

Figure 2.21 Physician's order sheet.

a. What is the route of administration for Nitroglycerine?

_____

b. Which drug(s) should be administered with breakfast?

_____

c. Which drugs are to be given daily?

_____

d. Which drugs were ordered on April 22, 2003?

_____

e. Which drug is to be given every eight hours?

_____

f. Identify the drug(s) which are to be administered before breakfast?

_____

8. Use the package insert and drug label shown in Figure 2.22 to answer the following questions.

DOSAGE AND ADMINISTRATION

Kefzol may be administered intramuscularly or intravenously after reconstitution. Total daily dosages are the same for either route of administration.

Intramuscular Administration—Reconstitute as directed by Table 3 with 0.9% Sodium Chloride Injection, Sterile Water for Injection, or Bacteriostatic Water for Injection. Shake well until dissolved. Kefzol should be injected into a large muscle mass. Pain on injection is infrequent with Kefzol.

TABLE 3. DILUTION TABLE

Vial Size	Diluent to Be Added	Approximate Available Volume	Approximate Average Concentration
250 mg	2 mL	2 mL	125 mg/mL
500 mg	2 mL	2.2 mL	225 mg/mL
1 g*	2.5 mL	3 mL	330 mg/mL

*The 1-g vial should be reconstituted only with Sterile Water for Injection or Bacteriostatic Water for Injection.

Intravenous Administration—Kefzol may be administered by intravenous injection or by continuous or intermittent infusion.

Intermittent intravenous infusion: Kefzol can be administered along with primary intravenous fluid management programs in a volume control set or in a separate, secondary IV bottle. Reconstituted 500 mg or 1 g of Kefzol may be diluted in 50 to 100 mL of 1 of the following intravenous solutions: 0.9% Sodium Chloride Injection, 5% or 10% Dextrose Injection, 5% Dextrose in Lactated Ringer's Injection, 5% Dextrose and 0.9% Sodium Chloride Injection (also may be used with 5% Dextrose and 0.45% or 0.2% Sodium Chloride Injection), Lactated Ringer's Injection, 5% or 10% Invert Sugar in Sterile Water for Injection, Ringer's Injection, Normosol®-M in D5-W, Ionosol® B with Dextrose 5%, or Plasma-Lyte® with 5% Dextrose.

ADD-Vantage Vials of Kefzol are to be reconstituted _only_ with 0.9% Sodium Chloride Injection or 5% Dextrose Injection in the 50-mL or 100-mL Flexible Diluent Containers.

Intravenous injection (Administer solution directly into vein or through tubing): Dilute the reconstituted 500 mg or 1 g of Kefzol in a minimum of 10 mL of Sterile Water for Injection. Inject solution slowly over 3 to 5 minutes. Do not inject in less than 3 minutes. (NOTE: ADD-VANTAGE VIALS ARE NOT TO BE USED IN THIS MANNER.)

Dosage—The usual adult dosages are given in Table 4.

TABLE 4. USUAL ADULT DOSAGE

Type of Infection	Dose	Frequency
Pneumococcal pneumonia	500 mg	q12h
Mild infections caused by susceptible gram-positive cocci	250 to 500 mg	q8h
Acute uncomplicated urinary tract infections	1 g	q12h
Moderate to severe infections	500 mg to 1 g	q6 to 8h
Severe, life-threatening infections (eg, endocarditis, and septicaemia)*	1 g to 1.5 g	q6h

*In rare instances, doses up to 12 g of cefazolin per day have been used.

(a)

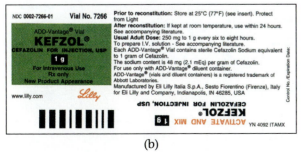

(b)

Figure 2.22 (a) Package insert (excerpt) for Kefzol and (b) Kefzol label. (Courtesy of Eli Lilly and Company.)

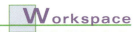
Workspace

a. What is the generic name of the drug?

_____

b. If 2.5 mL of diluent is added to the 1 gram vial, what is the approximate average concentration?

_____

c. Identify the route of administration for Kefzol?

_____

d. What is the usual adult dosage for Pneumococcal pneumonia?

_____

Additional Exercises

Now, on your own, test yourself! The answers to the *Additional Exercises* can be found on the companion Website or ask your instructor.

Study the drug labels shown in Figure 2.23, and supply the following information.

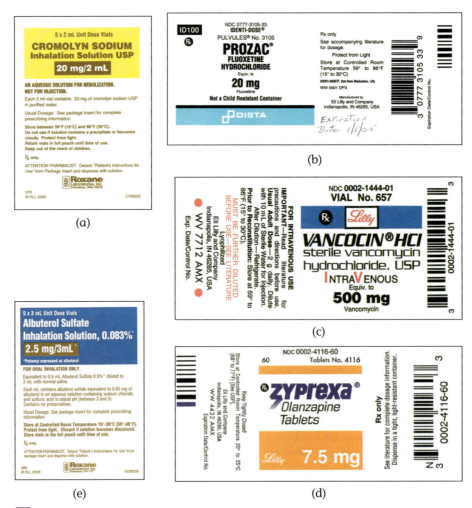

Figure 2.23 Drug labels.

((a, e) Used with permission of Roxane Laboratories, Inc. (b–d) Courtesy of Eli Lilly and Company.)

1. Write the trade name for vancomycin hydrochloride.

_____

2. Write the trade name for olanzapine.

_____

3. Which drug can be administered intravenously?

_____

4. What is the route of administration for Cromolyn sodium?

_____

5. Write a trade name for the drug whose NDC number is 0777-3105-33.

_____

6. Study the MAR in Figure 2.24. Fill in the following chart and answer the questions.

Name of Drug	Dose	Route of Administration	Time of Administration	Date Started	Date Discontinued
Isoproterenol					
Procardia					
Indomethacin					
digoxin					
Diuril					
Carafate					

a. Identify the drugs administered on July 18, 2003.

_____

b. Identify the drugs administered po on July 20, 2003.

_____

c. How many drugs were administered at 9 P.M. on July 20, 2003?

_____

d. Which drugs were administered daily for 6 consecutive days?

_____

e. Who administered the indomethacin at 5:00 P.M. on July 20?

_____

GENERAL HOSPITAL

YEAR 2003 MONTH July		DAY	18	19	20	21	22	23
SOLUTION MEDICATION ADDED DOSAGE AND INTERVAL			INITIALS* AND HOURS	INITIALS AND HOURS	INITIALS AND HOURS	INITIALS AND HOURS	INITIALS AND HOURS	INITIALS AND HOURS
Date Started 7/18/03		I	JO	JO	JO	JO		
Isoproterenol		AM	9	9	9	9		
15 mg SL tid		I	LA LA	LA LA	LA LA	LA LA		
Discontinued 7/21/03		PM	1 5	1 5	1 5	1 5		
Date Started 7/18/03		I	JO	JO	JO	JO		
Procardia		AM	9	9	9	9		
20 mg po bid		I	LA	LA	LA	LA		
Discontinued 7/21/03		PM	5	5	5	5		
Date Started 7/18/03		I	JO	JO	JO	JO		
indomethacin		AM	9	9	9	9		
25 mg bid po		I	LA	LA	LA	LA		
Discontinued 7/21/03		PM	5	5	5	5		
Date Started 7/18/03		I	JO	JO	JO	JO	JO	JO
digoxin 0.25 mg		AM	9	9	9	9	9	9
qd po		I						
Discontinued 7/23/03		PM						
Date Started 7/18/03		I	JO	JO	JO	JO	JO	JO
Diuril 500 mg		AM	9	9	9	9	9	9
qd po		I						
Discontinued 7/23/03		PM						
Date Started 7/20/03		I			JO	JO	JO	
Carofate		AM			9	9	9	
1g qid po ac & hs		I			LA LA LA	LA LA LA	LA LA LA	
Discontinued 7/22/03		PM			1 5 9	1 5 9	1 5 9	
Date Started		I						
		AM						
		I						
Discontinued		PM						

ALLERGIES: (Specify) None

Init.	Signature
JO	Jane Olsen LPN
LA	Leon Ablon RN
SG	Susan Green RN

*INITIALS – Nurses must sign name & title

PATIENT IDENTIFICATION

7286531   7/18/03

TYRELL JOHNSON   3/12/34
755 Bay Ridge Ave
Brooklyn, NY   Jewish
11209   Blue Cross

Dr. Anthony Giangrasso

Figure 2.24 Medication administration record.

f. Identify the drug for which the patient received 0.25 mg.

_____

g. How many doses of Carafate were received by Mr. Johnson on July 22?

_____

7. Study the physician's order sheet in Figure 2.25; then answer the following questions.

a. What is the dose of Declomycin?

_____

⊕ GENERAL HOSPITAL ⊕

PRESS HARD WITH BALLPOINT PEN. WRITE DATE & TIME AND SIGN EACH ORDER

DATE	TIME	A.M.
Oct 12, 2003	6	P.M.

Declomycin 300 mg po q6h

vitamin C 2 g po bid

Inderal 120 mg po qd

Esmolol 500 mg in

500 ml of 0.9% NS

infuse at rate of 15 mL/hr

SIGNATURE   L. Ablon   M.D.

IMPRINT

731122   10/12/03
Jose Sanchez   3/2/45
24 Third Ave.
Chicago, IL 54312   Medicaid

Dr. Leon Ablon

ORDERS NOTED
DATE 10/12/03 TIME 6:30   A.M. P.M.
❑ MEDEX   ❑ KARDEX
NURSE'S SIG. June Olsen R.N.

FILLED BY   DATE

PHYSICIAN'S ORDERS

Figure 2.25 Physician's order sheet.

b. How many times a day do you administer vitamin C to Mr. Sanchez?

_____

c. If the last dose of Declomycin was given at 12 noon, at what time would you administer the next dose?

_____

d. How many milliliters of Esmolol will Mr. Sanchez receive in 60 minutes?

_____

e. What was the patient's date of admission?

_____

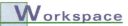
8. Use the package excerpt shown in Figure 2.26 to answer the following questions.

   a. What is the generic name of the drug?

   _____

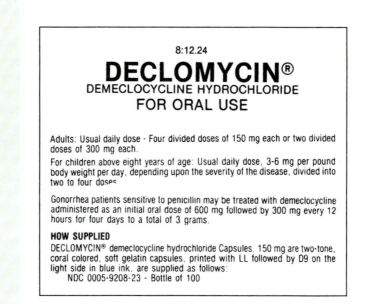

8:12.24

DECLOMYCIN®
DEMECLOCYCLINE HYDROCHLORIDE
FOR ORAL USE

Adults: Usual daily dose - Four divided doses of 150 mg each or two divided doses of 300 mg each.

For children above eight years of age: Usual daily dose, 3-6 mg per pound body weight per day, depending upon the severity of the disease, divided into two to four doses

Gonorrhea patients sensitive to penicillin may be treated with demeclocycline administered as an initial oral dose of 600 mg followed by 300 mg every 12 hours for four days to a total of 3 grams.

HOW SUPPLIED
DECLOMYCIN® demeclocycline hydrochloride Capsules. 150 mg are two-tone, coral colored, soft gelatin capsules. printed with LL followed by D9 on the light side in blue ink. are supplied as follows:
    NDC 0005-9208-23 - Bottle of 100

Figure 2.26 Package insert (excerpt) for Declomycin.
(Courtesy of Esi Lederle, a Business unit of Wyeth Pharmaceuticals, Philadelphia, PA.)

   b. What is the usual dose for an adult?

   _____

   c. What is the initial oral dose of Declomycin for patients with gonorrhea?

   _____

   d. How is this drug supplied?

   _____

Additional questions, web links, matching exercises, fill-in-the-blanks, and glossary for this chapter can be found on the companion Website at www.prenhall.com/olsen. Click on "Chapter 2" to select the activities for this chapter.

CHAPTER THREE

Dimensional Analysis

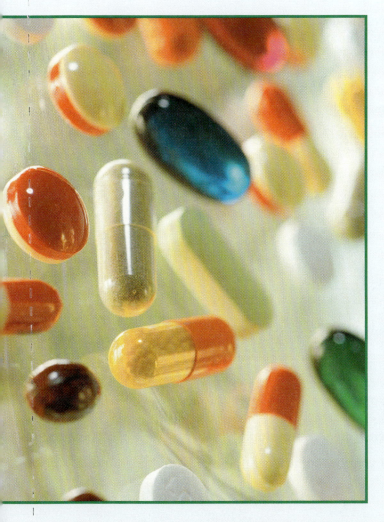

Objectives

After completing this chapter, you will be able to

- Solve a calculation problem using *dimensional analysis*.
- Identify some common units of measurement.
- Recognize the abbreviations for these units.
- State the equivalents for these units of measurement.
- Convert from one unit of measurement to another.

I n this chapter you will learn to use dimensional analysis to calculate drug dosages. **Dimensional analysis** is a commonsense approach to drug calculations that largely frees you from the need to memorize formulas. It is the method most commonly accepted in the physical sciences. Once you master this technique, you will be able to calculate drug dosages quickly and safely.

Getting Started

In order to use dimensional analysis you must know the equivalents involved. Some common equivalent measurements are listed in Table 3.1.

Table 3.1	

Equivalents for Common Units	
12 inches (in) =	1 foot (ft)
3 feet (ft) =	1 yard (yd)
16 ounces (oz) =	1 pound (lb)
60 seconds (sec) =	1 minute (min)
60 minutes (min) =	1 hour (h or hr)
24 hours (h or hr) =	1 day (d)
12 months (mon) =	1 year (yr)

You can use equivalents and dimensional analysis to solve problems. Suppose that you want to change 3 years into an equivalent number of months. The relationship is written as follows:

$$3 \, yr = ? \, mon$$

Whenever you divide something by itself, you get 1. For example, $5 \div 5 = 1$, or equivalently $\frac{5}{5} = 1$. Similarly, 7 days $\div$ 7 days = 1, or $\frac{7 \, days}{7 \, days} = 1$.

Since 7 days = 1 week,

$$7 \, days \div 1 \, week = 1 \quad or \quad \frac{7 \, days}{1 \, week} = 1$$

and

$$1 \, week \div 7 \, days = 1 \quad or \quad \frac{1 \, week}{7 \, days} = 1$$

Because 12 months is the same as 1 year, when you divide 12 months by 1 year, you get 1.

$$\frac{12 \, mon}{1 \, yr} = 1$$

Now see what happens when you multiply 3 years by $\frac{12 \, mon}{1 \, yr}$. The amount of time will not change, because you are really multiplying the time by 1.

$$3 \, yr = \frac{3 \, yr}{1} \times \frac{12 \, mon}{1 \, yr} = \frac{(3 \times 12) \, mon}{1} = 36 \, mon$$

So, 3 years is the same amount of time as 36 months.

Here is another problem. If a storm lasts for 72 hours, how many days does the storm last? You want to change 72 hours to days. The relationship is written as follows:

$$72\,h = ?\,d$$

Notice that $\dfrac{1\,d}{24\,h} = 1$, since 1 day is the same as 24 hours. Now you multiply 72 hours by $\dfrac{1\,d}{24\,h}$. The amount of time will not change, because you are really multiplying it by 1.

$$72\,h \times \frac{1\,d}{24\,h} = ?$$

$$\frac{\overset{3}{\cancel{72}}\,\cancel{h}}{1} \times \frac{1\,\textcircled{d}}{\underset{1}{\cancel{24}\,\cancel{h}}} = \frac{(3 \times 1)\,d}{1} = 3\,d$$

So, the 72-hour storm lasts for 3 days.

In both problems you canceled the original units and ended up with the desired units. You did this by multiplying a fraction that was equal to 1. The fraction had the old units on the bottom and the new units on the top. The method used to solve the previous two problems is called *dimensional analysis*.

Example 3.1

Change 2 feet to an equivalent number of inches.

$$2\,ft = ?\,in$$

You want to cancel the feet and get the answer in inches. Therefore, multiply 2 feet by a fraction that has feet on the bottom (in the denominator) and inches on the top (in the numerator).

$$2\,ft \times \frac{?\,in}{?\,ft} = ?\,in$$

Next, put in numbers that will make the fraction $\dfrac{?\,in}{?\,ft}$ equal to 1. Because 12 in = 1 ft, the fraction you want is $\dfrac{12\,in}{1\,ft}$. Now, multiply 2 feet by $\dfrac{12\,in}{1\,ft}$.

$$\frac{2\,\cancel{ft}}{1} \times \frac{12\,\textcircled{in}}{1\,\cancel{ft}} = \frac{(2 \times 12)\,in}{1} = 24\,in$$

So, 2 feet is the same as 24 inches.

Example 3.2

Change 36 inches to an equivalent number of feet.

$$36 \text{ in} = ? \text{ ft}$$

You want to cancel the inches and get the answer in feet. So you must multiply 36 inches by a fraction that has inches on the bottom (in the denominator) and feet on the top (in the numerator).

$$36 \text{ in} \times \frac{? \text{ ft}}{? \text{ in}} = ?$$

Note $\dfrac{1 \text{ ft}}{12 \text{ in}} = 1$, because 1 foot is the same as 12 inches. Now, multiply 36 inches by $\dfrac{1 \text{ ft}}{12 \text{ in}}$.

$$\overset{3}{\cancel{36}} \text{ in} \times \frac{1 \text{ ft}}{\underset{1}{\cancel{12}} \text{ in}} = \frac{3 \times 1 \text{ ft}}{1} = 3 \text{ ft}$$

So, 36 inches is the same as 3 feet.

Example 3.3

Change 15 yards to an equivalent length in feet.

$$15 \text{ yd} = ? \text{ ft}$$

You want to cancel the yards and get the answer in feet. So, multiply 15 yards by a fraction that has yards on the bottom (denominator). The answer must be in feet, so the fraction must have feet on the top (numerator).

$$15 \text{ yd} \times \frac{? \text{ ft}}{? \text{ yd}} = ? \text{ ft}$$

We must put in numbers that will make $\dfrac{? \text{ ft}}{? \text{ yd}}$ equal to 1. Because 3 ft = 1 yd, the fraction we want is $\dfrac{3 \text{ ft}}{1 \text{ yd}}$. Now multiply 15 yards by $\dfrac{3 \text{ ft}}{1 \text{ yd}}$.

$$15 \text{ yd} \times \frac{3 \text{ ft}}{1 \text{ yd}} = \frac{15 \times 3 \text{ ft}}{1} = 45 \text{ ft}$$

So, 15 yards is the same as 45 feet.

Example 3.4

Change 0.25 feet to an equivalent length in inches.

$$0.25 \text{ ft} = ? \text{ in}$$

You want to cancel feet and get the answer in inches. So, multiply 0.25 feet by a fraction that looks like $\dfrac{? \text{ in}}{? \text{ ft}}$.

$$0.25 \text{ ft} \times \frac{? \text{ in}}{? \text{ ft}} = ? \text{ in}$$

Because 12 in = 1 ft, the fraction we want is $\dfrac{12\text{ in}}{1\text{ ft}}$.

$$0.25\ \cancel{\text{ft}} \times \frac{12\,\textcircled{\text{in}}}{1\ \cancel{\text{ft}}} = \frac{0.25 \times 12\text{ in}}{1} = 3\text{ in}$$

So, 0.25 feet is the same as 3 inches.

Example 3.5

Change 64 ounces to pounds.

$$64\text{ oz} = ?\text{ lb}$$

You want to cancel ounces and get the answer in pounds. So, multiply 64 ounces by a fraction that looks like $\dfrac{?\text{ lb}}{?\text{ oz}}$.

$$64\text{ oz} \times \frac{?\text{ lb}}{?\text{ oz}} = ?\text{ lb}$$

Because 16 oz = 1 lb, the fraction we want is $\dfrac{1\text{ lb}}{16\text{ oz}}$.

$$\overset{4}{\cancel{64}}\ \cancel{\text{oz}} \times \frac{1\,\textcircled{\text{lb}}}{\underset{1}{\cancel{16}\ \cancel{\text{oz}}}} = 4\text{ lb}$$

So, 64 ounces is the same as 4 pounds.

Dimensional analysis can also be applied to other problems in everyday life. Here are some examples.

Example 3.6

If the exchange rate in a country is 9 pesos for 1 dollar, how many pesos will be exchanged for $45?

$$\$45 = ?\text{ pesos}$$

You want to cancel dollars and get the answer in pesos. So, multiply $45 by a fraction that looks like $\dfrac{?\text{ pesos}}{\$?}$.

$$\$45 \times \frac{?\text{ pesos}}{\$?} = ?\text{ pesos}$$

Because $1 = 9 pesos, the fraction we want is $\dfrac{9\text{ pesos}}{\$1}$.

$$\cancel{\$}\,45 \times \frac{9\,\textcircled{\text{pesos}}}{\cancel{\$}\,1} = 405\text{ pesos}$$

So, $45 will be exchanged for 405 pesos.

Example 3.7

There are 6 cans of soda in a package. A case of soda contains 4 packages. How many cans of soda are in 2 cases?

This problem involves two steps. Two-step problems are discussed in Chapter 6.

Step 1 Change cases to packages. Since 4 packages are in 1 case, the fraction to change cases to packages is $\frac{4\ packages}{1\ case}$.

$$2\ cases \times \frac{4\ packages}{1\ case} = 8\ packages$$

Step 2 Change 8 packages to cans. Since 6 cans are in 1 package, the fraction to change packages to cans is $\frac{6\ cans}{1\ package}$.

$$8\ packages \times \frac{6\ cans}{1\ package} = 48\ cans$$

These steps could be combined in a single step as follows:

$$2\ cases \times \frac{4\ packages}{1\ case} \times \frac{6\ cans}{1\ package} = 48\ cans$$

So, 2 cases contain 48 cans.

Example 3.8

Kim is having a party for 24 people, each person will have 2 hot dogs. If a package of hot dog buns contains 8 buns, how many packages of hot dog buns must Kim buy?

Step 1 Change people to hot dogs. Since 1 person has 2 hot dogs, the fraction is $\frac{2\ hot\ dogs}{1\ person}$.

$$24\ people \times \frac{2\ hot\ dogs}{1\ person} = 48\ hot\ dogs$$

Step 2 48 hot dogs require 48 buns. Now, change 48 buns to packages. Since 1 package has 8 buns, the fraction is $\frac{1\ package}{8\ buns}$.

$$\overset{6}{48}\ buns \times \frac{1\ package}{\underset{1}{8}\ buns} = 6\ packages$$

So, Kim must buy 6 packages of hot dog buns.

You will find the answers to *Try These for Practice* and to *Exercises* in Appendix A at the back of the book. The answers to the *Additional Exercises* can be found on the companion Website or ask your instructor.

Try These for Practice

Test your comprehension after reading the chapter.

1. How many minutes are in $3\frac{1}{4}$ hours? _____

2. An infant weighs 6 lb 8 oz. What is this weight in ounces? _____

3. A man is 72 inches tall. How tall is he in feet? _____

4. How many yards does 60 feet equal? _____

5. If it takes 78 months to pay off an automobile loan, how many years is that? _____

Exercises

Reinforce your understanding in class or at home.

1. 540 sec = _____ min

2. 1.25 yr = _____ mon

3. 4 d = _____ h

4. 4 lb = _____ oz

5. $\frac{3}{4}$ min = _____ sec

6. $1\frac{2}{3}$ yr = _____ mo

7. $1\frac{1}{2}$ yd = _____ ft

8. 12 oz = _____ lb

9. 480 in = _____ ft

10. 6 ft = _____ yd

11. An infant weighs 8 pounds at birth. What is the weight in ounces?

12. Convert 18 hours to days.

13. If your patient measures 48 inches in height, what does the patient measure in feet?

14. What part of an hour is 50 minutes?

15. How many years are there in 30 months?

16. Change 2.25 hours to minutes.

17. An IV solution has been infusing for 55 minutes. How many seconds is that?

18. What is the height of a 5-foot-tall patient in inches?

19. An infant weighs $2\frac{1}{2}$ pounds. What is the equivalent in ounces?

20. Convert 9 days to hours.

Additional Exercises

Now, on your own, test yourself! Ask your instructor to check your answers.

1. 2.5 yr = _____ mon   2. 7 d = _____ h

3. 3 lb = _____ oz   4. 360 sec = _____ min

5. 240 in = _____ ft   6. 9 ft = _____ yd

7. 4 oz = _____ lb   8. $1\frac{1}{2}$ yd = _____ ft

9. $1\frac{3}{4}$ yr = _____ mon   10. $\frac{1}{2}$ min = _____ sec

11. What is the height of a 6-foot-tall patient in inches? _____

12. An IV solution has been infusing for 5 minutes. How many seconds is that? _____

13. Change 3.75 hours to minutes. _____

14. How many years are there in 18 months? _____

15. What part of an hour is 45 minutes? _____

16. If your patient measures 66 inches in height, what does the patient measure in feet? _____

17. Convert 80 hours to days. _____

18. An infant weighs 6 pounds at birth. What is its weight in ounces? _____

19. A person is 5 feet 8 inches tall. Express this height in inches. _____

20. If an infant weighs $7\frac{1}{2}$ pounds, what is the equivalent in ounces? _____

Additional questions, web links, matching exercises, fill-in-the-blanks, and glossary for this chapter can be found on the companion Website at www.prenhall.com/olsen. Click on "Chapter 3" to select the activities for this chapter.

UNIT TWO

Systems of Measurement for Dosage Calculations

CHAPTER FOUR

The Apothecary, Household, and Metric Systems

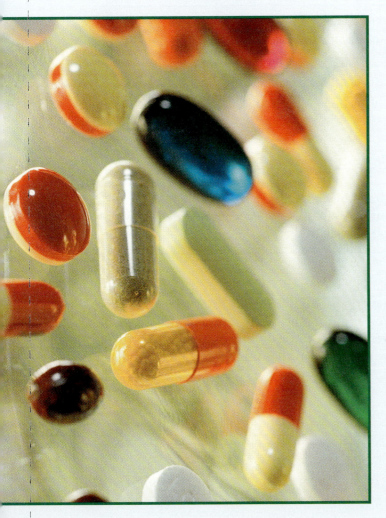

Objectives

After completing this chapter, you will be able to

- Identify units of measurement in the apothecary, household, and metric systems.

- Recognize the abbreviations for the units of measurement in the three systems.

- State the equivalents for the units of volume for liquids.

- State the equivalents for the units of weight for solids.

- Convert from one unit to another among the three systems.

At present, there are three systems used to measure drugs: the **apothecary system**, the **household system**, and the **International System of Units (SI)**. The SI, commonly known as the **metric system**, is replacing the other systems of measurement. However, the other systems are still in use, so you must understand all three systems and learn how to convert from one to another. In this chapter you will be introduced to the three systems. You will notice that the apothecary and household systems use fractions, such as $\frac{1}{2}$ and $2\frac{3}{4}$, whereas the metric system uses decimal numbers, such as 0.5 and 2.75.

The Apothecary System

The apothecary system is one of the oldest systems of drug measurement. Although it is infrequently used, you must nevertheless understand the apothecary system in order to administer medications safely. Apothecary units are rarely used on drug labels, but when they are, the metric equivalents are also provided.

Liquid Volume in the Apothecary System

Drugs in liquid form are measured by volume. The volume of a liquid is the amount of space it occupies. The equivalents for the units of measurement for liquid volume in the apothecary system are shown in Table 4.1 along with their abbreviations.

Table 4.1

Common Equivalents for Apothecary Liquid Volume Units

quart (qt) 1	=	pints (pt) 2
quart (qt) 1	=	ounces (℥ or oz) 32
pint (pt) 1	=	ounces (℥ or oz) 16
ounce (℥ or oz) 1	=	drams (ℨ) 8
dram (ℨ) 1	=	minims (♏) 60

> **NOTE**
>
> In the apothecary system, the abbreviation or symbol for the unit is placed before the quantity (as in pt 2). However, it is sometimes written the other way (2 pt) as well.

You can use dimensional analysis to convert from one unit to an equivalent unit within the apothecary system the same way you converted units in Chapter 3. You multiply the old measurement by a fraction that is equal to 1; the fraction has the old units on the bottom (the denominator) and the new units on top (the numerator) as the following examples show.

Example 4.1

The order reads drams $\frac{1}{6}$ of tincture of opium. How many minims would you administer?

$$\text{drams}\,\frac{1}{6} = \text{minims?}$$

Cancel the drams and obtain the equivalent amount in minims.

$$\frac{dr\ 1}{6} \times \frac{\text{m}\ ?}{dr\ ?} = \text{m}\ ?$$

Because m 60 = dr 1, the fraction you want is $\frac{\text{m}\ 60}{dr\ 1}$.

$$\frac{dr\ 1}{6} \times \frac{\overset{10}{\text{m}\ 60}}{dr\ 1} = \text{m}\ 10$$

So, drams $\frac{1}{6}$ is the same as minims 10, and you would administer minims 10 of tincture of opium.

Example 4.2

The patient is to receive drams 4 of magaldrate (Riopan). How many ounces of this antacid would you administer?

$$\text{ʒ}\ 4 = \text{ʒ}\ ?$$

Cancel the drams and get the answer in ounces.

$$\text{ʒ}\ 4 \times \frac{\text{ʒ}\ ?}{\text{ʒ}\ ?} = \text{ʒ}\ ?$$

Because ʒ 8 = ʒ 1, the fraction you want is $\frac{\text{ʒ}\ 1}{\text{ʒ}\ 8}$.

$$\overset{1}{\text{ʒ}\ 4} \times \frac{\text{ʒ}\ 1}{\underset{2}{\text{ʒ}\ 8}} = \text{ʒ}\ \frac{1}{2}$$

So, drams 4 is the same as ounce $\frac{1}{2}$, and you would administer ounce $\frac{1}{2}$ of Riopan.

Weight in the Apothecary System

The grain (gr) is the only unit of weight in the apothecary system that is used in administering medications. You will be converting this unit to its equivalent in other systems of measurement in Chapter 5.

Roman Numerals

Dosages in the apothecary system are sometimes written using Roman numerals. Table 4.2 shows Roman numerals.

Table 4.2

Roman Numerals				Symbols	
1	I	7	VII	$\frac{1}{2}$	ss
2	II	8	VIII	$1\frac{1}{2}$	iss
3	III	9	IX	$7\frac{1}{2}$	viiss
4	IV	10	X		
5	V	15	XV		
6	VI	20	XX		

The Household System

Liquid Volume in the Household System

Occasionally household measurements are used in prescribing liquid medication. Table 4.3 lists equivalent values, with their abbreviations, for units of liquid measurement in the household system.

Table 4.3

Equivalent Measurements in the Household System		
1 glass (usually)	=	ounces (℥ or oz) 8
1 measuring cup	=	ounces (℥ or oz) 8
1 teacup	=	ounces (℥ or oz) 6
1 ounce (℥)	=	2 tablespoons (T)
1 tablespoon (T)	=	3 teaspoons (t)
1 teaspoon (t)	=	60 drops (gtt)

Since these units are measured using household utensils, which are not necessarily accurate, the equivalents listed in Table 4.3 are only *approximate*. Unlike the metric system, which uses decimal numbers such as 0.5 and 3.75, the household system uses fractions such as $\frac{1}{2}$ and $3\frac{3}{4}$.

Notice that the ounce is a unit of measurement in both the apothecary and household systems.

Example 4.3

The patient is to receive 15 drops of the gastrointestinal antispasmodic drug, paregoric. How many teaspoons would the patient receive?

15 gtt = ? t

Cancel drops and obtain the equivalent amount in teaspoons.

$$15 \, \text{gtt} \times \frac{?\,t}{?\,\text{gtt}} = ?\,t$$

Because 60 gtt = 1 t, the fraction is $\frac{1\,t}{60\,\text{gtt}}$.

$$\overset{1}{\cancel{15}} \, \cancel{\text{gtt}} \times \frac{\boxed{1\,t}}{\underset{4}{\cancel{60}} \, \cancel{\text{gtt}}} = \frac{1}{4}\,t$$

So, 15 drops is approximately the same as $\frac{1}{4}$ teaspoon, and the patient would receive $\frac{1}{4}$ teaspoon of paregoric.

Example 4.4

The prescriber directs the patient to take 12 ounces of a laxative agent, GoLytely. How many teacups would the patient take?

$$12 \, \text{oz} = ? \, \text{teacups}$$

Cancel the ounces and obtain the equivalent amount in teacups.

$$12 \, \text{oz} \times \frac{?\,\text{teacups}}{?\,\text{oz}} = ?\,\text{teacups}$$

Because 1 teacup = 6 ounces, the fraction is $\frac{1\,\text{teacup}}{6\,\text{oz}}$.

$$\overset{2}{\cancel{12}} \, \cancel{\text{oz}} \times \frac{\boxed{1\,\text{teacup}}}{\cancel{6} \, \cancel{\text{oz}}} = 2 \, \text{teacups}$$

So, 12 ounces is approximately the same as 2 teacups, and the patient would take 2 teacups of GoLytely.

Weight in the Household System

The only units of weight used in the household system are ounces (oz) and pounds (lb), as shown in Table 4.4.

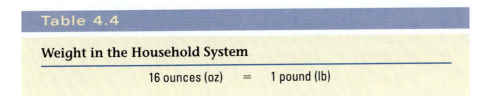

Table 4.4
Weight in the Household System
16 ounces (oz) = 1 pound (lb)

Example 4.5

An infant weighs 6 pounds 3 ounces. What is the weight of the infant in ounces?

First change the 6 pounds to ounces.

$$6\,\text{lb} = ?\,\text{oz}$$

Cancel the pounds and obtain the equivalent amount in ounces.

$$6\,\text{lb} = \frac{?\,\text{oz}}{?\,\text{lb}} = ?\,\text{oz}$$

Because 16 oz = 1 lb, the fraction is $\dfrac{16\,\text{oz}}{1\,\text{lb}}$.

$$6\,\cancel{\text{lb}} \times \frac{16\,\text{oz}}{1\,\cancel{\text{lb}}} = 96\,\text{oz}$$

Now add the extra 3 ounces.

$$96\,\text{oz} + 3\,\text{oz} = 99\,\text{oz}$$

So, the 6-pound, 3-ounce infant weighs 99 ounces.

The Metric System

Liquid Volume in the Metric System

The equivalents for the units of measurement for liquid volume in the metric system are shown in Table 4.5, along with their abbreviations.

Table 4.5

Metric Equivalents of Liquid Volume

1 cubic centimeter (cc or cm³)	=	1 milliliter (mL or ml)
1000 milliliters (mL or ml)	=	1 liter (L)
1000 cubic centimeters (cc or cm³)	=	1 liter (L)

NOTE

The prefix "milli" means "$\dfrac{1}{1000}$". So a milliliter is $\dfrac{1}{1000}$ of a liter.

The milliliter (mL) and cubic centimeter (cc) are equivalent measurements. A 30 mL vial of meperidine hydrochloride (Demerol) is, therefore, the same as a 30 cc vial of meperidine hydrochloride.

Using dimensional analysis and the information in Table 4.5, you can convert a quantity written in one unit of metric volume to another. The next examples show how to do this.

Example 4.6

If the prescriber ordered 0.75 liters of 5% dextrose in water (D/W), how many cubic centimeters were ordered?

$$0.75 \, L = ? \, cc$$

Cancel the liters and obtain the equivalent amount in cubic centimeters.

$$0.75 \, L \times \frac{? \, cc}{? \, L} = ? \, cc$$

Since 1000 cc = 1 L, the fraction you want is $\dfrac{1000 \, cc}{1 \, L}$.

$$0.75 \, \cancel{L} \times \frac{1000 \, \cancel{cc}}{1 \, \cancel{L}} = 750 \, cc$$

So the prescriber ordered 750 cubic centimeters of 5% D/W.

NOTE

Write 0.75 liters instead of $\dfrac{75}{100}$ or $\dfrac{3}{4}$ liters because in the metric system quantities are written as decimal numbers instead of fractions.

Example 4.7

Your patient is to receive 1750 milliliters of 10% dextrose (D) in normal saline (NS). What is the same dose in liters?

$$1750 \, mL = ? \, L$$

Cancel the milliliters and obtain the equivalent amount in liters.

$$1750 \, mL \times \frac{? \, L}{? \, mL} = ? \, L$$

Because 1000 mL = 1 L, the fraction you want is $\dfrac{1 \, L}{1000 \, mL}$.

$$1750 \, \cancel{mL} \times \frac{1 \, \cancel{L}}{1000 \, \cancel{mL}} = \frac{1750 \, L}{1000} = 1.75 \, L$$

So, 1750 milliliters of 10% D/NS is the same dose as 1.75 liters of 10% D/NS.

Weight in the Metric System

Drugs in dry form are measured by weight in the metric system. Metric equivalents for weight are shown in Table 4.6, along with their abbreviations.

Table 4.6

Metric Equivalents of Weight

1 kilogram (kg)	=	1000 grams (g)
1 gram (g)	=	1000 milligrams (mg)
1 milligram (mg)	=	1000 micrograms (μg or mcg)

> **NOTE**
>
> "Kilo" means "thousand" (1000). So, a kilogram is 1000 grams. "Milli" means "one thousandth" $\left(\dfrac{1}{1000}\right)$. So, a milligram is $\dfrac{1}{1000}$ of a gram.
>
> "Micro" means "one millionth" $\left(\dfrac{1}{1,000,000}\right)$. So, a microgram is $\dfrac{1}{1,000,000}$ of a gram.

Using dimensional analysis and the information in Table 4.6, you can convert a quantity written in one unit of metric weight to an equivalent quantity in another unit of metric weight. The following examples show you how to do this.

Example 4.8

The prescriber has ordered 1500 micrograms of Nembutal. How many milligrams in this dose?

$$1500\,\mu g = ?\,mg$$

Cancel the micrograms and obtain the equivalent amount in milligrams.

$$1500\,\mu g \times \frac{?\,mg}{?\,\mu g} = ?\,mg$$

Because $1000\,\mu g = 1\,mg$, the fraction you want is $\dfrac{1\,mg}{1000\,\mu g}$.

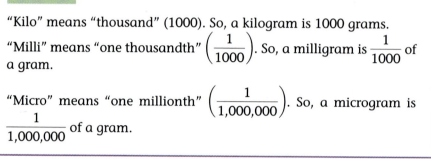

So, 1500 micrograms is the same as 1.5 milligrams.

Example 4.9

The order reads 125 micrograms of digoxin (Lanoxin). How many milligrams of this anti-arrythmic medication would you administer to the patient?

$$125 \text{ mcg} = ? \text{ mg}$$

Cancel the micrograms and obtain the equivalent amount in milligrams.

$$125 \text{ mcg} \times \frac{? \text{ mg}}{? \text{ mcg}} = ? \text{ mg}$$

Because 1000 mcg = 1 mg, you have:

$$125 \text{ mcg} \times \frac{1 \text{ mg}}{1000 \text{ mcg}} = 0.125 \text{ mg}$$

So, 125 micrograms is the same as 0.125 milligram, and you would administer 0.125 milligram of digoxin.

Example 4.10

The order reads 0.015 gram of Glucotrol, an oral hypoglycemic agent. How many milligrams would you administer?

$$0.015 \text{ g} = ? \text{ mg}$$

Cancel the grams and obtain the equivalent amount in milligrams.

$$0.015 \text{ g} \times \frac{? \text{ mg}}{? \text{ g}} = ? \text{ mg}$$

$$0.015 \text{ g} \times \frac{1000 \text{ mg}}{1 \text{ g}} = 15 \text{ mg}$$

So, 0.015 gram is the same as 15 milligrams, and you would administer 15 milligrams of Glucotrol.

BY THE WAY

A dose is always expressed in the form of a number and a unit of measure. Both are important. For example:

15 cc	dram 1
2.5 mg	1.5 mL
3 tablets	0.5 L

When you write your answer, be sure to include the appropriate unit.

PRACTICE SETS

The answers to *Try These for Practice, Exercises,* and *Cumulative Review* appear in Appendix A at the back of the book. The answers to the *Additional Exercises* can be found on the companion Website or ask your instructor.

Try These for Practice

Test your comprehension after reading the chapter.

1. You need to memorize all the apothecary, household, and metric equivalents. To test yourself, fill in the missing numbers in the following chart.

Apothecary System

    a. qt 1   =   pt _____

    b. pt 1   =   ℥ _____

    c. ℥ 1   =   ℨ _____

    d. ℨ 1   =   ℳ _____

Household System

    e. 1 glass   =   ℥ _____

    f. 1 measuring cup   =   ℥ _____

    g. 1 teacup   =   ℥ _____

    h. 1 oz   =   _____ T

    i. 1 T   =   _____ t

    j. 1 t   =   _____ gtt

    k. 1 lb   =   _____ oz

Metric System

    l. 1 L   =   _____ cc

    m. 1 mL   =   _____ cc   =   _____ cm^3

    n. 1 L   =   _____ mL

    o. 1 kg   =   _____ g

    p. 1 g   =   _____ mg

    q. 1 mg   =   _____ μg

    r. 1 mg   =   _____ mcg

    s. 1 μg   =   _____ mcg

2. According to the label in Figure 4.1, each capsule of Sinequan contains 75 mg. Convert 75 milligrams to grams.

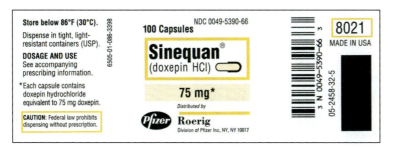

Figure 4.1 Drug label for Sinequan.
(Registered Trademark of Pfizer Inc. Reproduced with permission.)

3. The prescriber ordered 0.05 mg of Sandostatin po, a hormone. How many micrograms are in this dose? _____

4. Prescriber order: 2000 milliliters of H_2O q24 h po. Change milliliters to ounces. _____

5. You have an order for 2 ounces of castor oil po. How many drams will you give the patient? _____

Exercises

Reinforce your understanding in class or at home.

1. ʒ 32 = ℥ _____

2. 0.05 g = _____ mg

3. 0.04 g = _____ mg

4. 4.75 L = _____ cc

5. ʒ 3 = ℳ _____

6. ℥ 64 = ʒ _____

7. 120 mL = _____ cc

8. 100,000 mcg = _____ mg

9. $3\frac{1}{2}$ t = ℳ _____

10. 6 T = _____ t

11. 8 pt = _____ qt

12. 0.26 kg = _____ g

13. The label in Figure 4.2 indicates the quantity of Wellbutrin in one tablet. Change milligrams to grams.

100 Tablets NDC 0173-0178-55

Each film-coated tablet contains

100 mg

WELLBUTRIN®
(bupropion hydrochloride)
Tablets

WARNING: Do not use in combination with ZYBAN®, or any other medicines that contain bupropion hydrochloride.
Store at 15° to 25°C (59° to 77°F).
Protect from moisture.
Dispense in a tight, light-resistant container as defined in the USP.

Rx only

GlaxoWellcome
Manufactured by
Catalytica Pharmaceuticals, Inc.
Greenville, NC 27834
for Glaxo Wellcome Inc.
Research Triangle Park, NC 27709

646123

LOT
EXP

NDC 0173-0178-55

100 Tablets

Each film-coated
tablet contains

100 mg

WELLBUTRIN®
(bupropion hydrochloride)
Tablets

See package insert
for Dosage and
Administration.

NSN 6505-01-314-6640

4117565   Rev. 9/99

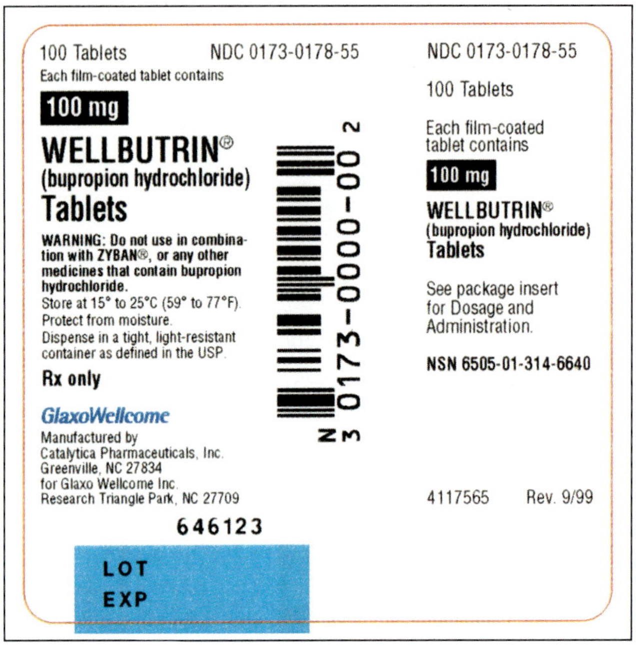

Figure 4.2 Drug label for Wellbutrin.
(Reproduced with permission of GlaxoSmithKline.)

14. The physician ordered 30 mg of ProBanthine po. Change milligrams to grams.

15. According to the physician's order sheet in Figure 4.3, what is the dose of theophylline in milligrams?

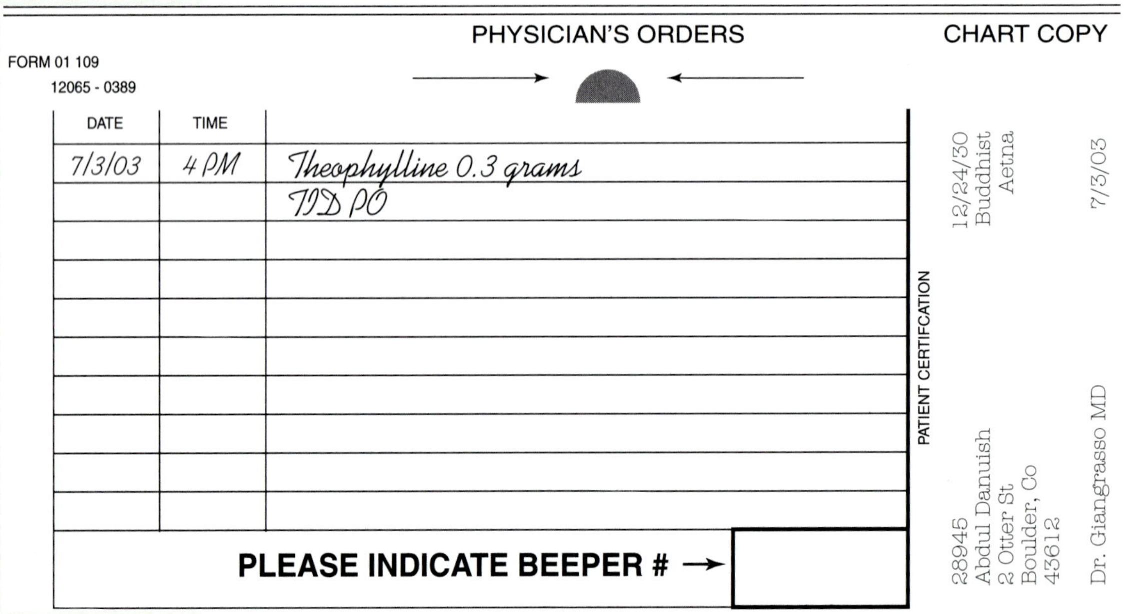

PHYSICIAN'S ORDERS   CHART COPY

FORM 01 109
12065 - 0389

DATE	TIME		
7/3/03	4 PM	Theophylline 0.3 grams TID PO	

PLEASE INDICATE BEEPER # →

PATIENT CERTIFCATION

12/24/30 Buddhist Aetna

28945 Abdul Danuish 2 Otter St. Boulder, Co 43612

Dr. Giangrasso MD

7/3/03

Figure 4.3 Physician's order sheet.

16. The prescriber ordered the following:

Orange juice $\frac{1}{2}$ pint po q2h

How many ounces of orange juice should be given q2h?

17. Xanax 0.5 mg po stat has been ordered for a client. Read the label in Figure 4.4. What is the equivalent dose in grams?

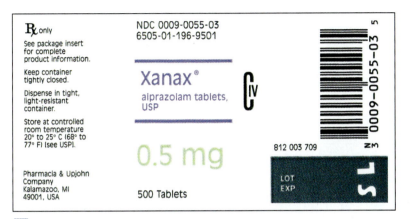
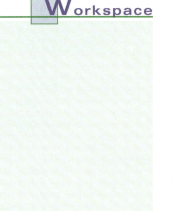

Figure 4.4 Drug label for Xanax.
(Courtesy of Pharmacia Corporation.)

18. The label in Figure 4.5 indicates the amount of Zantac in each tablet. Convert milligrams to grams.

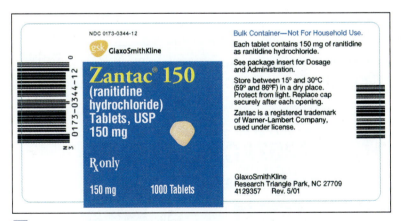

Figure 4.5 Drug label for Zantac.
(Reproduced with permission of GlaxoSmithKline.)

19. An infant weighs 2.8 kg. How much does the infant weigh in grams?

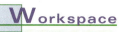

20. Read the order on the physician's order sheet in Figure 4.6. Convert the grams to milligrams.

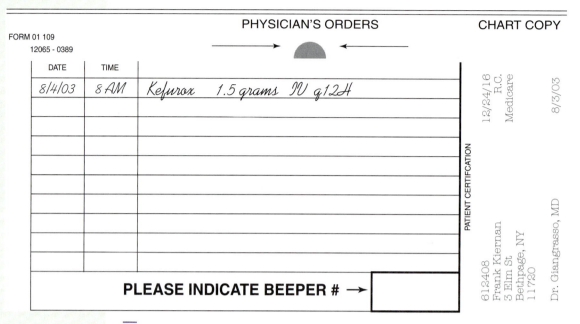

PHYSICIAN'S ORDERS   CHART COPY

FORM 01 109
12065 - 0389

DATE	TIME		
8/4/03	8 AM	Kefurox 1.5 grams IV q12H	

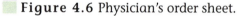

PLEASE INDICATE BEEPER # →

PATIENT CERTIFCATION

12/24/16
R.C.
Medicare

8/3/03

612408
Frank Kiernan
3 Elm St
Bethpage, NY
11720

Dr. Giangrasso, MD

Figure 4.6 Physician's order sheet.

Additional Exercises

Now, on your own, test yourself! Ask your instructor to check your answers.

1. 2500 g = _____ kg   **2.** 3.5 L = _____ cc

3. ♏ 120 = dr _____   **4.** ʒ 32 = ʒ _____

5. 0.006 g = _____ mg   **6.** ʒ 24 = ʒ _____

7. 0.4 kg = _____ g   **8.** qt 4 = pt _____

9. ʒ 30 = ♏ _____   **10.** 3 t = _____ gtt

11. 25,000 mcg = _____ mg   **12.** 50 mL = _____ cc

13. The label in Figure 4.7 indicates the quantity of Prozac in 1 pulvule. Indicate the number of grams of Prozac in 1 pulvule. _____

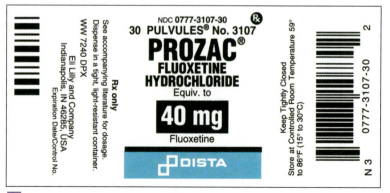

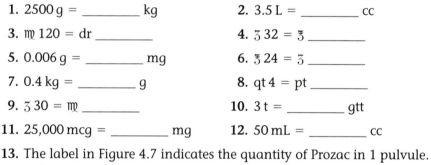

Figure 4.7 Drug label for Prozac.
(Courtesy of Eli Lilly and Company.)

14. How many milligrams would you administer po to the patient if the order for the sedative drug, triazolam (Halcion), was 0.075 gram?_____

15. According to the physician's order sheet in Figure 4.8, what is the dose of guaifenesin (Robitussin) in ounces?_____

✚ GENERAL HOSPITAL ✚

PRESS HARD WITH BALLPOINT PEN. WRITE DATE & TIME AND SIGN EACH ORDER

DATE	TIME	A.M. / P.M.
3/8/03	11	

Robitussin dr 4 po q6h

IMPRINT
273189   3/7/03
James Cane   2/1/75
2 Elm St.   Buddhist
Silver Springs, CO   Aetna
43612
Anthony Giangrasso, M.D.

ORDERS NOTED
DATE _3/8/03_ TIME _11:20_ A.M./P.M.

❑ MEDEX ❑ KARDEX

NURSE'S SIG. _J. Olsen R.N._

FILLED BY   DATE

SIGNATURE   A. Giangrasso M.D.

PHYSICIAN'S ORDERS

Figure 4.8 Physician's order sheet.

16. The prescriber ordered 5% D/W 0.7 L IV q8h. How many milliliters are contained in this amount of solution? _____

17. The prescriber ordered the following:

$$H_2O \ \frac{1}{4} \ pt \ po \ q1h$$

How many ounces should be given every hour? _____

18. The patient must receive 0.75 milligram of dexamethasone po stat ("immediately"). What is the equivalent dose in micrograms? _____

19. Read the label in Figure 4.9. How many grams of this anti-anginal drug are in 1 tablet of Atenolol?

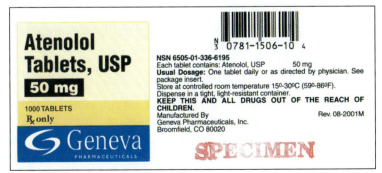

Atenolol Tablets, USP
50 mg
1000 TABLETS
℞ only
ⓒ Geneva
PHARMACEUTICALS

N 3 0781-1506-10 4

NSN 6505-01-336-6195
Each tablet contains: Atenolol, USP   50 mg
Usual Dosage: One tablet daily or as directed by physician. See package insert.
Store at controlled room temperature 15º-30ºC (59º-86ºF).
Dispense in a tight, light-resistant container.
KEEP THIS AND ALL DRUGS OUT OF THE REACH OF CHILDREN.
Manufactured By   Rev. 08-2001M
Geneva Pharmaceuticals, Inc.
Broomfield, CO 80020

SPECIMEN

Figure 4.9 Drug label for Atenolol.
(Courtesy of Geneva Pharmaceuticals.)

W orkspace

14. How many milligrams would you administer po to the patient if the order for the sedative drug, triazolam (Halcion), was 0.075 gram?_____

15. According to the physician's order sheet in Figure 4.8, what is the dose of guaifenesin (Robitussin) in ounces?_____

✚ GENERAL HOSPITAL ✚

PRESS HARD WITH BALLPOINT PEN. WRITE DATE & TIME AND SIGN EACH ORDER

DATE 3/8/03   TIME 11   A.M. / P.M.

Robitussin dr 4 po q6h

IMPRINT
273189   3/7/03
James Cane   2/1/75
2 Elm St.   Buddhist
Silver Springs, CO   Aetna
43612
Anthony Giangrasso, M.D.

ORDERS NOTED
DATE _3/8/03_ TIME _11:20_ A.M./P.M.

❑ MEDEX ❑ KARDEX

NURSE'S SIG. _J. Olsen R.N._

FILLED BY   DATE

SIGNATURE   A. Giangrasso M.D.

PHYSICIAN'S ORDERS

Figure 4.8 Physician's order sheet.

16. The prescriber ordered 5% D/W 0.7 L IV q8h. How many milliliters are contained in this amount of solution? _____

17. The prescriber ordered the following:

$$H_2O \ \frac{1}{4} \ pt \ po \ q1h$$

How many ounces should be given every hour? _____

18. The patient must receive 0.75 milligram of dexamethasone po stat ("immediately"). What is the equivalent dose in micrograms? _____

19. Read the label in Figure 4.9. How many grams of this anti-anginal drug are in 1 tablet of Atenolol?

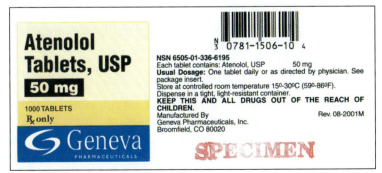

Figure 4.9 Drug label for Atenolol.
(Courtesy of Geneva Pharmaceuticals.)

Practice Sets   73

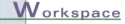
20. Read the label in Figure 4.10. How many micrograms of Paxil are contained in 1 tablet?

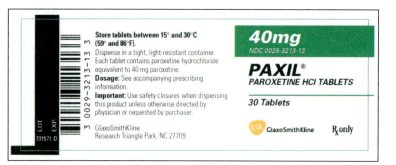

Figure 4.10 Drug label for Paxil.
(Reproduced with permission of GlaxoSmithKline.)

CUMULATIVE REVIEW EXERCISES

Review your mastery of earlier chapters.

1. 7.8 g = _____ mg

2. 0.25 mg = _____ μg

3. ℳ 240 = ℨ _____

4. ℨ 28 = ℨ _____

5. ℳ 60 = _____ t

6. 7.6 kg = _____ g

7. Convert 750 milliliters of urine to liters.

8. How many teaspoons are contained in 4 tablespoons?

9. The order reads 1 gram of Carafate. Convert this dose to milligrams.

10. The patient must receive 250 milligrams of Cloxacillin po. Change to grams.

11. Change 0.65 milligrams to micrograms.

12. The physician ordered 2 tablespoons of Mylanta po, an antacid medication. How many teaspoons would you prepare?

13. The order is 15 drops of tincture of belladonna po stat for your patient. How many teaspoons would you prepare?

14. Change 250 milliliters to liters.

15. The order reads 0.032 gram of a drug. How many milligrams would you administer?

Additional questions, web links, matching exercises, fill-in-the-blanks, and glossary for this chapter can be found on the companion Website at www.prenhall.com/olsen. Click on "Chapter 4" to select the activities for this chapter.

CHAPTER FIVE

Converting from One System of Measurement to Another

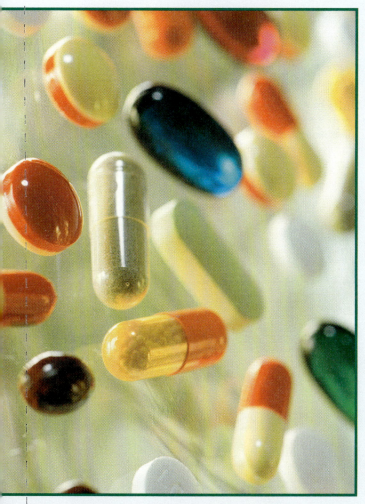

Objectives

After completing this chapter, you will be able to

- State the equivalent units of weight for the metric, apothecary, and household systems.

- State the equivalent units of volume for the metric, apothecary, and household systems.

- State the equivalent units of length for the metric and household systems.

- Convert from one unit to its equivalent among the three systems.

When calculating drug dosages, you will sometimes need to convert a quantity expressed in one system of measurement to an equivalent quantity expressed in another. For example, you might need to convert a quantity measured in drams to the same quantity measured in milliliters. This chapter will show you how to use dimensional analysis to accomplish this conversion.

Equivalents of Common Units of Measurement

To get started, you will need to learn some basic equivalent values of the various units in the different systems. Tables 5.1 through 5.3 list some common equivalent values for weight, volume, and length in the metric, apothecary, and household systems of measurement. Although these equivalents are considered standards, many of them are approximations.

Table 5.1

Equivalent Values for Units of Weight

Metric		Apothecary		Household
60 milligrams (mg)	=	grain (gr) 1		
1 gram (g)	=	grains (gr) 15		
1 kilogram (kg)			=	2.2 pounds (lb)
0.45 kilogram (kg)			=	1 pound (lb)

Table 5.2

Equivalent Values for Units of Volume

Metric		Apothecary		Household
		minim (♏) 1	=	1 drop (gtt)
1 milliliter (mL)	=	minims (♏) 15 or 16	=	15 or 16 drops (gtt)
4 or 5 milliliters (mL)	=	dram (ʒ) 1	=	1 teaspoon (t)
		minims (♏) 60	=	1 teaspoon (t)
		minims (♏) 60	=	60 drops (gtt)
15 milliliters (mL)	=	ounce (ʒ) $\frac{1}{2}$	=	1 T
30 milliliters (mL)	=	ounce (ʒ) 1	=	1 ounce (ʒ) or 2 T
500 milliliters (mL)	=	ounces (ʒ) 16	=	1 pint (pt)
1000 milliliters (mL)	=	ounces (ʒ) 32	=	1 quart (qt) or 2 pints (pt)

Table 5.3

Equivalent Values for Units of Length

Metric		Household
1 centimeter (cm)	=	0.4 inch (in)
2.5 centimeters (cm)	=	1 inch (in)

You can use dimensional analysis to convert from one system to another in exactly the same way you converted from one unit to another within the same system. Multiply the original measurement by a fraction that is equal to 1. This fraction will have the original units on the bottom and the new units on the top. Figure 5.1 depicts some useful equivalents of volume measurements among the three systems.

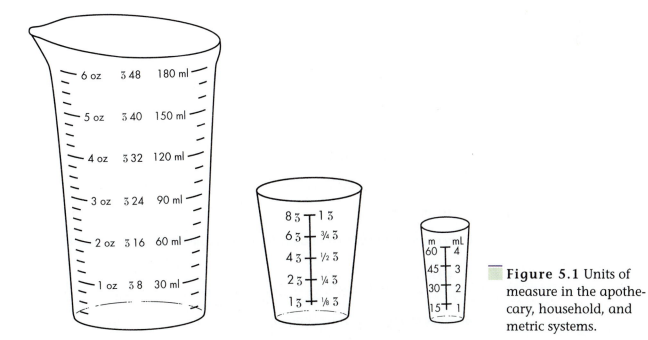

Figure 5.1 Units of measure in the apothecary, household, and metric systems.

The surface of a liquid in a medication cup is not flat (see Figure 5.2). It is curved. We read the amount of liquid at the level of the bottom of the meniscus.

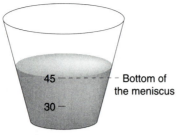

Figure 5.2
Medication cup
with 45 mL.

45 ---- -- Bottom of
          the meniscus

30 —

Metric-to-Apothecary Conversions

Example | **5.1**

Convert 600 milligrams to grains.

$$600\,\text{mg} = \text{gr}\,?$$

You want to cancel the milligrams and obtain the equivalent amount in grains.

$$600\,\text{mg} \times \frac{\text{gr}\,?}{?\,\text{mg}} = \text{gr}\,?$$

Because 60 mg = gr 1, the fraction is $\dfrac{\text{gr}\,1}{60\,\text{mg}}$

$$600\,\cancel{\text{mg}} \times \frac{\text{gr}\,1}{60\,\cancel{\text{mg}}} = \frac{\text{gr}\,60}{6} = \text{gr}\,10$$

So, 600 milligrams are equivalent to grains 10.

Example | **5.2**

Convert 40 milligrams to grains.

$$40\,\text{mg} = \text{gr}\,?$$

Cancel the milligrams and obtain the equivalent amount in grains.

$$40\,\text{mg} \times \frac{\text{gr}\,?}{?\,\text{mg}} = \text{gr}\,?$$

Because 60 mg = gr 1, the fraction is $\dfrac{\text{gr}\,1}{60\,\text{mg}}$

$$\overset{2}{\cancel{40}}\,\cancel{\text{mg}} \times \frac{\text{gr}\,1}{\underset{3}{\cancel{60}}\,\cancel{\text{mg}}} = \text{gr}\,\frac{2}{3}$$

So, 40 milligrams are equivalent to grain $\dfrac{2}{3}$.

Example 5.3

The label for dexamethasone is shown in Figure 5.3. Convert the milligrams in 1 tablet to grains.

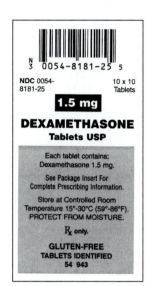

Figure 5.3 Drug label for dexamethasone. (Courtesy of ESI Lederle a Business Unit of Wyeth Pharmaceutical. Philadelphia, PA.)

$$1.5 \, mg = gr \, ?$$

You want to cancel the milligrams and get the answer in grains.

$$1.5 \, mg \times \frac{gr \, ?}{? \, mg} = gr \, ?$$

Because gr 1 = 60 mg, the fraction is $\dfrac{gr \, 1}{60 \, mg}$

$$1.5 \, \cancel{mg} \times \frac{gr \, 1}{60 \, \cancel{mg}} = \frac{gr \, 1.5}{60} \times \frac{10}{10} = gr \, \frac{15}{600} = gr \, \frac{1}{40}$$

So, 1.5 mg is equivalent to grain $\dfrac{1}{40}$.

In Example 5.3, we multiplied both the numerator and the denominator of the fraction $\dfrac{gr \, 1.5}{60}$ by 10 to eliminate the decimal number.

Example 5.4

Convert 0.2 grams to grains.

$$0.2 \, g = gr \, ?$$

You want to cancel the grams and obtain the equivalent amount in grains.

$$0.2 \, g \times \frac{gr \, ?}{? \, g} = gr \, ?$$

Because 1 g = gr 15, the fraction is $\dfrac{\text{gr }15}{1\text{ g}}$

$$0.2\ \cancel{\text{g}} \times \dfrac{\text{gr }15}{1\ \cancel{\text{g}}} = \text{gr }3$$

So, 0.2 gram is are equivalent to grains 3.

Example 5.5

Convert 0.12 milligrams to grains.

$$0.12\text{ mg} = \text{gr }?$$

You want to cancel the milligrams and get the equivalent amount in grains.

$$0.12\text{ mg} \times \dfrac{\text{gr }?}{?\text{ mg}} = \text{gr }?$$

Because 60 mg = gr 1, the fraction is $\dfrac{\text{gr }1}{60\text{ mg}}$

$$0.12\ \cancel{\text{mg}} \times \dfrac{\text{gr }1}{60\ \cancel{\text{mg}}} = \text{gr}\dfrac{0.12}{60} \times \dfrac{100}{100} = \text{gr}\dfrac{12}{6000} = \text{gr}\dfrac{1}{500}$$

So, 0.12 mg is equivalent to grains $\dfrac{1}{500}$.

Example 5.6

Read the information on the label in Figure 5.4 and convert the quantity of drug in the vial to grains.

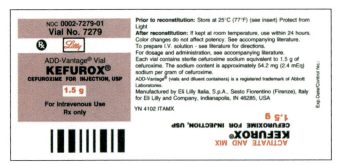

Figure 5.4 Drug label for Kefurox.

(Courtesy of Eli Lilly, and Company.)

$$1.5\text{ g} = \text{gr }?$$

You want to cancel the grams and obtain the equivalent amount in grains.

$$1.5\text{ g} \times \dfrac{\text{gr }?}{?\text{ g}} = \text{gr }?$$

Because 1 g = gr 15, the fraction is $\dfrac{\text{gr }15}{1\text{ g}}$

$$1.5 \, g \times \frac{gr \, 15}{1 \, g} = gr \, 22.5 \quad \text{or} \quad gr \, 22\frac{1}{2}$$

So, 1.5 grams is equivalent to grains $22\frac{1}{2}$.

NOTE

Grains are expressed in fractions and whole numbers. Therefore, grains 22.5 should be expressed as grains $22\frac{1}{2}$.

Apothecary-to-Metric Conversions

Example **5.7**

Convert grain $\frac{1}{300}$ to milligrams.

$$gr \, \frac{1}{300} = ? \, mg$$

You want to cancel the grain and obtain the equivalent amount in milligrams.

$$gr \, \frac{1}{300} \times \frac{? \, mg}{gr \, ?} = ? \, mg$$

Because 60 mg = gr 1, the fraction is $\frac{60 \, mg}{gr \, 1}$

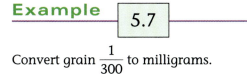

So, grain $\frac{1}{300}$ is equivalent to 0.2 milligrams.

Example **5.8**

Convert grains 20 to milligrams.

$$gr \, 20 = ? \, mg$$

You want to cancel the grains and obtain the equivalent amount in milligrams.

$$gr \, 20 \times \frac{? \, mg}{gr \, ?} = ? \, mg$$

Because 60 mg = gr 1, the fraction is $\dfrac{60\,\text{mg}}{\text{gr}\,1}$

$$\text{gr}\,20 \times \dfrac{60\,\text{mg}}{\text{gr}\,1} = 1200\,\text{mg}$$

So, grains 20 are equivalent to 1200 milligrams.

Example 5.9

Convert grains $7\dfrac{1}{2}$ to grams.

$$\text{gr}\,7\dfrac{1}{2} = ?\,\text{g}$$

You want to cancel the grains and obtain the equivalent amount in grams.

$$\text{gr}\,\dfrac{15}{2} \times \dfrac{?\,\text{g}}{\text{gr}\,?} = ?\,\text{g}$$

Since 1 g = gr 15, the fraction is $\dfrac{1\,\text{g}}{\text{gr}\,15}$

$$\text{gr}\,\dfrac{\overset{1}{\cancel{15}}}{2} \times \dfrac{1\,\text{g}}{\cancel{\text{gr}\,15}\,\underset{1}{}} = \dfrac{1}{2}\,\text{g} = 0.5\,\text{g}$$

So, grains $7\dfrac{1}{2}$ are equivalent to 0.5 gram.

> **NOTE**
>
> Grams are expressed in decimals or whole numbers. Therefore, $\dfrac{1}{2}$ gram is expressed as 0.5 gram.

Example 5.10

Convert grain $\dfrac{3}{4}$ to grams.

$$\text{gr}\,\dfrac{3}{4} = ?\,\text{g}$$

You want to cancel the grains and obtain the equivalent amount in grams.

$$\text{gr}\,\dfrac{3}{4} \times \dfrac{?\,\text{g}}{\text{gr}\,?} = ?\,\text{g}$$

Because 1 g = gr 15, the fraction is $\dfrac{1\,\text{g}}{\text{gr}\,15}$

$$\text{gr}\,\dfrac{\overset{1}{\cancel{3}}}{4} \times \dfrac{1\,\text{g}}{\underset{5}{\cancel{\text{gr}\,15}}} = \dfrac{1}{20}\,\text{g} = 0.05\,\text{g}$$

So, grain $\dfrac{3}{4}$ is equivalent to 0.05 gram.

Household-to-Apothecary or Household-to-Metric Conversions

Example 5.11

Convert 8 teaspoons to milliliters.

$$8\,t = ?\,mL$$

You want to cancel the teaspoons and obtain the equivalent in milliliters.

$$8\,t \times \frac{?\,mL}{?\,t} = ?\,mL$$

You can either use $4\,mL = 1\,t$ or $5\,mL = 1\,t$. For this calculation, use $5\,mL = 1\,t$; the fraction is therefore $\dfrac{5\,mL}{1\,t}$

$$8\,\cancel{t} \times \frac{5\,mL}{1\,\cancel{t}} = 40\,mL$$

So, 8 teaspoons are equivalent to 40 milliliters.

> ### BY THE WAY
>
> If you used the equivalent $4\,mL = 1\,t$ in this example, the answer would be 32 milliliters instead of 40 milliliters. This illustrates the approximate nature of the equivalents among systems. The equivalent $5\,mL = 1\,t$ is the more commonly used.

Example 5.12

Change $\dfrac{1}{3}$ teaspoon to drops.

$$\frac{1}{3}\,t = ?\,gtt$$

You want to cancel the teaspoon and obtain the equivalent amount in drops.

$$\frac{1}{3}\,t \times \frac{?\,gtt}{?\,t} = ?\,gtt$$

Since $60\,gtt = 1\,t$, the fraction is $\dfrac{60\,gtt}{1\,t}$

$$\frac{1}{\underset{1}{\cancel{3}}}\,\cancel{t} \times \frac{\overset{20}{\cancel{60}}\,gtt}{\cancel{t}} = 20\,gtt$$

So, $\dfrac{1}{3}$ teaspoon is equivalent to 20 drops.

Example 5.13

Susan is 5 feet 3 inches tall. What is her height in centimeters?

5 ft 3 in   means   5 ft + 3 in

First determine Susan's height in inches. To do this, convert 5 feet to inches.

5 ft = ? in

You want to cancel feet and obtain the equivalent height in inches.

$$5 \, ft \times \frac{? \, in}{? \, ft} = ? \, in$$

Because 1 ft = 12 in, the fraction is $\dfrac{12 \, in}{1 \, ft}$

$$5 \, ft \times \frac{12 \, in}{1 \, ft} = 60 \, in$$

Second, add the extra 3 inches.

60 in + 3 in = 63 in

Now convert 63 inches to centimeters.

63 in = ? cm

You want to cancel inches and obtain the equivalent length in centimeters.

$$63 \, in \times \frac{? \, cm}{? \, in} = ? \, cm$$

Because 1 in = 2.5 cm, the fraction is $\dfrac{2.5 \, cm}{1 \, in}$

$$63 \, in \times \frac{2.5 \, cm}{1 \, in} = 157.5 \, cm$$

So, Susan is 157.5 centimeters tall.

Example 5.14

Jennifer weighs 103 pounds 8 ounces. What is her weight in kilograms?

103 lb 8 oz   means   103 lb + 8 oz

First determine Jennifer's weight in pounds. To do this, convert 8 ounces to pounds.

8 oz = ? lb

You want to cancel ounces and obtain the equivalent amount in pounds.

$$8 \text{ oz} \times \frac{? \text{ lb}}{? \text{ oz}} = ? \text{ lb}$$

Because 1 lb = 16 oz, the fraction is $\dfrac{1 \text{ lb}}{16 \text{ oz}}$

$$\overset{1}{\cancel{8}} \text{ oz} \times \frac{1 \text{ lb}}{\underset{2}{\cancel{16}} \text{ oz}} = \frac{1}{2} \text{ lb}$$

So, Jennifer weighs 103 lb $+ \dfrac{1}{2}$ lb or 103.5 pounds.

Second, convert 103.5 pounds to kilograms.

$$103.5 \text{ lb} = ? \text{ kg}$$

You want to cancel pounds and obtain the equivalent amount in kilograms.

$$103.5 \text{ lb} \times \frac{? \text{ kg}}{? \text{ lb}} = ? \text{ kg}$$

Because 1 kg = 2.2 lb, the fraction is $\dfrac{1 \text{ kg}}{2.2 \text{ lb}}$

$$103.5 \cancel{\text{ lb}} \times \frac{1 \text{ kg}}{2.2 \cancel{\text{ lb}}} = 47.0 \text{ kg}$$

So, Jennifer weighs 47 kilograms.

If we use the equivalent 1 lb = 0.45 kg instead of 2.2 lb = 1 kg, then our calculations would be

$$103.5 \cancel{\text{ lb}} \times \frac{0.45 \text{ kg}}{1 \cancel{\text{ lb}}} = 46.575 \text{ kg}$$

This answer is different from the previous result because of the approximate nature of the equivalents among systems.

PRACTICE SETS

The answers to *Try These for Practice, Exercises,* and *Cumulative Review* appear in Appendix A at the back of the book. The answers to the *Additional Exercises* can be found on the companion Website or ask your instructor.

Try These for Practice

Test your comprehension after reading the chapter.

1. In order to do the exercises at the end of this chapter, you need to memorize all the equivalents presented so far. To test yourself, fill in the missing numbers in the following chart.

Metric System

a. 1 mL   =   1 cc   =   _____ cm^3

b. 1 L   =   _____ mL

c. 1 kg   =   _____ g

d. 1000 mg   =   _____ g

e. 1000 μg   =   _____ mg

f. 1 μg   =   _____ mcg

Household System

g. 1 glass   =   ʒ _____

h. 1 teacup   =   ʒ _____

i. ʒ 1   =   _____ T

j. 1 T   =   _____ t

k. 1 t   =   _____ gtt

l. 1 lb   =   _____ oz

m. 1 ft   =   _____ in

Apothecary System

n. 1 qt   =   _____ pt

o. 1 pt   =   ʒ _____

p. ʒ 1   =   ʒ _____

q. ʒ 1   =   ℳ _____

Mixed Systems

r. ʒ 1 = _____ t   = ℳ _____   = _____ gtt = _____ mL

s. ʒ 1   = _____ T   = ʒ _____   = _____ mL

t. 1 measuring cup = _____ glass = ℥ _____ = _____ pt

u. gr 1 = _____ mg

v. 1 g = gr _____

w. 1 mL = _____ gtt

x. 1 kg = _____ lb

y. 1 lb = _____ kg

z. 1 in = _____ cm

2. The prescriber ordered Ery-Tab 666 milligrams po. Read the label in Figure 5.5. How many grains of Ery-Tab are contained in 2 tablets?

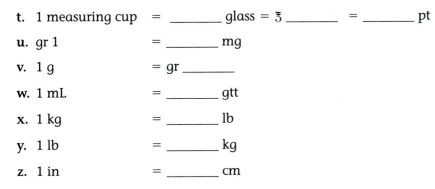

Figure 5.5 Drug label for Ery-Tab.
(Reproduced with permission of Abbott Laboratories.)

3. An adult weighs 172 pounds. Convert this weight to kilograms.

4. Using the information in Figure 5.6, calculate the number of grains in 1 tablet.

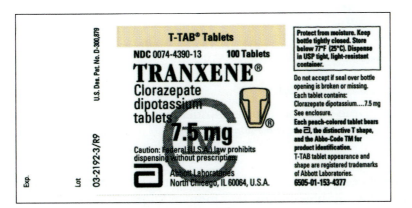

Figure 5.6 Drug label for Tranxene.
(Reproduced with permission of Abbott Laboratories.)

5. The prescriber ordered atropine sulfate gr $\frac{1}{250}$ s/c stat. How many milligrams will you prepare?

Workspace

Exercises

Reinforce your understanding in class or at home.

1. Convert 3200 micrograms to milligrams.

2. How many milligrams are contained in 250 grams?

3. 0.005 g = _____ mg

4. 0.004 mg = _____ mcg

5. gr $7\frac{1}{2}$ = _____ g

6. 0.006 mg = gr _____

7. 0.7 mg = _____ g

8. 8.25 L = _____ mL

9. 10,075 mL = _____ L

10. gr $3\frac{3}{4}$ = _____ mg

11. Read the label in Figure 5.7. How many milligrams of codeine are contained in one milliliter?

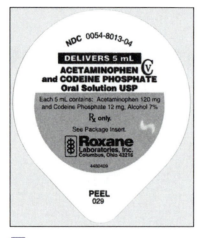

Figure 5.7 Drug label for codeine phosphate and acetaminophen.
(Used with permission of Roxane Laboratories, Inc.)

12. A capsule of acetaminophen (Tylenol), an antipyretic drug, contains 0.5 gram. One capsule contains how many milligrams?

13. A prescriber ordered

    Chlorpromazine 150 mg po stat

    From the label in Figure 5.8, determine the number of milliliters of this antianxiety drug you would give your client.

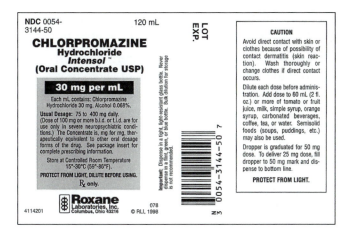

Figure 5.8 Drug label for Chlorpromazine.
(Used with permission of Roxane Laboratories, Inc.)

14. A prescriber ordered fluoxetine hydrochloride (Prozac) 30 mg po bid. Read the label in Figure 5.9. How many milliliters will you give your client?

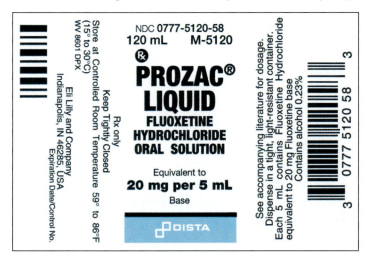

Figure 5.9 Drug label for Prozac.
(Courtesy of Eli Lilly and Company.)

15. A prescriber ordered erythromycin (Ery-Tab) 500 mg po q12h. Read the information in Figure 5.10 to determine the number of tablets which you would administer to your client.

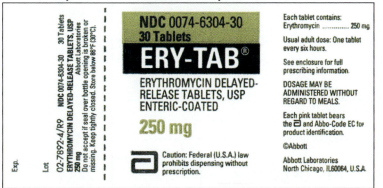

Figure 5.10 Drug label for Ery-Tab.
(Reproduced with permission of Abbott Laboratories.)

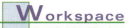

16. The patient is to receive 10 mL po of Benadryl 25 mg, an antihistamine drug. How many teaspoons will you administer to your patient?

17. Order: Elixir of Digoxin 150 μg stat po. Read the information in Figure 5.11 and calculate the number of milliliters of Digoxin you will prepare.

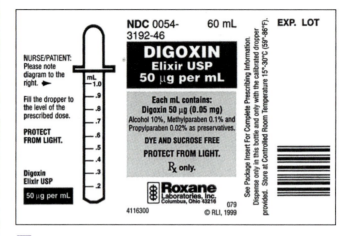

Figure 5.11 Drug label for Digoxin.
(Used with permission of Roxane Laboratories, Inc.)

18. Read the information on the physician's order sheet in Figure 5.12. If each tablet of clonidine hcl contains 0.1 mg, how many tablets will the patient receive in a day?

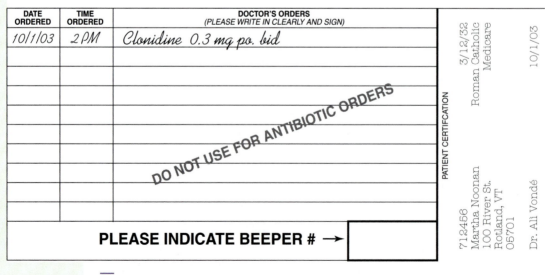
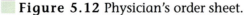

Figure 5.12 Physician's order sheet.

19. Diabinese (chlorpropamide) has been prescribed for your patient. The order is 200 mg po qd. Read the label in Figure 5.13 and calculate the number of tablets you will give the patient.

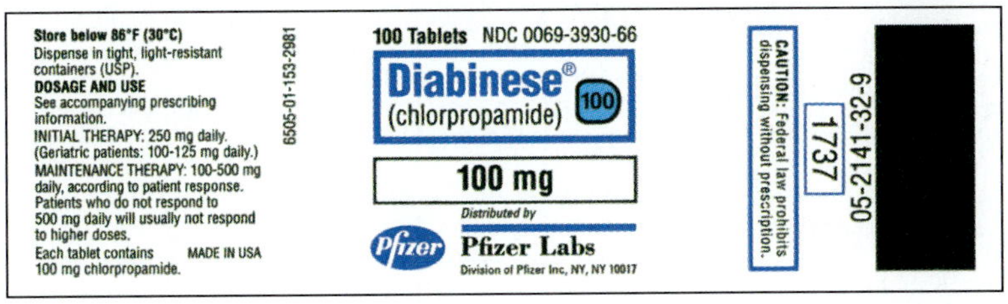

Figure 5.13 Drug label for Diabinese.
(Registered Trademark of Pfizer Inc. Reproduced with permission.)

20. Convert grains 45 to grams.

Additional Exercises

Now, on your own, test yourself! The answers to the *Additional Exercises* can be found on the companion Website or ask your instructor.

1. Convert 75 micrograms to milligrams. _____

2. How many grams does 2.25 kilograms equal? _____

3. 0.003 g = _____ mg

4. 0.005 mg = _____ mcg

5. 6.25 L = _____ mL

6. 0.6 mg = gr _____

7. 0.4 mg = _____ g

8. 0.2 mg = _____ mcg

9. 2400 mL = _____ L

10. gr $3\frac{3}{4}$ = _____ mg

11. $2\frac{1}{2}$ t = _____ gtt

12. gr $\frac{1}{600}$ = _____ mg

13. The prescriber ordered atropine sulfate 0.2 mg sc q6h prn. What is the equivalent dose in micrograms? _____

14. The order reads grains 4 of a drug. Change this order to grams. _____

15. A prescriber has ordered 25 milligrams of captopril (Capoten) po. What is the equivalent quantity in micrograms? _____

16. According to the medication administration record in Figure 5.14, how many milligrams of glipizide will you give the patient each day? _____

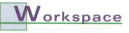

✚ GENERAL HOSPITAL ✚

Year 2003	Month *February*	Day	12	13	14	15	16	
Medication Dosage and Interval			Initials* and Hours	Initials and Hours	Initials and Hours	Initials and Hours	Initials and Hours	Initials and Hours
Date started: *2/12/03*		I	*JO*					
glipizide gr $\frac{1}{3}$ *po qd*		AM	*10*					
		I						
Discontinued		PM						

Allergies: (Specified)
none

Init*	Signature
JO	*June Olsen R.N.*

PATIENT IDENTIFICATION

```
78901                        2/12/03
Jairo Rodriquez
40 Water Street             6/16/60
Merrymount, NY 10301           Prot
                               BCBS


L. Ablon, M.D.
```

MEDICATION ADMINISTRATION RECORD

Figure 5.14 Medication administration record.

17. Using the information in Figure 5.15, calculate the number of grams in each tablet. _____

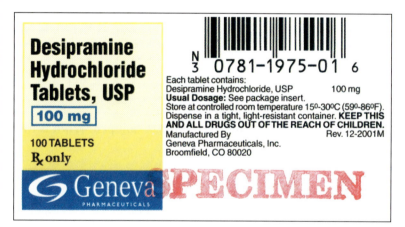

Figure 5.15 Drug label for Desipramine.
(Courtesy of Geneva Pharmaceuticals.)

18. Read the label in Figure 5.16 and change the milligrams to grains. _____

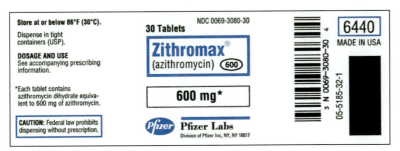

Figure 5.16 Drug label for Zithromax.
(Registered Trademark of Pfizer Inc. Reproduced with permission.)

19. Using the information in Figure 5.17, calculate the number of grams in 1 tablet. _____

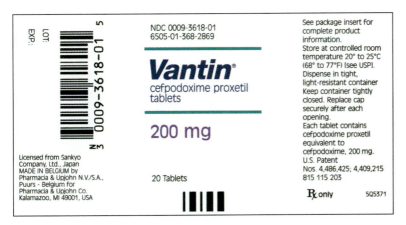

Figure 5.17 Drug label for Vantin.
(Courtesy of Pharmacia Corporation.)

20. The prescriber ordered potassium chloride 60 mEq po. Calculate the number of packets needed for this dose from the label in Figure 5.18. _____

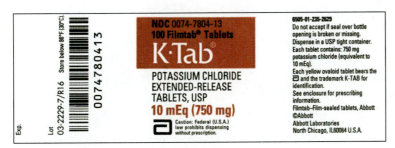

Figure 5.18 Drug label for K-Lor.
(Reproduced with permission of Abbott Laboratories.)

Workspace

CUMULATIVE REVIEW EXERCISES

Review your mastery of earlier chapters.

1. Convert 0.125 milligrams to micrograms.
2. 0.009 g = ________ mg
3. How many grams are contained in 5.65 kilograms?
4. 0.1 mg = ________ mcg
5. 0.06 g = ________ mg
6. gr $3\frac{3}{4}$ = ________ mg
7. 7.75 L = ________ mL
8. 0.6 mg = ________ mcg
9. 1250 mL = ________ L
10. 30 mg = gr ________
11. Read the label in Figure 5.19. How many grains of Agenerase are contained in 3 capsules?

NDC 0173-0679-00
Agenerase®
(amprenavir)
Capsules 50 mg
480 Capsules
Each capsule contains 50 mg of amprenavir.
Rx only
ALERT
Find out about medicines that should NOT be taken with AGENERASE.
Note to Pharmacist: Do not cover ALERT box with pharmacy label.
3 N 0173-0679-00 0
Store at controlled room temperature of 25°C (77°F) (see USP).
See package insert for Dosage and Administration.
AGENERASE (amprenavir) Capsules are not interchangeable on a mg/mg basis with AGENERASE (amprenavir) Oral Solution.
US Patent Nos. 5,585,397; 5,723,490; and 5,646,180
Licensed from Vertex Pharmaceuticals Incorporated Cambridge, MA 02139
AGENERASE is a registered trademark of the Glaxo Wellcome group of companies.
Manufactured by R.P. Scherer Beinheim, France for Glaxo Wellcome Inc. Research Triangle Park, NC 27709 Made in France
GlaxoWellcome
VERTEX™
4128648 Rev. 2/01

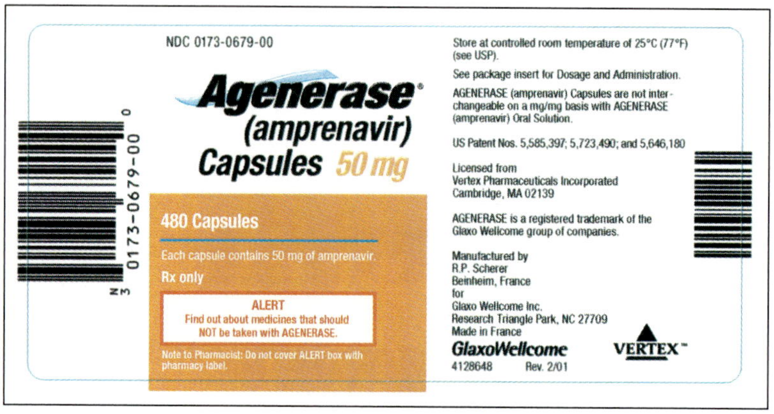

Figure 5.19 Drug label for Agenerase.
(Reproduced with permission of Glaxosmithkline.)

12. Read the label in Figure 5.19. How many grams of Agenerase are contained in 3 capsules?
13. Read the label in Figure 5.20. Calculate the number of grams in each tablet.

Store below 86°F (30°C).
Dispense in tight, light-resistant containers (USP).
DOSAGE AND USE
See accompanying prescribing information.
USUAL DOSAGE: ADULTS: 25 mg t.i.d. to 100 mg q.i.d.
CHILDREN: Under 6 years–50 mg daily in divided doses.
Over 6 years–50 to 100 mg daily in divided doses.
Each tablet contains 10 mg of hydroxyzine hydrochloride.
CAUTION: Federal law prohibits dispensing without prescription.
MADE IN USA
NDC 0049-5600-66
100 Tablets
Atarax® 10
(hydroxyzine HCl)
10 mg
Pfizer
Roerig
Division of Pfizer Inc, NY, NY 10017
3 N 0049-5600-66 3
05-2190-32-1
4341

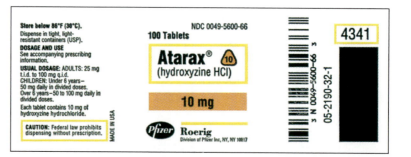

Figure 5.20 Drug label for Atarax.
(Registered Trademark of Pfizer Inc. Reproduced with permission.)

14. How many grams are equal to the number of milligrams contained in 2 mL of the drug Pancuronium shown in Figure 5.21?

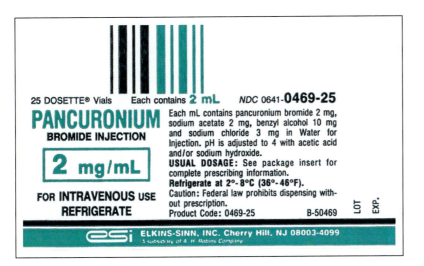

Figure 5.21 Drug label for Pancuronium.
(Courtesy of ESI Ledele, a Business Unit of Wyeth Pharmaceuticals, Philadephia, PA.)

15. The label for Procardia XL is shown in Figure 5.22. Convert the milligrams and one tablet to grams.

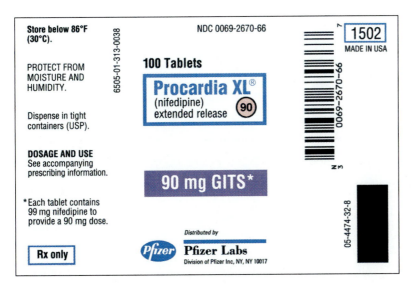

Figure 5.22 Drug label for Procardia XL.
(Registered Trademark of Pfizer Inc. Reproduced with permission.)

Additional questions, web links, matching exercises, fill-in-the-blanks, and glossary for this chapter can be found on the companion Website at www.prenhall.com/olsen. Click on "Chapter 5" to select the activities for this chapter.

UNIT THREE

Common Medication Preparations

Calculating Oral Medication Doses

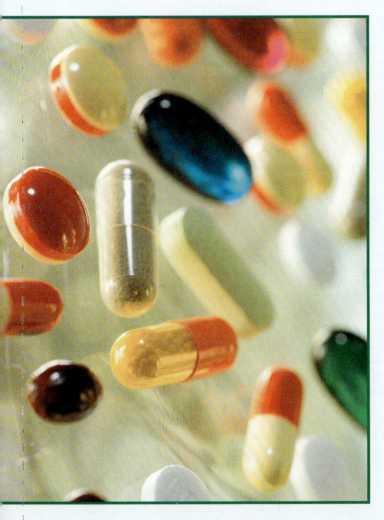

Objectives

After completing this chapter, you will be able to

- Calculate doses by body weight.
- Calculate doses by body surface area.
- Do multistep conversion problems.
- Calculate doses for oral medications in liquid form.
- Calculate doses for oral medications in tablet, capsule, and caplet form.
- Calculate doses for oral medications from the information given on drug labels.

In this chapter you will learn the computations necessary to calculate doses of oral medication in liquid, tablet (tab), capsule (cap), or caplet (cap) form.

One-Step Conversions

In the calculations you have done in previous chapters, all the equivalents have come from standard tables. For example, 60 mg = gr 1. In this section, the equivalent used will depend on the strength of the drug that is available, for example 1 tab = 15 mg. In the following examples, the equivalent used is found on the label of the drug container.

Example  6.1

The order reads 150 milligrams of Pamelor po, a tricylic antidepressant drug. Read the drug label in Figure 6.1 and determine how many capsules you would administer to the patient.

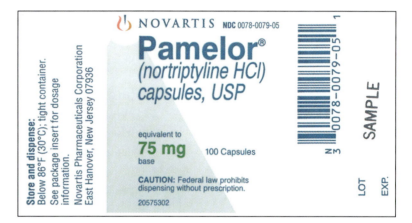

Figure 6.1 Drug label for Pamelor.

(Copyright Novartis Pharmaceuticals Corporation. Reprinted with permission.)

First convert the order, 150 milligrams, to capsules.

$$150 \, \text{mg} = ? \, \text{cap}$$

Then cancel the milligrams and obtain the equivalent amount in capsules.

$$150 \, \text{mg} \times \frac{? \, \text{cap}}{? \, \text{mg}} = ? \, \text{cap}$$

Because the label states that 1 cap = 75 mg, the fraction is $\dfrac{1 \, \text{cap}}{75 \, \text{mg}}$.

$$150 \, \cancel{\text{mg}} \times \frac{1 \, \text{cap}}{75 \, \cancel{\text{mg}}} = 2 \, \text{cap}$$

So, 150 milligrams is equivalent to 2 capsules, and you would give 2 capsules of Pamelor to the patient.

Example 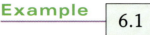 6.2

The order reads as follows:

Geodon 120 mg po

The label is shown in Figure 6.2. How many capsules will you administer to the patient?

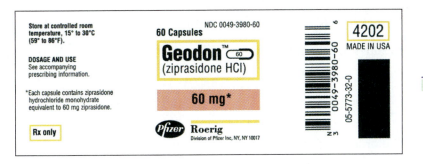

Figure 6.2 Drug label for Geodon.

(Registered Trademark of Pfizer, Inc. Reproduced with permission.)

You want to convert 120 milligrams to capsules

$$120\,\text{mg} = ?\,\text{cap}$$

You want to cancel the milligrams and calculate the equivalent amount in capsules.

$$120\,\text{mg} \times \frac{?\,\text{cap}}{?\,\text{mg}} = ?\,\text{cap}$$

Because the label indicates that each capsule contains 60 milligrams, you use the equivalent $\dfrac{1\,\text{cap}}{60\,\text{mg}}$

$$\overset{2}{\cancel{120\,\text{mg}}} \times \frac{1\,\text{cap}}{\underset{1}{\cancel{60\,\text{mg}}}} = 2\ \text{capsules of Geodon.}$$

Example 6.3

How many tablets should you give a patient if the order is for grain $\dfrac{1}{2}$ of codeine sulfate and each tablet contains grain $\dfrac{1}{4}$?

In this problem you want to convert the order grain $\dfrac{1}{2}$ to tablets.

$$\text{gr}\,\frac{1}{2} = ?\,\text{tab}$$

Then cancel the grain and determine the equivalent amount in tablets.

$$\text{gr}\,\frac{1}{2} \times \frac{?\,\text{tab}}{\text{gr}\,?} = ?\,\text{tab}$$

Because $1\,\text{tab} = \text{gr}\,\dfrac{1}{4}$, the fraction is $\dfrac{1\,\text{tab}}{\text{gr}\,\dfrac{1}{4}}$.

$$\cancel{\text{gr}}\,\frac{1}{2} \times \frac{1\,\text{tab}}{\cancel{\text{gr}}\,\dfrac{1}{4}} = \frac{1\,\text{tab}}{\dfrac{2}{4}} = 1\,\text{tab} \div \frac{2}{4} = 1\,\text{tab} \times \frac{4}{2} = 2\,\text{tab}$$

So, grain $\frac{1}{2}$ is equivalent to 2 tablets, and you should give the patient 2 tablets of codeine sulfate.

Example 6.4

The order reads 8 milligrams of the antihypertensive drug Cardura. Read the label in Figure 6.3. How many tablets should be given to the patient po?

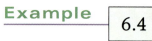

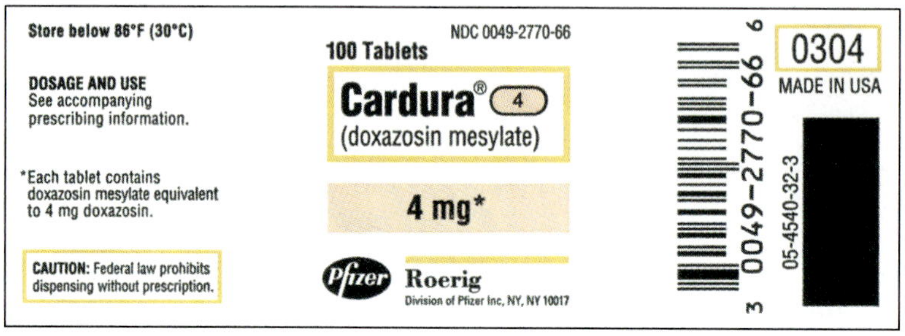

Figure 6.3 Drug label for Cardura.

(Registered Trademark of Pfizer Inc. Reproduced with permission.)

First convert the order, 8 milligrams, to tablets.

$$8\,mg = ?\,tab$$

Then cancel the milligrams and obtain the equivalent amount in tablets.

$$8\,mg \times \frac{?\,tab}{?\,mg} = ?\,tab$$

Since each tablet contains 4 milligrams, the equivalent fraction is $\frac{1\,tab}{4\,mg}$.

$$8\,mg \times \frac{1\,tab}{4\,mg} = 2\,tab$$

So, 8 milligrams is equivalent to 2 tablets, and the patient should be given 2 tablets of Cardura.

Example 6.5

The prescriber orders 75 mg of Viagra for a patient with erectile disfunction. Read the drug label shown in Figure 6.4 and determine how many of these tablets you would give the patient.

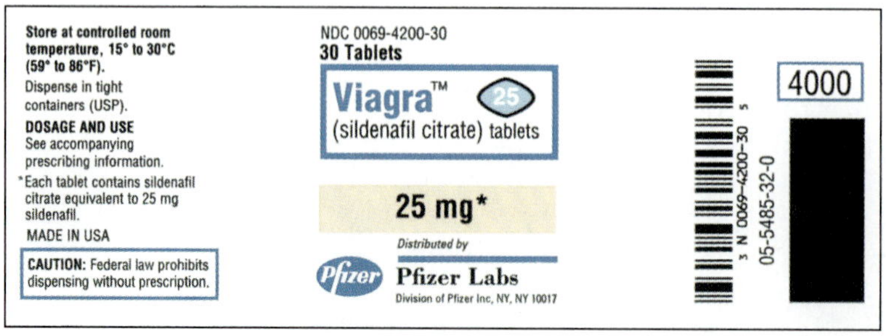

Figure 6.4 Drug label for Viagra.

(Registered Trademark of Pfizer Inc. Reproduced with permission.)

You want to convert 75 milligrams to tablets.

75 mg = ? tab

You want to cancel the milligrams and obtain the equivalent amount in tablets.

$$75 \text{ mg} \times \frac{?\text{ tab}}{?\text{ mg}} = ?\text{ tab}$$

Because 1 tab = 25 mg, the equivalent fraction is $\dfrac{1 \text{ tab}}{25 \text{ mg}}$.

$$\overset{3}{\cancel{75}} \text{ mg} \times \frac{1 \text{ tab}}{\underset{1}{\cancel{25}} \text{ mg}} = 3 \text{ tab}$$

So, 75 milligrams is equivalent to 3 tablets, and you would give 3 tablets of Viagra to the patient.

Example 6.6

Read the label in Figure 6.5. The physician ordered 5 mg po qd. How many tablets are taken daily?

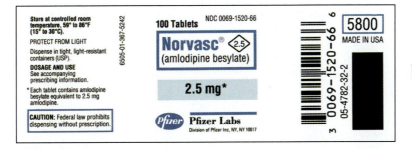

Figure 6.5 Drug label for Norvasc.
(Registered Trademark of Pfizer Inc. Reproduced with permission.)

Convert 5 mg to tablets.

5 mg = ? tab

Cancel the milligrams and obtain the equivalent amount in tablets.

$$5 \text{ mg} \times \frac{?\text{ tab}}{?\text{ mg}} = ?\text{ tab}$$

Because 1 tab = 2.5 mg, the equivalent fraction is $\dfrac{1 \text{ tab}}{2.5 \text{ mg}}$.

$$5 \text{ mg} \times \frac{1 \text{ tab}}{2.5 \text{ mg}} = 2 \text{ tab}$$

So, 2 tablets is equivalent to 5 mg, and 2 tablets are taken daily.

Dosage by Body Weight

Sometimes the amount of medication prescribed depends on the patient's body weight. A patient, who weighs more, will receive more of the drug, and a patient, who weighs less, will receive less of the drug.

Example 6.7

The prescriber orders 15 milligrams per kilogram of methsuximide (Celontin) for a patient who weighs 80 kilograms. How much of this anticonvulsant drug should the patient receive?

> **NOTE**
>
> The expression 15 mg/kg means that the patient is to receive 15 milligrams of the drug for each kilogram of body weight. So you will use the equivalent 15 mg (of drug) = 1 kg (of body weight).

Convert body weight to dosage.

$$80 \text{ kg (of body weight)} = ? \text{ mg (of drug)}$$

$$80 \text{ kg (of body weight)} \times \frac{? \text{ mg (of drug)}}{? \text{ kg (of body weight)}} = \text{mg (of drug)}$$

So, you use the fraction $\dfrac{15 \text{ mg}}{1 \text{ kg}}$, which relates dosage to body weight.

$$80 \text{ kg} \times \frac{15 \text{ mg}}{1 \text{ kg}} = 1200 \text{ mg}$$

The patient should receive 1200 milligrams of methsuximide.

Example 6.8

The order is 6.6 milligrams per kilogram of the antibiotic drug, Biaxin (clarithromycin). How many milligrams would you administer to a patient, who weighs 75 kilograms?

Convert body weight to dosage.

$$75 \text{ kg} = ? \text{ mg}$$

$$75 \text{ kg} \times \frac{? \text{ mg}}{? \text{ kg}} = ? \text{ mg}$$

Use the equivalent 6.6 mg = 1 kg. So, the fraction you use is $\dfrac{6.6 \text{ mg}}{1 \text{ kg}}$.

$$75 \text{ kg} \times \frac{6.6 \text{ mg}}{1 \text{ kg}} = 495 \text{ mg}$$

The patient should receive 495 milligrams of Biaxin.

Calculating Dosage by Body Surface Area

In many cases, body surface area (BSA) is a more important factor than weight in determining appropriate drug dosages. This is particularly true of pediatric drugs and drugs that are used for cancer therapy.

A patient's BSA, which is measured in square meters (m^2), can be determined by using either of the mathematical formulas below or by using a nomogram.

Formula for metric units

$$BSA = \sqrt{\frac{weight\ in\ kg \times height\ in\ cm}{3600}}$$

Formula for household units

$$BSA = \sqrt{\frac{weight\ in\ pounds \times height\ in\ inches}{3131}}$$

Example 6.9

Find the BSA of an adult who is 183 cm tall and weighs 92 kg.
Because we are using metric units (kg and cm), we use the formula

$$BSA = \sqrt{\frac{weight\ in\ kg \times height\ in\ cm}{3600}}$$

$$= \sqrt{\frac{92 \times 183}{3600}}$$

At this point we need a calculator with a square root key.

$$= \sqrt{4.6767}$$

$$= 2.16\ m^2$$

> **NOTE**
>
> In this book, we will round off BSA to two decimal places.

Example 6.10

What is the BSA of a man who is 4 feet 10 inches tall and weighs 142 pounds?
First you convert 4 feet 10 inches to 58 inches.

Because we are using household units (lb and in), we use the formula

$$BSA = \sqrt{\frac{weight\ in\ pounds \times height\ in\ inches}{3131}}$$

$$= \sqrt{\frac{142 \times 58}{3131}}$$

$$= \sqrt{2.6305}$$

$$= 1.62\ m^2$$

Nomogram

BSA can also be approximated by using nomograms. As Figure 6.6 shows, if a straight line is drawn on the nomogram from the patient's height (left column) to the patient's weight (right column), the line will cross the center column at the approximate BSA of this patient.

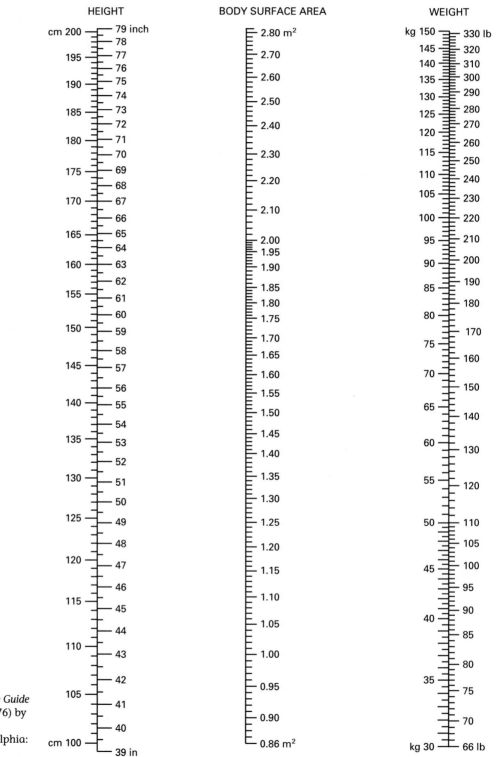

Figure 6.6 Adult nomogram.
Source: From *Davis's Drug Guide for Nurses*, 5th ed. (p. 1276) by J. H. Deglin and A. H. Vallerand, 1997, Philadelphia: Davis.

In Example 6.9, we used the formula to calculate the BSA of a 183 cm, 92 kg patient to be 2.16 m². Now let's use the adult nomogram to do the same problem. In Figure 6.7, you can see that the line from 183 cm to 92 kg intersects the BSA column at about 2.20 m².

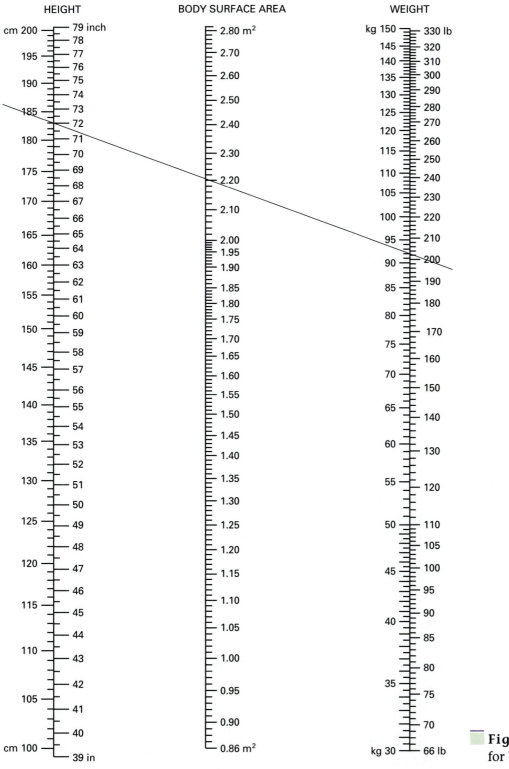

HEIGHT   **BODY SURFACE AREA**   **WEIGHT**

Figure 6.7 Nomogram for Example 6.9.

> ### NOTE
>
> Whether formulas or nomograms are used to obtain body surface area, the results are only approximations. This explains why we obtained both 2.16 m² (using the formula) and 2.20 m² (using the nomogram) as BSA for the same patient.

In Example 6.10, using the formula we calculated the BSA of a 4 ft 10 in, 142 lb patient to be 1.62 m². If we use the adult nomogram to determine the BSA (see Figure 6.8), we get 1.59 m².

Example 6.11

The order is 40 mg/m² of the corticosteroid prednisone (Deltasone). How many milligrams of this adrenocorticoid drug would you administer to an adult patient weighing 88 kg with a height of 150 cm?

The first step is to determine the BSA of the patient. This can be done by formula or nomogram.
Using the formula, you get

$$\text{BSA} = \sqrt{\frac{88 \times 150}{3600}}$$

$$= \sqrt{3.6667}$$

$$= 1.91 \, \text{m}^2$$

With the adult nomogram, you get 1.81 m². So, you can use either 1.91 m² or 1.81 m² as the BSA. If you choose to use 1.81 m², you want to convert BSA to dosage in mg.

$$1.81 \, \text{m}^2 = ? \, \text{mg}$$

$$1.81 \, \text{m}^2 \times \frac{? \, \text{mg}}{\text{m}^2} = ? \, \text{mg}$$

You use the equivalent 40 mg/m², so the fraction you use is $\dfrac{40 \, \text{mg}}{\text{m}^2}$.

$$1.81 \, \text{m}^2 \times \frac{40 \, \text{mg}}{\text{m}^2} = 72.4 \, \text{mg}$$

If you use the BSA of 1.91 m², the calculations are similar and the last step is

$$1.91 \, \text{m}^2 \times \frac{40 \, \text{mg}}{\text{m}^2} = 76.4 \, \text{mg}$$

So, you would administer between 72.4 mg and 76.4 mg of prednisone to the patient.

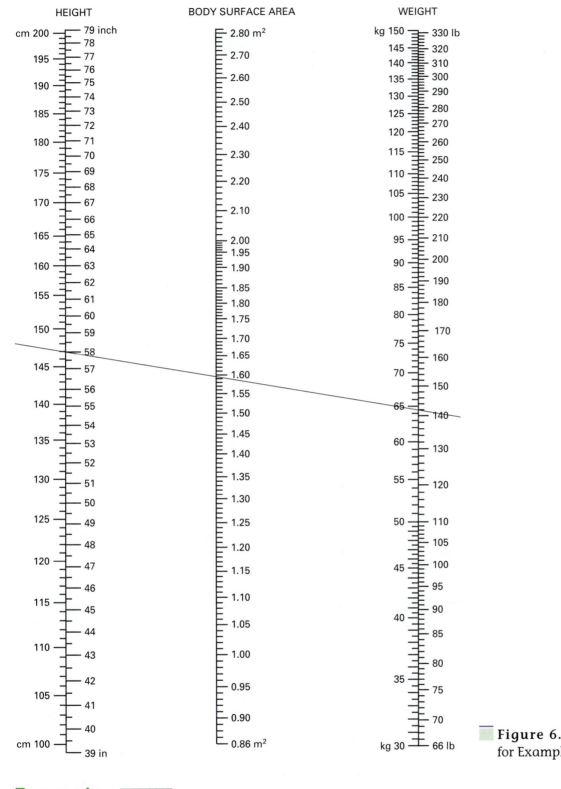

HEIGHT	BODY SURFACE AREA	WEIGHT

Figure 6.8 Nomogram for Example 6.10.

Example 6.12

The prescriber ordered 30 mg/m² of Nembutal for a patient, who has a BSA of 1.65 m². Read the label in Figure 6.9 and determine how many capsules of this sedative drug you would administer to your patient.

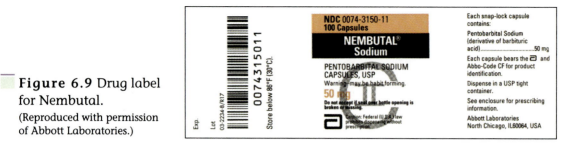

Figure 6.9 Drug label for Nembutal.

(Reproduced with permission of Abbott Laboratories.)

In this case, you know the BSA. You want to convert the BSA of 1.65 m² to the dosage.

$$1.65 \, \text{m}^2 = ? \, \text{mg (of drug)}$$

$$1.65 \, \text{m}^2 \times \frac{? \, \text{mg}}{\text{m}^2} = ? \, \text{mg (of drug)}$$

Use the fraction $\dfrac{30 \, \text{mg}}{\text{m}^2}$, which relates dosage (in milligrams) to BSA.

$$1.65 \, \cancel{\text{m}^2} \times \frac{30 \, \text{mg}}{\cancel{\text{m}^2}} = 49.5 \, \text{mg}$$

The drug label in Figure 6.9 indicates that each capsule contains 50 mg. Therefore, you would administer 1 capsule of Nembutal.

Multistep Conversions

Sometimes drug dosage calculations involve more than one step. For example, suppose you want to find out how many seconds are in 2 hours. You can do this conversion in two steps.

Step 1 Change hours to minutes. Because 60 minutes is 1 hour, the fraction to change hours to minutes is $\dfrac{60 \, \text{min}}{1 \, \text{hr}}$.

$$2 \, \text{hr} \times \frac{60 \, \text{min}}{1 \, \text{hr}}$$

Step 2 Change minutes to seconds. Because 60 seconds is 1 minute, the fraction to change minutes to seconds is $\dfrac{60 \, \text{sec}}{1 \, \text{min}}$.

$$2 \, \text{hr} \times \frac{60 \, \text{min}}{1 \, \text{hr}} \times \frac{60 \, \text{sec}}{1 \, \text{min}}$$

Cancel hours and minutes.

$$2 \, \cancel{\text{hr}} \times \frac{60 \, \cancel{\text{min}}}{1 \, \cancel{\text{hr}}} \times \frac{60 \, \text{sec}}{1 \, \cancel{\text{min}}} = \frac{2 \times 60 \times 60}{1} \, \text{sec} = 7200 \, \text{sec}$$

This is the method you will use in the following examples. **When you do this kind of calculation, you must make sure that each equivalent fraction you use is equal to 1 and that it gives the units needed.**

Example 6.13

The order is 600 milligrams of acetylsalicylic acid (aspirin); grains 5 caplets are available. How many caplets of this antipyretic should be given to the patient?

In this problem, you need to convert 600 milligrams to grains and then convert grains to caplets.

$$600\,\text{mg} \longrightarrow \text{gr}? \longrightarrow ?\,\text{cap}$$

This is done in two steps as follows:

Step 1 Change milligrams to grains.

$$600\,\text{mg} \times \frac{\text{gr}?}{?\,\text{mg}}$$

Step 2 Change grains to caplets.

$$600\,\text{mg} \times \frac{\text{gr}?}{?\,\text{mg}} \times \frac{?\,\text{cap}}{\text{gr}?} = ?\,\text{cap}$$

Because gr 1 = 60 mg, the first fraction is $\dfrac{\text{gr}\,1}{60\,\text{mg}}$. Since 1 cap = gr 5, the second fraction is $\dfrac{1\,\text{cap}}{\text{gr}\,5}$.

$$\overset{10}{\cancel{600}}\,\cancel{\text{mg}} \times \frac{\cancel{\text{gr}}\,1}{\cancel{60}\,\cancel{\text{mg}}} \times \frac{1\,\text{cap}}{\cancel{\text{gr}}\,5} = 2\,\text{cap}$$

So, 600 milligrams are equivalent to 2 caplets, and 2 caplets of aspirin should be given to the patient.

> **NOTE**
>
> Equivalent values for units of weight are given in Table 5.1. By this point, however, you should have all the equivalent values memorized.

Example 6.14

The order is 0.8 milligram per kilogram bid of piroxicam (Feldene) for a patient who weighs 50 kilograms. Read the drug label in Figure 6.10 and

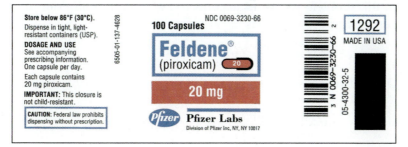

Figure 6.10 Drug label for Feldene.

(Registered Trademark of Pfizer Inc. Reproduced with permission.)

determine the number of capsules of this anti-inflammatory drug you would give to the patient.

In this problem you want to convert 50 kilograms to milligrams and then convert milligrams to capsules.

$$50\,kg \longrightarrow ?\,mg \longrightarrow ?\,cap$$

This is done in two steps.

Step 1   Change body weight in kilograms to dosage in milligrams.

$$50\,kg \times \frac{?\,mg}{?\,kg}$$

Step 2   Change milligrams to capsules.

$$50\,kg \times \frac{?\,mg}{?\,kg} \times \frac{?\,cap}{?\,mg} = ?\,cap$$

Because the patient is to receive 0.8 milligram of piroxicam per kilogram of body weight, the first equivalent fraction is $\frac{0.8\,mg}{1\,kg}$. Because the label indicates that 1 cap = 20 mg, the second equivalent fraction is $\frac{1\,cap}{20\,mg}$.

$$50\,\cancel{kg} \times \frac{0.8\,\cancel{mg}}{1\,\cancel{kg}} \times \frac{1\,cap}{20\,\cancel{mg}} = \frac{40}{20}\,cap = 2\,cap$$

So, the patient should receive 2 capsules of piroxicam.

Example 6.15

The order is 0.4 gram of the antifungal drug, Diflucan (fluconazole). Read the label shown in Figure 6.11 and calculate how many tablets should be given.

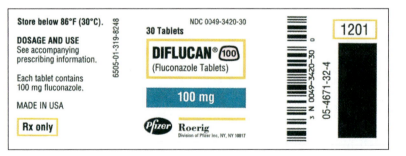

Figure 6.11 Drug label for Diflucan.

(Registered Trademark of Pfizer Inc. Reproduced with permission.)

In this problem you want to convert 0.4 gram to milligrams and then convert milligrams to tablets.

$$0.4\,g \longrightarrow ?\,mg \longrightarrow ?\,tab$$

Do the two steps on one line as follows:

$$0.4\,g \times \frac{?\,mg}{?\,g} \times \frac{?\,tab}{?\,mg} = ?\,tab$$

Because 1000 mg = 1 g, the first equivalent fraction is $\dfrac{1000\,mg}{1\,g}$. Because

100 mg = 1 tab, the second equivalent fraction is $\dfrac{1\,tab}{100\,mg}$.

$$0.4\,\cancel{g} \times \frac{1000\,\cancel{mg}}{1\,\cancel{g}} \times \frac{1\,tab}{100\,\cancel{mg}} = 4\,tab$$

So, 0.4 gram is equivalent to 4 tablets, and 4 tablets of Diflucan should be given to the patient.

NOTE

Sometimes prescribed oral medications are in liquid form. The calculations for these drugs follow the same format you have been using. The label will always state how much drug is contained in a certain amount of liquid.

Example 6.16

The prescriber orders 0.02 gram of the diuretic, furosemide. Study the label shown in Figure 6.12 and calculate how many milliliters you will administer.

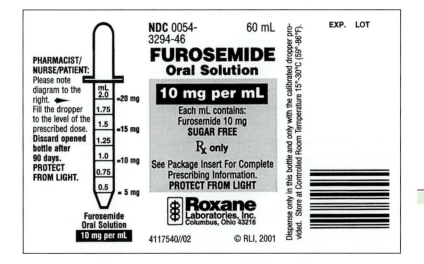

Figure 6.12 Drug label for furosemide.
(Used with permission of Roxane Laboratories, Inc.)

In this problem you convert 0.02 gram to milligrams and then convert milligrams to milliliters.

$$0.02\,g \longrightarrow ?\,mg \longrightarrow ?\,mL$$

You do the two steps on one line as follows:

$$0.02\,g \times \frac{?\,mg}{?\,g} \times \frac{1\,mL}{?\,mg} = ?\,mL$$

Because $1000 \, \text{mg} = 1 \, \text{g}$, the first equivalent fraction is $\dfrac{1000 \, \text{mg}}{1 \, \text{g}}$. The label on the bottle indicates that 1 mL contains 10 milligrams of furosemide. So, the second equivalent fraction is $\dfrac{1 \, \text{mL}}{10 \, \text{mg}}$.

$$0.02 \, \cancel{\text{g}} \times \frac{1000 \, \cancel{\text{mg}}}{1 \, \cancel{\text{g}}} \times \frac{1 \, \text{mL}}{10 \, \cancel{\text{mg}}} = 2 \, \text{mL}$$

So, you would administer 2 mL of furosemide.

Example 6.17

The patient is to receive 0.625 gram of calcium carbonate. Read the information on the drug label in Figure 6.13 and determine how many milliliters you would administer.

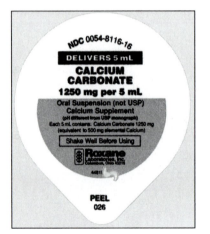

Figure 6.13 Drug label for calcium carbonate.
(Used with permission of Roxane Laboratories, Inc.)

The label on the bottle reads 1250 milligrams per 5 milliliters. This means that each 5 milliliters of liquid contains 1250 milligrams of calcium carbonate. In this problem you want to convert 0.625 gram to milligrams and then get its equivalent in milliliters.

$$0.625 \, \text{g} \longrightarrow ? \, \text{mg} \longrightarrow ? \, \text{mL}$$

Do this on one line as follows:

$$0.625 \, \text{g} \times \frac{? \, \text{mg}}{? \, \text{g}} \times \frac{? \, \text{mL}}{? \, \text{mg}} = ? \, \text{mL}$$

Because $1000 \, \text{mg} = 1 \, \text{g}$, the first equivalent fraction is $\dfrac{1000 \, \text{mg}}{1 \, \text{g}}$. Because $5 \, \text{mL} = 1250 \, \text{mg}$, the second equivalent fraction is $\dfrac{5 \, \text{mL}}{1250 \, \text{mg}}$.

$$0.625 \, \cancel{\text{g}} \times \frac{1000 \, \cancel{\text{mg}}}{1 \, \cancel{\text{g}}} \times \frac{5 \, \text{mL}}{1250 \, \cancel{\text{mg}}} = 2.5 \, \text{mL}$$

So, you would administer 2.5 milliliters of calcium carbonate.

Example 6.18

The prescriber orders 0.0025 gram po of olanzapine (Zyprexa), an antipsychotic drug. Study the information on the label shown in Figure 6.14 and calculate the number of tablets of this drug you would administer.

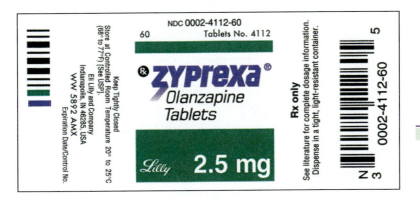

Figure 6.14 Drug label for Zyprexa.
(Courtesy of Eli Lilly and Company.)

The label on the bottle reads 2.5 milligrams per tablet. In this problem you want to convert 0.0025 gram to milligrams and then get its equivalent in tablets.

$$0.0025\,g \longrightarrow ?\,mg \longrightarrow ?\,tab$$

Do this on one line as follows:

$$0.0025\,g \times \frac{?\,mg}{?\,g} \times \frac{?\,tab}{?\,mg} = ?\,tab$$

Because 1000 mg = 1 g, the first equivalent fraction is $\dfrac{1000\,mg}{1\,g}$. Because 1 tab = 2.5 mg, the second equivalent fraction is $\dfrac{1\,tab}{2.5\,mg}$.

$$0.0025\,\cancel{g} \times \frac{1000\,\cancel{mg}}{1\,\cancel{g}} \times \frac{1\,tab}{2.5\,\cancel{mg}} = 1\,tab$$

So, you would administer 1 tablet of Zyprexa.

NOTE

In Example 6.19, the unit value is milliequivalents. Electrolytes are usually measured in milliequivalents, which is abbreviated mEq. Recently, pharmaceutical companies have begun to label their electrolytes in milligrams as well as milliequivalents. For example, oral potassium chloride might be labeled

10 mEq = 750 mg (see Figure 6.15)

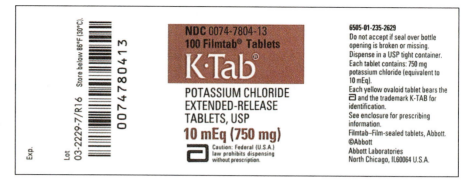

Figure 6.15 Drug label for K-Tab.

(Reproduced with permission of Abbott Laboratories.)

Example 6.19

The order for Mr. Jones is 20 milliequivalents of potassium chloride (K-Tab). Read the label in Figure 6.15 and determine how many tablets of this electrolyte to administer.

In this problem you want to change 20 milliequivalents to tablets.

$$20\,\text{mEq} = ?\,\text{tab}$$

$$20\,\text{mEq} \times \frac{?\,\text{tab}}{?\,\text{mEq}} = ?\,\text{tab}$$

Because the label indicates that each tablet contains 10 mEq, the fraction is $\dfrac{1\,\text{tab}}{10\,\text{mEq}}$.

$$\overset{2}{\cancel{20\,\text{mEq}}} \times \frac{1\,\text{tab}}{\underset{1}{\cancel{10\,\text{mEq}}}} = 2\,\text{tab}$$

So, you would administer 2 tablets of K-Tab.

Practice Reading Labels

Calculate the following doses using the labels shown. (You will find the answers to *Practice Reading Labels* in Appendix A at the back of the book.)

1. Piroxicam (Feldene) 0.01 g = _____ cap

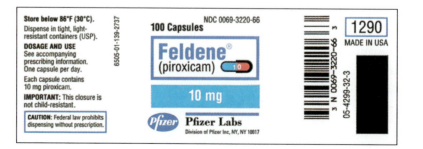

(Registered Trademark of Pfizer Inc. Reproduced with permission.)

2. Raloxifene (Evista) 0.12 g = _____ tab

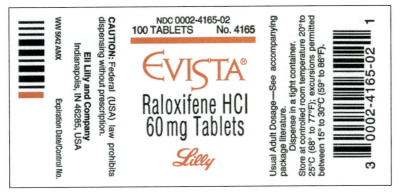

3. Nabumetone (Relafen) 0.5 g = _____ tab

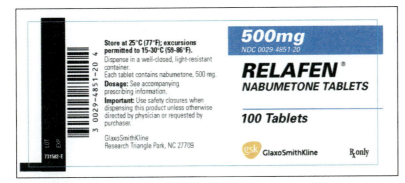

4. Cefaclor (Ceclor) 245 mg = _____ mL

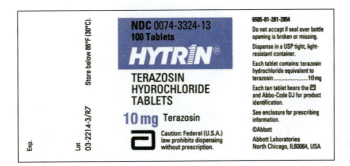

5. Terazosin (Hytrin) 0.01 g = _____ tab

6. Chlorpromazine HCl (Thorazine) 200 mg = _____ tab

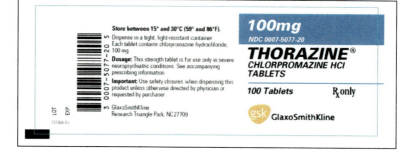

(Reproduced with permission of
GlaxoSmithKline.)

7. Cefaclor (Ceclor) 75 mg = _____ mL

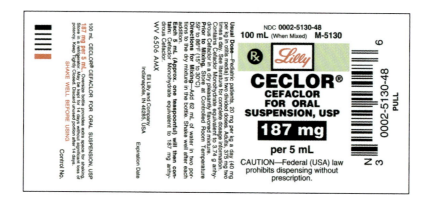

(Courtesy of Eli Lilly and
Company.)

8. Zovirax (acyclovir) gr 3 = _____ mL

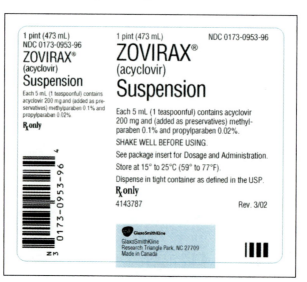

(Reproduced with permission of
GlaxoSmithKline.)

9. Alprazolam gr $\dfrac{1}{6}$ = _____ mL

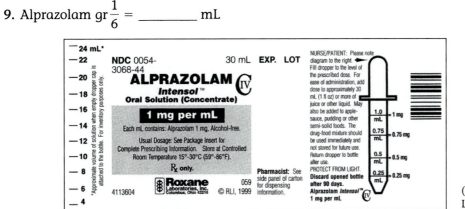

(Used with permission of Roxane Laboratories, Inc.)

10. Olanzapine (Zyprexa) 7500 μg = _____ tab

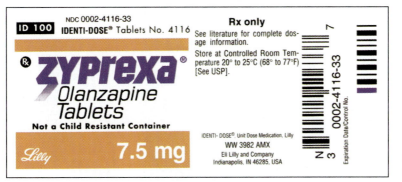

(Courtesy of Eli Lilly and Company.)

11. Clarithromycin (Biaxin) 0.5 g = _____ tab

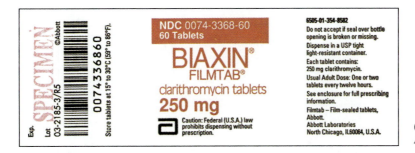

(Reproduced with permission of Abbott Laboratories.)

12. Erythromycin (Ery-Tab) 0.999 g = _____ tab

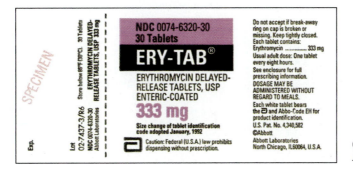

(Reproduced with permission of Abbott Laboratories.)

13. Tolterodine tartrate (Detrol LA) 6 mg = _____ cap

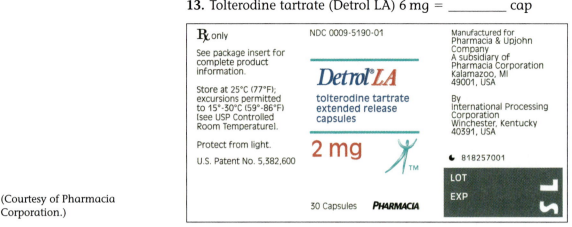

(Courtesy of Pharmacia Corporation.)

14. Zileuton (Zyflo) 1.2 g = _____ tab

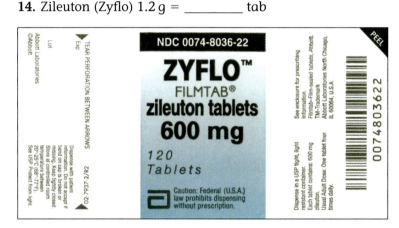

(Reprodeced with permission of Abbott Laboratories.)

15. Cefpodoxime proxetil (Vantin) 200 mg = _____ mL

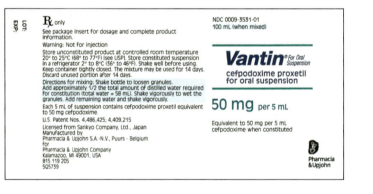

(Courtesy of Pharmacia Corporation.)

16. Methadone hcl (Dolophine HCL) 0.02 g = _____ tab

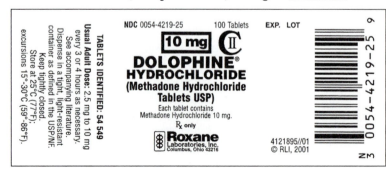

(Used with permission of Roxane Laboratories, Inc.)

17. Misoprostol (Cytotec) 0.2 mg = _____ tab

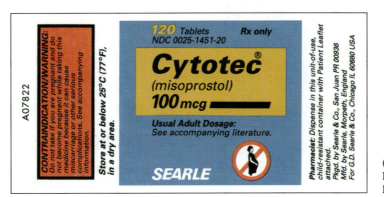

(Copyright Novartis Pharmaceuticals Corporation. Reprinted with permission.)

18. Codeine phosphate 15 mg = _____ mL

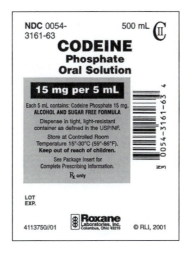

(Used with permission of Roxane Laboratories, Inc.)

19. Erythromycin (E.E.S. 400) 800 mg = _____ tab

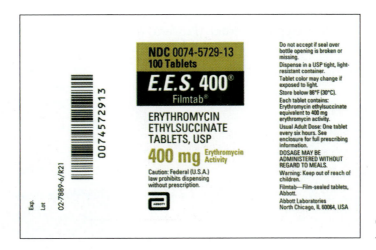

(Reproduced with permission of Abbott Laboratories.)

20. Diazepam 10 mg = _____ mL

NDC 0054-
3188-63   500 mL Ⓒ Ⓥ

DIAZEPAM
Oral Solution USP

5 mg per 5 mL

SUGAR FREE
Each 5 mL contains: Diazepam 5 mg.
Dilute before using to enhance palatability.

Dispense in tight, light-resistant
container as defined in the USP/NF.

Store at Controlled Room
Temperature 15°-30°C (59°-86°F)
Keep out of reach of children.

See Package Insert for Complete Prescribing Information.
Caution: Federal law prohibits dispensing
without prescription.

LOT
EXP.

4116001   ⊕ **Roxane**
                 Laboratories, Inc.
                 Columbus, Ohio 43216   033
                                           © RLI, 1993

(Used with permission of Roxane
Laboratories, Inc.)

21. Rifabutin (Mycobutin) 0.45 g = _____ cap

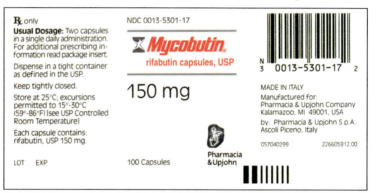

(Courtesy of Pharmacia
Corporation.)

22. Glipizide (Glucotrol XL) 0.01 g = _____ tab

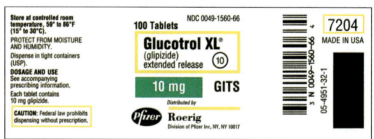

(Registered Trademark of Pfizer
Inc. Reproduced with permission.)

23. Medroxyprogesterone (Provera) gr $\frac{1}{6}$ = _____ tab

℞ only
See package insert
for complete
product information.
Dispense in
tight container.
Notice: Include one
patient insert with
each Rx.
Store at controlled
room temperature
20° to 25°C (68° to
77°F) [see USP].
813 415 504
Pharmacia &
Upjohn Company
Kalamazoo, MI
49001, USA

NDC 0009-0050-11
6505-01-289-9825

Provera®
medroxyprogesterone
acetate tablets, USP

10 mg

500 Tablets

(Courtesy of Pharmacia
Corporation.)

24. Pemoline (Cylert) 0.0375 g = _____ tab

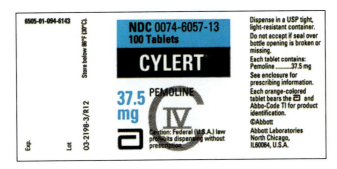

(Reproduced with permission of Abbott Laboratories.)

25. Azithromycin (Zithromax) 150 mg = _____ mL

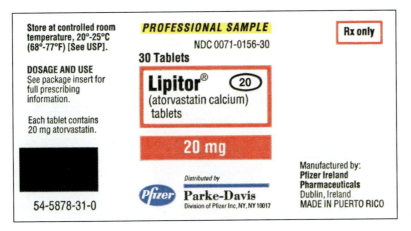

(Registered Trademark of Pfizer Inc. Reproduced with permission.)

26. Atorvastatin calcium (Lipitor) 0.02 g = _____ tab

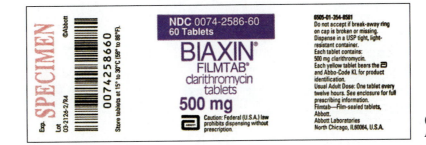

(Registered Trademark of Pfizer Inc. Reproduced with permission.)

27. Clarithromycin (Biaxin) 1 g = _____ tab

(Reproduced with permission of Abbott Laboratories.)

28. Terazosin hcl (Hytrin) 0.005 g = _____ tab

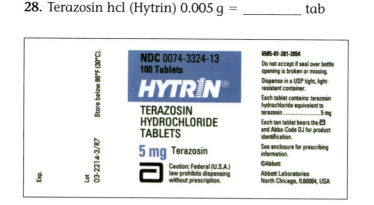

(Reproduced with permission of Abbott Laboratories.)

29. Erythromycin (EryPed Drops) 400 mg = _____ mL

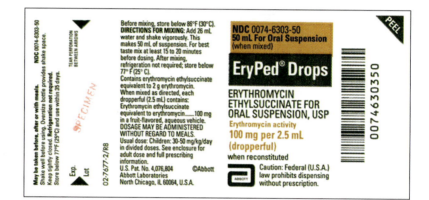

(Reproduced with permission of Abbott Laboratories.)

30. Cyclophosphamide 0.05 g = _____ tab

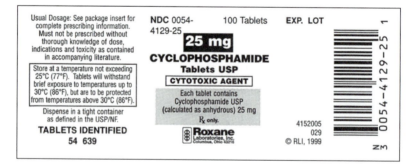

(Used with permission of Roxane Laboratories, Inc.)

31. Fluconazole (Diflucan) 60 mg = _____ mL

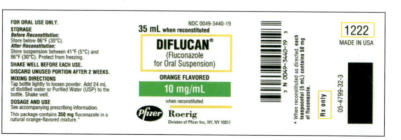

(Registered Trademark of Pfizer Inc. Reproduced with permission.)

32. Glipizide (Glucotrol XL) 0.01 g = _____ tab

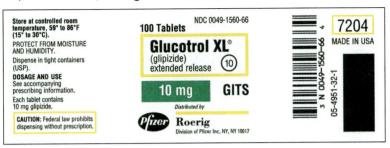

(Registered Trademark of Pfizer Inc. Reproduced with permission.)

33. Cefaclor (Ceclor) 375 mg = _____ mL

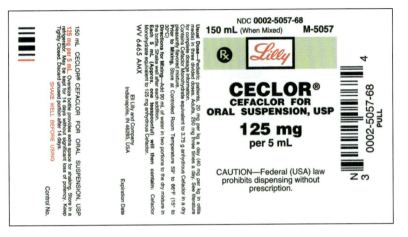

(Courtesy of Eli Lilly and Company.)

34. Doxazosin mesylate (Cardura) 0.004 g = _____ tab

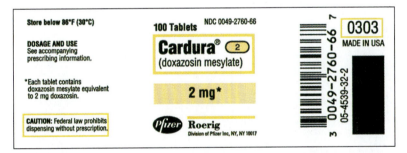

(Registered Trademark of Pfizer Inc. Reproduced with permission.)

35. Acetaminophen 60 mg and codeine 6 mg = _____ mL.

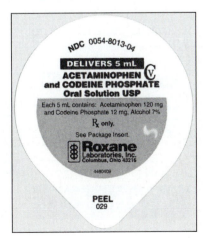

(Used with permission of Roxane Laboratories, Inc.)

36. Ethchlorvynol (Placidyl) 400 mg = _____ cap

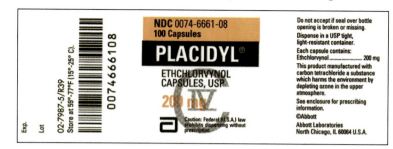

(Reproduced with permission of
Abbott Laboratories.)

37. Pentobarbital sodium (Nembutal) 0.2 g = _____ cap

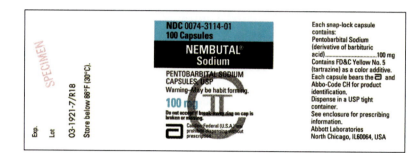

(Reproduced with permission of
Abbott Laboratories.)

38. Calcium carbonate 1.25 g = _____ mL

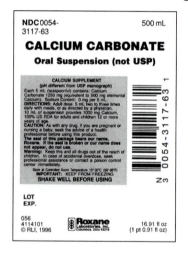

(Used with permission of Roxane
Laboratories, Inc.)

39. Amitriptyline HCl 50 mg = _____ tab

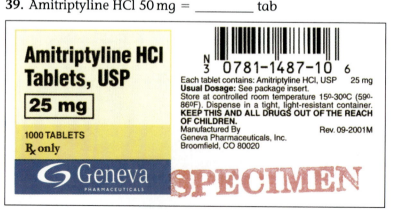

(Courtesy of Geneva
Pharmaceuticals.)

40. Terazosin (Hytrin) gr $\frac{1}{60}$ = _____ tab

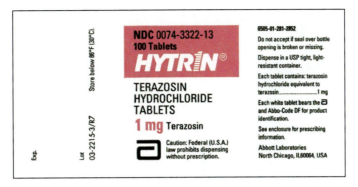

(Reproduced with permission of Abbott Laboratories.)

41. Zolpidem tartrate (Ambien) gr $\frac{1}{6}$ = _____ tab

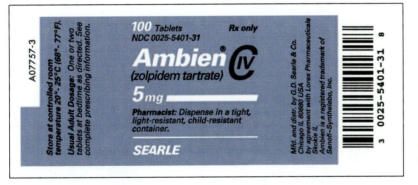

(Copyright Novartis Pharmaceuticals Corporation. Reprinted with permission.)

42. Pemoline (Cylert) 0.0375 g = _____ tab

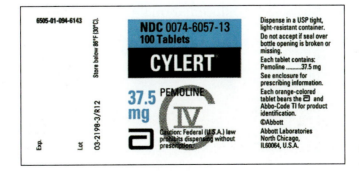

(Reproduced with permission of Abbott Laboratories.)

43. Furosemide 40 mg = _____ tab

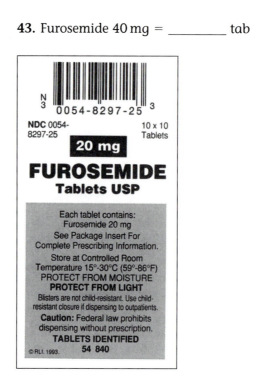

(Used with permission of Roxane
Laboratories, Inc.)

44. Sulfasalazine (Azulfidine) 2 g = _____ tab

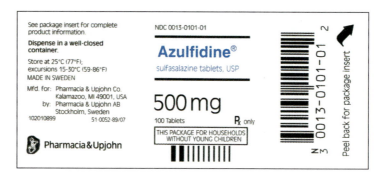

(Courtesy of Pharmacia
Corporation.)

45. Fluconazole (Diflucan) 60 mg = _____ mL

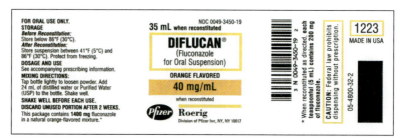

(Registered Trademark of Pfizer
Inc. Reproduced with permission.)

46. Hydrocortisone (Cortef) 50 mg = _____ mL

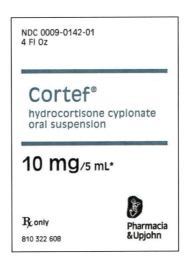

NDC 0009-0142-01
4 Fl Oz

Cortef®
hydrocortisone cypionate
oral suspension

10 mg/5 mL*

℞ only
810 322 608

Pharmacia
&Upjohn

(Courtesy of Pharmacia
Corporation.)

47. Glyburide (Micronase) 2500 mcg = _____ tab

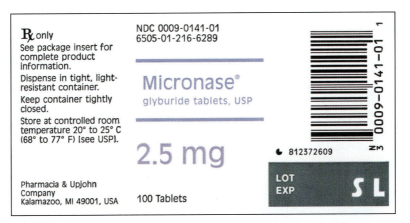

℞ only
See package insert for
complete product
information.
Dispense in tight, light-
resistant container.
Keep container tightly
closed.
Store at controlled room
temperature 20° to 25° C
(68° to 77° F) [see USP].

Pharmacia & Upjohn
Company
Kalamazoo, MI 49001, USA

NDC 0009-0141-01
6505-01-216-6289

Micronase®
glyburide tablets, USP

2.5 mg

● 812372609

100 Tablets

LOT
EXP

S L

0009-0141-01 1

(Courtesy of Pharmacia
Corporation.)

48. Benazepril (Lotensin HCT) 20 mg/25 mg = _____ tab

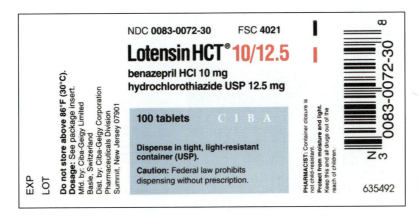

NDC 0083-0072-30   FSC 4021

Lotensin HCT® 10/12.5

benazepril HCl 10 mg
hydrochlorothiazide USP 12.5 mg

100 tablets   C I B A

Dispense in tight, light-resistant
container (USP).

Caution: Federal law prohibits
dispensing without prescription.

EXP
LOT

Do not store above 86°F (30°C).
Dosage: See package insert.
Mfd. by: Ciba-Geigy Limited
Basle, Switzerland
Dist. by: Ciba-Geigy Corporation
Pharmaceuticals Division
Summit, New Jersey 07901

PHARMACIST: Container closure is
not child-resistant.
Protect from moisture and light.
Keep this and all drugs out of the
reach of children.

0083-0072-30 8

635492

(Copyright Novartis
Pharmaceutical Corporation.
Reprinted with permission.)

49. Nifedipine (Procardia XL) 180 mg = _____ tab

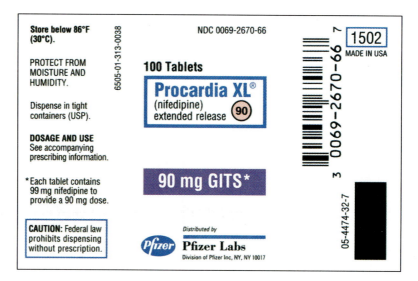

(Registered Trademark of Pfizer Inc. Reproduced with permission.)

50. Atenolol 0.1 g = _____ tab

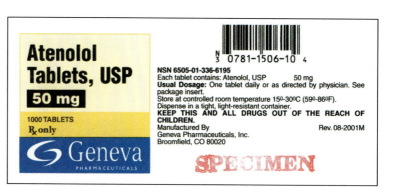

(Courtesy of Geneva Pharmaceuticals.)

51. Erythromycin (Ery-Tab) 500 mg = _____ tab

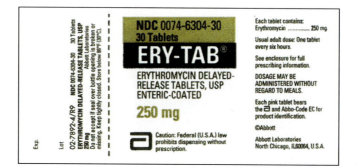

(Registered with permission of Abbott Laboratories.)

52. Triazolam (Halcion) 0.25 mg = _____ tab

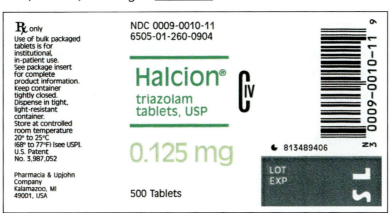

(Courtesy of Pharmacia Corporation.)

53. Linezolid (Zyvox) 1.8 g = _____ tab

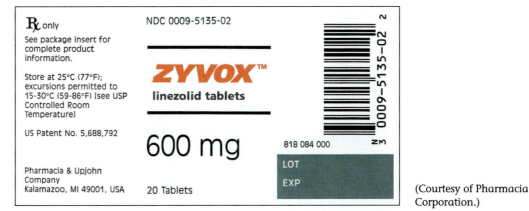

(Courtesy of Pharmacia Corporation.)

54. Ziprasidone (Geodon) gr $\frac{2}{3}$ = _____ cap

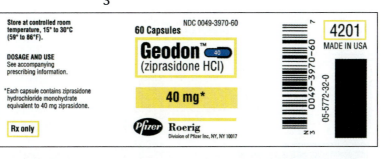

(Registered Trademark of Pfizer Inc. Reproduced with permission.)

55. Haloperidol 5000 μg = _____ tab

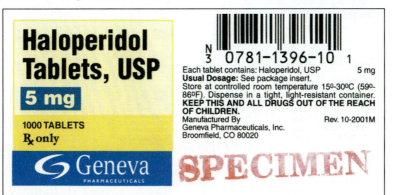

(Courtesy of Geneva Pharmaceuticals.)

56. Fluphenazine Hydrochloride 0.005 g = _____ tab

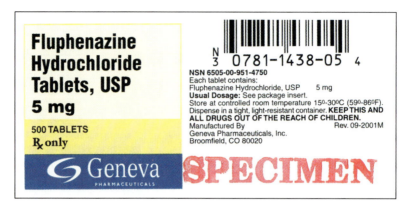

(Courtesy of Geneva Pharmaceutical.)

57. Misoprostol (Cytotec) 0.3 mg = _____ tab

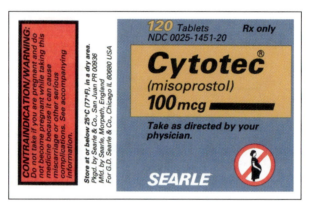

(Copyright Novartis Pharmaceuticals Corporation. Reprinted with permission.)

58. Delavirdine (Rescriptor) 0.1 g = _____ tab

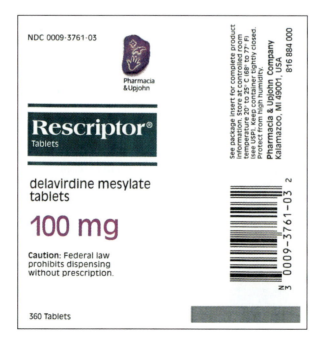

(Courtesy of Pharmacia Corporation.)

59. Sildenafil citrate (Viagra) 100 mg = _____ tab

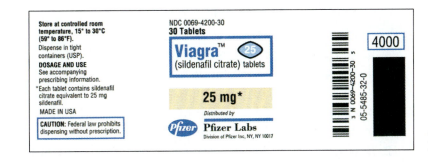

(Registered Trademark of Pfizer Inc. Reproduced with permission.)

60. Dexamethasone 4 mg = _____ mL

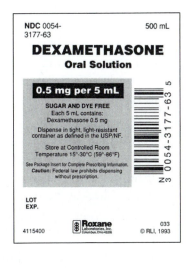

(Used with permission of Roxane Laboratories, Inc.)

Case Study 6.1

Mrs. S., an 88-year-old patient, is transferred from a nursing home to General Hospital with the following diagnoses: pneumonia, pressure ulcer, stage three in the coccygeal area, anorexia, dehydration, and diabetes mellitus Type II. The orders are:

- Chest X ray
- Culture and Sensitivity of pressure ulcer drainage
- Culture and Sensitivity of sputum × 3 days
- Soft diet
- Zithromax 500 mg q6h po
- Tikosyn 250 mcg qd po
- Famotidine 0.02 g po bid
- Atenolol 100 mg po qd
- Range-of-motion exercises to upper and lower extremities q4h when awake
- Bathroom privileges prn with assistance
- Colace 200 mg po bid
- Glucotrol 5 mg po ac breakfast
- Force fluids 100 mL q1h when awake
- Intake and Output

- Foley catheter to bedside drainage
- Diazepam 10 mg qhs prn po
- Zoloft 25 mg po bid

Refer to labels in Figure 6.16 when necessary to answer the following questions:

1. The patient receives 1200 milliliters of H_2O, 200 milliliters of cranberry juice, and 150 milliliters of ginger ale. How many milliliters of fluid does the patient receive?

2. How many capsules of azithromycin will you administer in 24 hours?

3. How many capsules of dofetilide, an antiarrhythmic drug, will you administer to Mrs. S. every day?

4. Colace, a stool-softening drug, is prepared as an oral liquid, 150 mg = 15 mL. How many milliliters contain the prescribed dose?

5. How many tablets of Atenolol contain the prescribed dose?

6. How many cubic centimeters of diazepam will you prepare for your patient?

7. How many tablets of Zoloft will the patient receive per day? How many tablets of Zoloft will the patient receive in three weeks?

8. The physician cancelled the order for azithromycin and ordered clarithromycin 0.5 g bid. How many tablets will you give this patient?

9. How many tablets of famotidine are contained in one bottle?

10. How many tablets of glipizide contain the prescribed dose?

11. The order for Zoloft has been cancelled. The new order is Tranxene 0.015 g bid po, an antianxiety drug. How many tablets will the patient receive in one day?

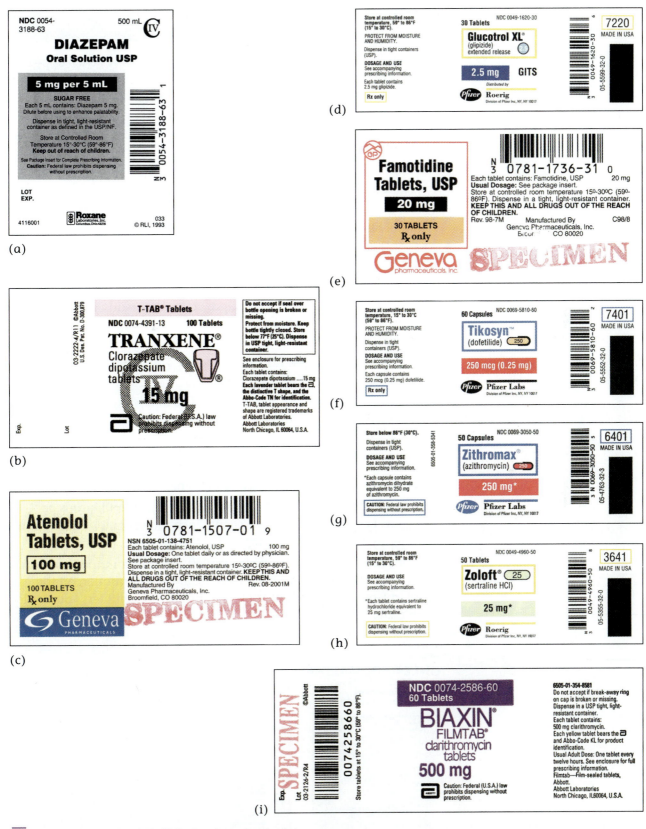

Figure 6.16 Drug labels for Case Study 6.1.

(a) Used with permission of Roxane Laboratories, Inc. (b, i) Reproduced with permission of Abbott Laboratories. (c, e) Courtesy of Geneva Pharmaceuticals. (d, f–h) Registered Trademark of Pfizer Inc. Reproduced with permission.

PRACTICE SETS

The answers to *Try These for Practice, Exercises,* and *Cumulative Review* appear in Appendix A at the back of the book. The answers to the *Additional Exercises* can be found on the companion Website or ask your instructor.

Try These for Practice

Test your comprehension after reading the chapter.

1. Prescriber order:

   Diltiazem (Cardizem) 0.06 g po q8h

   Each tablet contains 30 milligrams. How many tablets of this calcium channel blocker will you give this patient? _____

2. The physician ordered 800 milligrams of ibuprofen (Motrin, Advil, Aleve) po stat. The medication is labeled 0.1 g/5 ml. How many milliliters will you prepare? _____

3. The order is Dilantin 300 mg po q8h. The label reads 125 mg/5 ml oral suspension. How many milliliters will you administer to the patient? _____

4. Augmentin 0.5 g po q8h has been ordered. The tablets are labeled 125 mg. How many tablets are needed? _____

5. The order for Cardura is 6 mg po daily. The following tablets are available: 1 mg; 2 mg; 4 mg; 8 mg. Which tablets would be the best choice for this dose?

Exercises

Reinforce your understanding in class or at home.

1. Paroxetine HCl (Paxil), an antidepressant drug, 40 milligrams po daily has been ordered for your client. Each tablet contains 0.02 gram. How many tablets will you prepare?

2. The physician ordered Chlorpromazine 0.55 milligrams per kilogram po. The patient weighs 65 kilograms. Read the information on the label in Figure 6.17 and calculate the number of milliliters you would administer.

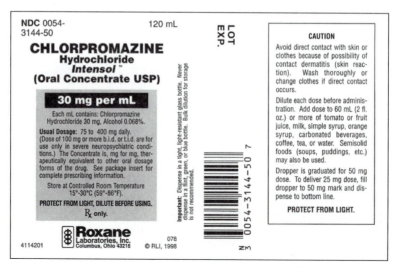

Figure 6.17 Drug label for Chlorpromazine.
(Used with permission of Roxane Laboratories, Inc.)

3. Glucophage 0.85 gram po ac breakfast and dinner has been prescribed for your client. Each tablet contains 850 milligrams. How many tablets will you give your client ac breakfast?

4. Prescriber's order:

>   *Glyburide (Micronase) 5 milligrams po ac breakfast.*

Each tablet contains 2.5 milligrams. How many tablets will you prepare?

5. Glycopyrrolate (Robinol), an anticholinergic medication, has been prescribed for a patient who weighs 66 kilograms. The order is 0.015 milligrams per kilogram po. Each tablet contains 1 milligram. How many tablets will the patient receive?

6. Norvasc 0.005 gram po has been ordered for a patient with Prinzmetal's angina. The tablet contains 2.5 milligrams. How many tablets will you administer to this patient?

7. Vasotec, an ACE inhibiting drug, used to treat hypertension and symptomatic heart failure, 7.5 milligrams po has been prescribed. Tablets available are 2.5 mg; 5 mg; 10 mg; and 20 mg. Which tablets would you select for this order?

8. Alprazolam 0.5 milligrams po has been prescribed for your client. Read the information on the label in Figure 6.18. How many milliliters of this antianxiety drug will you administer to your patient.

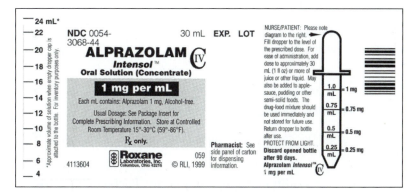

Figure 6.18 Drug label for Alprazolam.
(Used with permission of Roxane Laboratories, Inc.)

9. Ambien 0.01 gram po qhs has been ordered for a patient with insomnia. Each tablet contains 0.005 gram. How many tablets will you administer to your patient?

10. Order: Coumadin 2.5 mg po Monday, Wednesday, and Friday and 1 mg po Tuesday, Thursday, Saturday, and Sunday. How many milligrams of Coumadin will your patient receive in one week?

11. Ticlopidine (Ticlid) 0.5 gram po stat, has been ordered for your patient. Each tablet contains 0.25 gram. How many tablets of this platelet aggregator inhibitor drug will you give to your patient?

12. Dexamethasone (Decadron), a steroid, 3 milligrams po q12 h has been ordered for a patient. Read the information on the label in Figure 6.19 and calculate the number of tablets that the patient will receive in 24 hours.

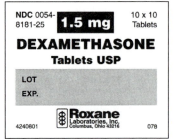

Figure 6.19 Drug label for Dexamethasone.
(Used with permission of Roxane Laboratories, Inc.)

13. Order: furosemide 0.08 gram po qd. Read the label in Figure 6.20 and determine how many tablets you will give this patient.

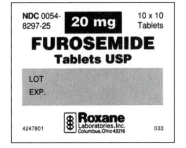

Figure 6.20 Drug label for Furosemide.
(Used with permission of Roxane Laboratories, Inc.)

14. Physician's order:

    Papaverine (Pavabid) 200 mg bid po

    Each tablet contains 0.2 gram. Calculate the number of tablets required for this order.

15. Order: Motrin 0.8 gram q8h po for five days only. Each caplet contains 400 milligrams. How many caplets will you give this patient in the 5 days?

16. The antigout medication, Colchicine, grain 1/100 po q1h for 8 doses has been ordered. Each tablet contains 0.6 milligrams. How many milligrams of Colchicine will the patient receive in eight hours?

17. Order: Zidovudine 100 milligrams po q4h around the clock. The drug label states: 50 mg/5 ml. How many milliliters will you prepare?

18. The physician ordered Ganciclovir (Cytovene) po, an antiviral drug used for the treatment of CMV retinitis. The order is 500 mg/m^2 q8h for 21 days. The client weighs 90 kg and is 160 cm in height. How many milligrams of this drug will you give the patient per day? (Use the formula for BSA.)

19. Cyclophosphamide (Cytoxan) 3 mg/kg po daily. The client weighs 148 pounds. Read the label in Figure 6.21. How many tablets will you prepare?

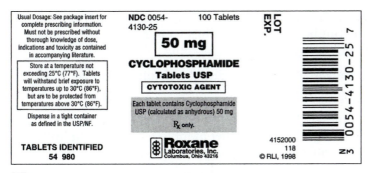

Figure 6.21 Drug label for Cyclophosphamide.
(Used with permission of Roxane Laboratories, Inc.)

20. Physician's order: prednisone 30 mg/m² po stat for a patient with an onset of hives. The BSA is 1.65 m² and each tablet contains 50 milligrams. How many tablets will you give this patient?

Additional Exercises

Now, on your own, test yourself! The answers to the *Additional Exercises* can be found on the companion Website or ask your instructor.

1. Amantadine hydrochloride (Symmetrel) is an antiviral drug, and 0.2 gram po has been ordered for a patient. Each capsule contains 100 milligrams. How many capsules will you administer to the patient? _____

2. If the patient is unable to swallow Symmetrel capsules, the patient must receive the oral suspension labeled 50 milligrams per 5 milliliters. How many milliliters equal 200 milligrams? _____

3. The order reads 0.4 gram of cyclosporine (Sandimmune) po. If each capsule contains 100 milligrams, how many capsules of this immunosuppressant drug equals the prescribed dose? _____

4. The patient has been prescribed 0.01 gram po of the antihistamine drug loratadine (Claritin). Each tablet contains 10 milligrams. How many tablets will you administer? _____

5. The order reads as follows:

   Estradiol 0.004 g transdermal

   See Figure 6.22. How many patches would you apply? _____

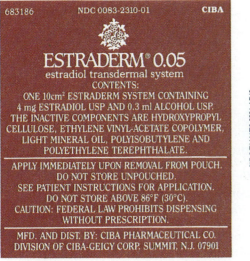

Figure 6.22 Drug label for Estraderm.

6. Ten milligrams of the antihypertensive drug amlodipine (Norvasc) is ordered po for your patient. If each tablet contains 0.005 grams, how many tablets will you give your patient? _____

7. The order in Problem 6 has been reduced to 5 milligrams po. How many tablets equal this dose? _____

8. Read the first order on the medication administration record in Figure 6.23. Name the drug and the number of tablets you will administer to the patient if the label reads 100 milligrams per tablet. _____

✛ GENERAL HOSPITAL ✛

Year 2003	Month December	Day	17	18	19	20	21	22
Medication Dosage and Interval			Initials* and Hours	Initials and Hours	Initials and Hours	Initials and Hours	Initials and Hours	Initials and Hours
Date started: 12/17/03		I	LA	LA				
Zoloft 0.2 g po qd		AM	10	10				
		I						
Discontinued:		PM						
Date started: 12/18/03		I						
Dalmane 15 mg po hs		AM						
		I		JO				
Discontinued:		PM		10				

Allergies: (Specify)

penicillin, codeine

Init*	Signature
LA	Leon Ablon R.N.
JO	June Olsen R.N.

PATIENT IDENTIFICATION

```
226310                          12/17/03

Susan Jackson                   1/30/63
80 Martin Ave.                  Epis
Little Rock, AR                 HIP
76412

Dr. Anthony Giangrasso
```

MEDICATION ADMINISTRATION RECORD

Figure 6.23 Medication administration record.

9. Read the second order from the MAR in Figure 6.23. Name the drug and the number of capsules you will administer if each capsule contains 0.015 g of this sedative drug? _____

10. Your patient is to receive 0.125 milligram of the cardiac glycoside digoxin (Lanoxin) po. Each scored tablet contains 0.25 milligram. How many tablets will you administer to the patient? _____

11. The order reads Tenormin 50 mg qd po. Each tablet contains 25 milligrams. How many tablets equal 50 mg? _____

12. A patient with tuberculosis has an order for the antitubercular drug, ethambutol hydrochloride (Myambutol). Each tablet contains 400 milligrams. If the order is 1.6 grams po, how many tablets will you administer to the patient? _____

13. The prescriber has ordered 20 milligrams of piroxicam (Feldene) po. Each capsule contains 0.01 gram. How many capsules of this nonsteroidal anti-inflammatory drug (NSAID) will you give the patient? _____

14. The order in Problem 13 was changed to 0.375 gram po of the NSAID naproxen (Naprosyn). Each scored tablet containes 250 milligrams. How many tablets would you administer to the patient? _____

15. The order reads trimethadione 13 mg/kg po qd. The patient weighs 46 kilograms. Each capsule contains 300 milligrams. How many capsules of this anticonvulsant drug will equal the prescribed dose? _____

16. The prescriber has ordered 0.01 gram tid po of the anti-anginal medication nifedipine (Cardalate MR) for a patient. If each tablet contains 5 milligrams, how many tablets equal this dosage? _____

17. A patient is 5 feet 3 inches tall and weighs 150 pounds. Use the adult nomogram to estimate her BSA. The order is 60 mg/m^2 po of the antibiotic doxycycline (Vibramycin), and the oral suspension is labeled 25 milligrams per 5 milliliters. How many milliliters would you give to the patient? _____

18. The patient has been prescribed 0.0009 g of clonidine hydrochloride (Catapres) po, an antihypertensive drug. The drug is available in 0.3 mg tablets. How many tablets equals the prescribed dose?

_____

19. A patient is 183 centimeters tall and weighs 80 kilograms. The prescriber has written the order for clozapine (Clozaril) 50 mg/m^2 po. Each tablet contains 100 mg of clozapine. How many tablets would you administer to this patient? (Use the formula to estimate the BSA.) _____

20. The order reads: azithromycin 7.2 mg/kg po qd. Each capsule contains 250 milligrams. How many capsules will you prepare of this antiviral drug for a patient weighing 154 pounds? _____

CUMULATIVE REVIEW EXERCISES

Review your mastery of earlier chapters.

1. Prescriber's order:

Atropine SO$_4$ gr 1/150 po

Each tablet contains 0.4 mg. How many tablets will you prepare for your patient? _____

2. Lorabid 400 mg po q12h. The label reads 200 mg in 5 ml. How many milliliters will you give your patient? _____

3. Azithromycin 0.2 g po has been ordered. Convert this dose to grains. _____

4. 0.4 g = _____ mg

5. gr $\dfrac{1}{500}$ = _____ mg

6. grains viiss = _____ mg

7. ℥ 40 = ℈ _____

8. The order reads 267 mg/m² of cefpodoxime po. The patient weighs 72 kg and is 70 in. tall. The label reads 50 mg/ml. How many milliliters will you administer to this patient? Use the nomogram to estimate the BSA.

9. Order: Aminophylline gr $3\dfrac{3}{4}$ po q8h. The label reads each capsule contains 250 mg. How many capsules will you give this patient?

10. The order reads Tenormin 100 mg po daily. Each tablet contains 0.025 g. How many tablets will you prepare?

11. The physician ordered bromocriptine mesylate (Parlodel), an antiparkinsonian drug, 7.5 mg po bid with meals. Each tablet contains 2.5 mg. How many tablets will you prepare?

12. A patient must receive 60 mEq of potassium chloride po stat. Each tablet is labeled 20 mEq/tab. How many tablets will you prepare?

13. 200 mg = _____ g

14. A patient must receive Videx 2.2 mg/kg po. The patient weighs 90 kg. How many tablets will the patient receive if each tablet contains 100 mg?

15. 1 t = _____ mL

Additional questions, web links, matching exercises, fill-in-the-blanks, and glossary for this chapter can be found on the companion Website at www.prenhall.com/olsen. Click on "Chapter 6" to select the activities for this chapter.

CHAPTER SEVEN

Syringes

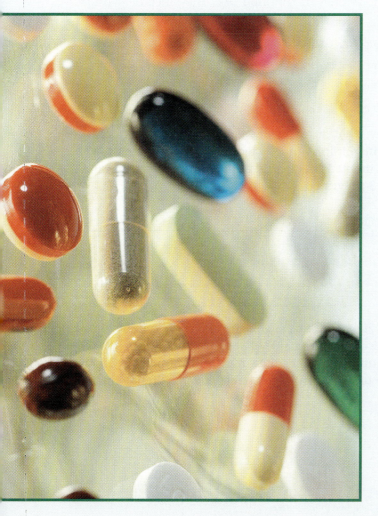

Objectives

After completing this chapter, you will be able to

- Identify the various types of syringes.
- Identify the parts of a syringe.
- Determine the amount of solution in a syringe.
- Describe prepackaged cartridges.
- Read and use USP units.

A *hypodermic syringe* is an instrument used in parenteral therapy to administer sterile liquid medications by injection. The medication is introduced into a body space, such as a vein, a muscle, subcutaneous tissue, cardiac muscle, subarachnoid space, or bone tissue. Figure 7.1 illustrates the parts of a syringe: the plunger, barrel, and hollow needle, which must all be connected separately. The plunger, needle, and the inside of the barrel must always be sterile.

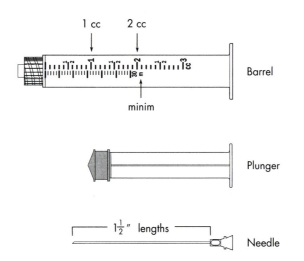

Figure 7.1 A needle, plunger, and barrel.

Common Types of Syringes

There are many types of syringes in common use. They include syringes with such capacities as

1 cc	10 cc	30 cc	100 cc
3 cc	12 cc	35 cc	
5 cc	20 cc	50 cc	
6 cc	25 cc	60 cc	

The circumference and length of a syringe increase with its capacity. Many syringes are calibrated in minims and in tenths of a cubic centimeter. These two scales of measurement frequently appear together on the same syringe, particularly the 3 cc syringe.

> **BY THE WAY**
>
> A cubic centimeter is the same as a milliliter:
>
> 1 cc = 1 mL

The syringe shown in Figure 7.2 has a capacity of 3 cubic centimeters or minims 30. The minims scale is on one side of the barrel, where each marking represents minim 1 and the longer lines represent minims 5. On the other side is the milliliter or cubic centimeter scale. Each line represents 0.1

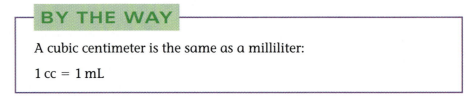

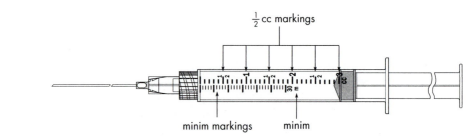

Figure 7.2 A 3 cc syringe.

milliliter or 0.1 cubic centimeter, and the longer lines represent 0.5 milliliter or $\frac{1}{2}$ cubic centimeter (more commonly written as 0.5 cc). The 3 cc syringe is the most commonly used syringe for subcutaneous (sc) and intramuscular (IM) injections.

Figure 7.3 shows a 10 cc syringe. Notice that this syringe has neither incremental markings of 0.5 cubic centimeter nor a minims scale. Each line represents 0.2 cubic centimeter, and the longer lines represent 1 cubic centimeter. This syringe can be used to draw venous or arterial blood as well as to add sterile diluent to a vial or ampule of powdered medication.

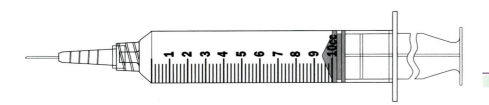

Figure 7.3 A 10 cc syringe.

A 20 cc syringe is shown in Figure 7.4. Each line on the scale represents 1 cubic centimeter, and the longer line indicates 5 cubic centimeters. The 20 cc syringe can be used to inject large volumes of sterile liquids.

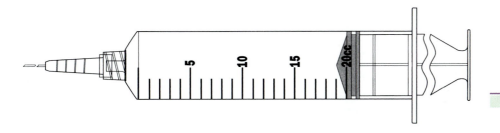

Figure 7.4 A 20 cc syringe.

Figure 7.5 shows a 20 cc syringe filled with liquid up to the 12 cc mark.

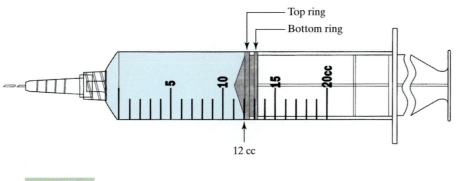

Figure 7.5 A 20 cc syringe containing 12 cc of liquid.

NOTE

The liquid volume in a syringe is read from the *top ring*, **not** the bottom ring or the raised section in the middle of the plunger tip.

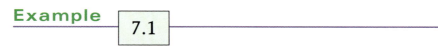

Example 7.1

How much liquid is in the 10 cc syringe in Figure 7.6?

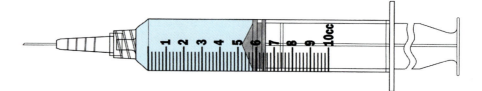

Figure 7.6 A partially filled 10 cc syringe.

The top ring of the plunger is at the fourth line above 5 cubic centimeters. Because each line measures 0.2 cubic centimeter, the fourth line measures 0.8 cubic centimeter. So, the amount of fluid in the syringe is 5.8 cubic centimeters.

Example 7.2

How much liquid is in the 3 cc syringe in Figure 7.7?

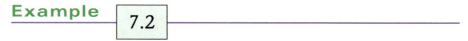

Figure 7.7 A partially filled 3 cc syringe.

The top ring of the plunger is at the second line above 2 cubic centimeters. Because each line measures 0.1 cubic centimeter, the two lines measure 0.2 cubic centimeter. So, the amount of liquid in the syringe is 2.2 cubic centimeters.

Example 7.3

How much liquid is in the 3 cc syringe in Figure 7.8?

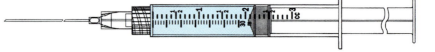

Figure 7.8 A partially filled 3 cc syringe.

The top ring of the plunger is at the second line above $\frac{1}{2}$ cubic centimeter.

Because each short line measures 0.1 cubic centimeter, the two lines measure 0.2 cubic centimeter. So, the amount of liquid in the syringe is 0.7 cubic centimeter.

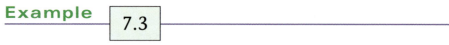
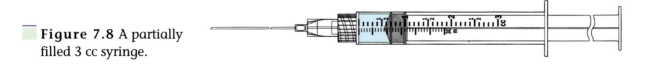

Example

7.4

A physician ordered 9 mg IV of fluconazole (Diflucan). Read the label in Figure 7.9 and place an arrow at the appropriate level of measurement on the syringe to indicate the correct dose.

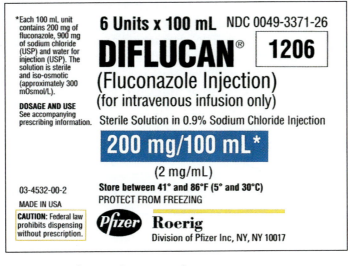

The order is 9 mg. You must change 9 mg to mL.

$$9 \text{ mg} \times \frac{? \text{ mL}}{? \text{ mg}} = ? \text{ mL}$$

The label reads 200 mg/100 mL, and 2 mg/mL, so the fraction is

$$\frac{100 \text{ mL}}{200 \text{ mg}} \quad \text{or} \quad \frac{1 \text{ mL}}{2 \text{ mg}}$$

$$9 \text{ mg} \times \frac{1 \text{ mL}}{2 \text{ mg}} = \frac{9}{2} \text{ mL} = 4.5 \text{ mL}$$

If you use the 5 cc syringe in Figure 7.10, each line on the syringe represents 0.2 cubic centimeters.

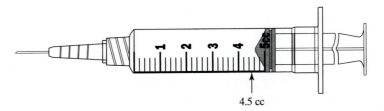

4.5 cc

Figure 7.10 A 5 cc syringe.

On the 5 cc syringe 4.4 cc is 2 lines more than 4 cc, and 4.6 cc is 3 lines more than 4 cc. Therefore, 4.5 cc would be between these two lines, as shown in Figure 7.11.

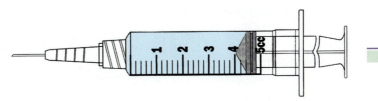

Figure 7.11 A 5 cc syringe with 4.5 cc of fluconazole.

Other Types of Syringes

Other types of syringes that are available for administering medications include the prepackaged cartridge, the tuberculin syringe, and the insulin syringe.

A **prepackaged cartridge** is a syringe that is prefilled with medication. If the medication order is for the exact amount of drug in the prepackaged cartridge, the possibility of measurement error by the medication administrator is eliminated. The prepackaged cartridge syringe shown in Figure 7.12 is calibrated so that each line measures 0.1 milliliter and the thicker lines measure 0.5 milliliter. Note that the prepackaged cartridges are measured in millimeters rather than cubic centimeters.

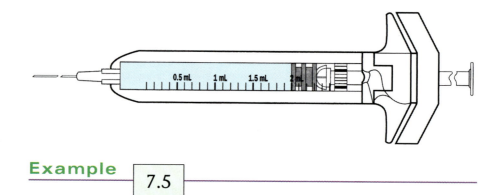

Figure 7.12 A prepackaged cartridge.

Example 7.5

How much medication is in the prepackaged cartridge shown in Figure 7.13? The top of the plunger is at two lines above 1.5 milliliters. Because each line measures 0.1 milliliter, the two lines measure 0.2 milliliter. So the prepackaged cartridge contains 1.7 milliliters.

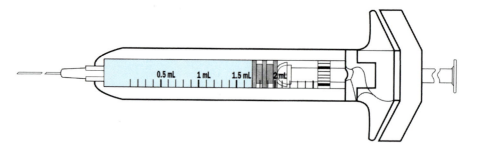

Figure 7.13 A partially filled prepackaged 2 mL syringe.

The **tuberculin syringe** shown in Figure 7.14 is a small, slender syringe used to inject small quantities of liquids. It has a capacity of 1 cubic centimeter. Each line on the syringe represents 0.01 cubic centimeter, and the longer lines represent 0.05 cubic centimeter. This syringe is used for intradermal injection (injection directly beneath the skin) as well as for injection of small quantities of medication that might be prescribed for pediatric or adult patients.

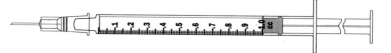

Figure 7.14 A tuberculin syringe.

Example 7.6

How much liquid is in the tuberculin syringe shown in Figure 7.15?

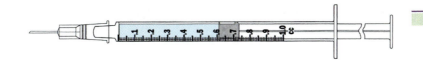

Figure 7.15 A partially filled tuberculin syringe.

The top ring of the plunger is at one line above 0.60 milliliter. Because each line represents 0.01 milliliter, the amount of liquid in the syringe is 0.61 milliliter.

The **insulin syringe** is used to measure insulin. Insulin is a hormone used to treat patients with insulin-dependent diabetes mellitus (IDDM). It is available in both short-acting and long-acting preparations. Insulin can also be prescribed for patients who are hyperglycemic as a result of certain medical therapies. Insulin is supplied in standardized units of potency rather than by weight or volume. These standardized units are called **USP units**, which is often shortened to **units** and sometimes abbreviated **u**. However in order to avoid dosage errors, it is safer to write out the word **units**.

The insulin syringe is calibrated in units. Figure 7.16 shows an insulin syringe with a capacity of 100 units (1 cubic centimeter or 1 milliliter), where each line on the scale measures 2 units (0.02 cubic centimeter).

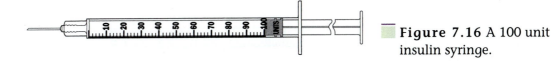

Figure 7.16 A 100 unit insulin syringe.

A 50 unit insulin syringe is shown in Figure 7.17. Each line on its scale measures 1 unit (0.01 cubic centimeter).

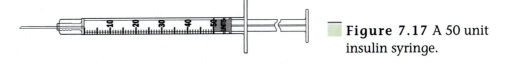

Figure 7.17 A 50 unit insulin syringe.

A 30 unit insulin (Lo-Dose®) syringe is shown in Figure 7.18. Each line represents 1 unit (0.01 cubic centimeter).

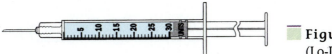

Figure 7.18 A 30 unit (Lo-Dose) syringe.

The top ring of an insulin syringe plunger is flat. As mentioned earlier, other types of syringes have a peak in the center of the top ring. With both types of syringes, the liquid volume is measured from the *top ring*.

Example 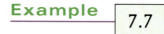 7.7

How much liquid is in the 50 unit insulin syringe shown in Figure 7.19?

Figure 7.19 A partially filled 50 unit insulin syringe.

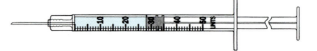

The top ring of the plunger is at three lines above 25. Because each line represents 1 unit, the amount of liquid in the syringe is 28 units.

Example 7.8

How much liquid is in the 100 unit insulin syringe shown in Figure 7.20?

Figure 7.20 A partially filled 100 unit insulin syringe.

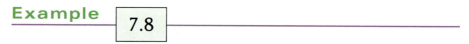

The top ring of the plunger is at one line above 70. Because each line represents 2 units, the amount of liquid in the syringe is 72 units.

Example 7.9

Explain what you would do to fill a medication order for 55 units of NPH insulin.

There are no calculations necessary. You would simply draw 55 units of NPH insulin into an insulin syringe as shown in Figure 7.21.

Figure 7.21 The correctly filled insulin syringe.

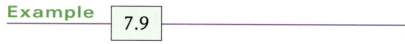

Example

7.10

The physician prescribed 26 units of Lente insulin. Read the label in Figure 7.22 and place an arrow at the appropriate level of measurement on the syringe.

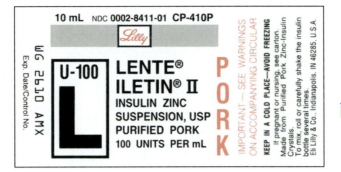

Figure 7.22 Drug label for Lente insulin.
(Courtesy of Eli Lilly and Company.)

There are no calculations necessary. You would draw 26 units of Lente insulin into the insulin syringe as shown in Figure 7.23.

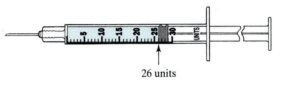

26 units

Figure 7.23 The correctly filled 30 unit (Lo-Dose) insulin syringe.

Example

7.11

The prescriber ordered 15 units of regular insulin and 45 units of NPH insulin in the same syringe for a total of 60 units sc. Explain how you would fill this order.

The steps are shown in Figure 7.24.

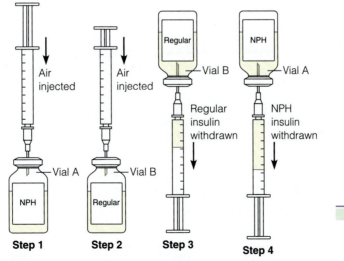

Figure 7.24 Mixing regular insulin and NPH insulin in one syringe.

Step 1 Inject 45 units of air into the vial with NPH insulin.

Step 2 Inject 15 units of air into the vial with regular insulin.

Step 3   Withdraw 15 units of regular insulin into the 100 unit syringe.

Step 4   Withdraw 45 units of NPH insulin into the same syringe.

BY THE WAY

It is recommended that regular insulin be drawn into the syringe first.

The most common types of syringes are summarized in figure 7.25.

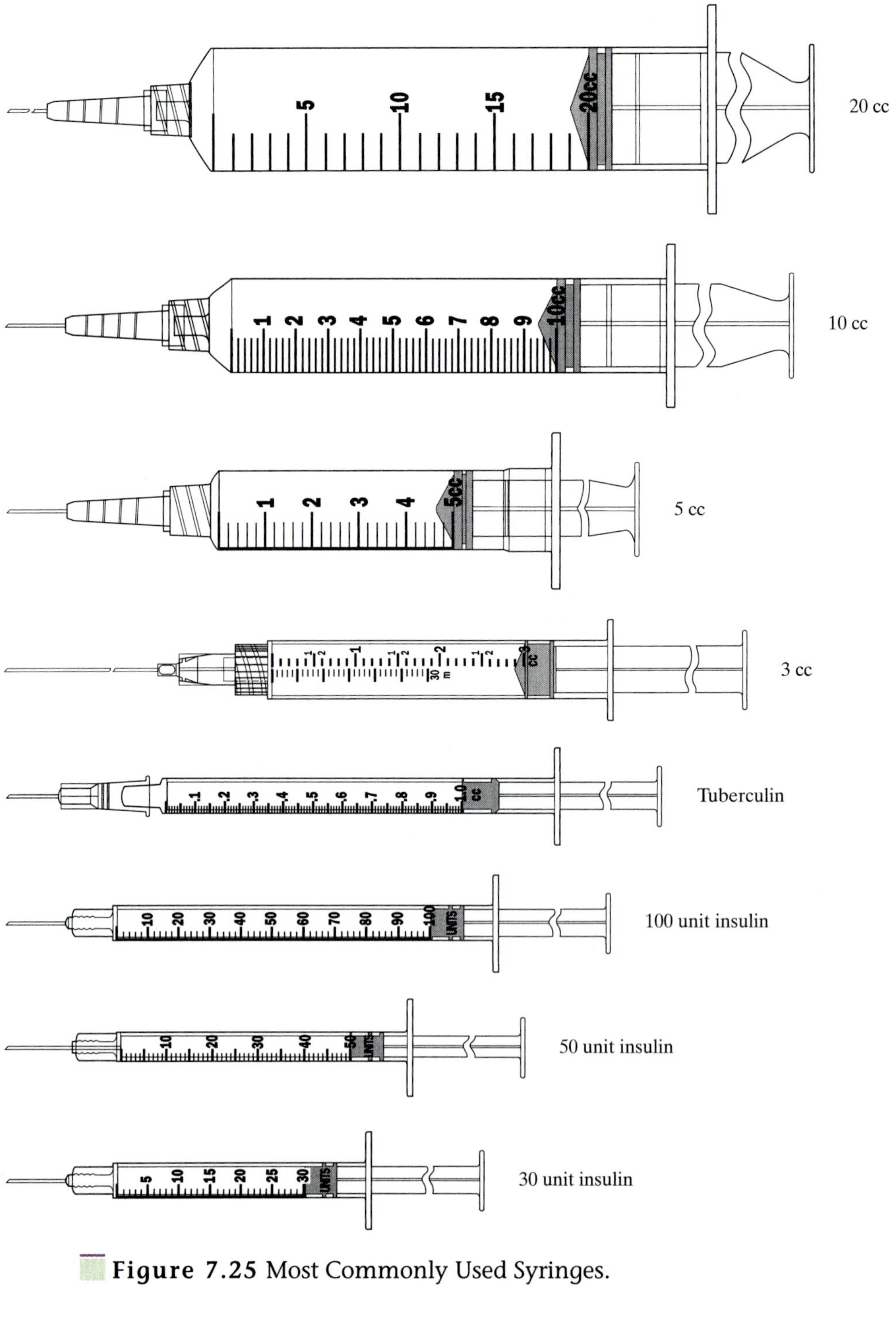

Figure 7.25 Most Commonly Used Syringes.

Case Study 7.1

A 75-year-old female with a medical history of diabetes mellitus, depression, hypertension, and osteoarthritis is brought to the emergency room after falling in a supermarket. Her right leg is externally rotated and shorter than the left leg. She is diaphoretic and complains of severe pain (10/10 on the pain scale) in her right leg. Xray confirms a fracture of the right femur and she is admitted for surgery. She weighs 154 pounds and is allergic to peanuts and penicillin. Vital signs are: T, 101°, BP, 152/90; P, 110; R, 26.

- *Pre-op orders:*
- NPO
- V/S q4h
- Neurovascular checks q4h
- Morphine 10 mg sc q4h prn for acute pain
- IV N/S @ 83 cc/h
- Pre-op meds: Atropine sulfate 0.4mg IM one hour before surgery
- Demerol 50 mg and Versed 0.07 mg/kg IM one hour before surgery
- *Post-op orders:*
- NPO progress to clear diet as tolerated
- Neurovascular checks q4h
- V/S q4h
- IV N/S @ 125 cc/h
- Compazine (prochlorperazine) 0.005g IM q4h prn nausea
- Demerol (meperidine hcl) 50 mg and Vistaril (hydroxyzine) 25 mg IM q3–4h prn pain
- Mefoxin (cefoxitin) 1g IVPB q8h × 3 days
- Lovenox (enoxaparin) 30 mg sc bid

1. The label on the Morphine vial reads 10mg/mL.

   a. Draw a line indicating the appropriate measurement on each of the following syringes.

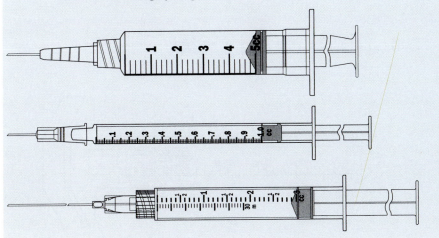

b. Which is the best syringe to use in administering this medication?

2. The label on the vial of Atropine reads gr $\frac{1}{150}$ per mL.

   a. How many milliliters are needed?

   b. Choose the best syringe to use in administering this medication and draw a line indicating the correct dose.

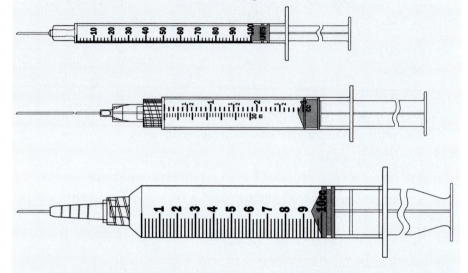

3. a. Calculate the dose of Versed.

   b. The Versed is supplied in 1 mg/mL and 5 mg/mL vials. The Demerol is available in prepackaged 2 mL syringes labeled 10 mg/mL; 25 mg/mL; 50 mg/mL; 75 mg/mL; and 100 mg/mL. Draw a line on the appropriate syringe indicating the dose of these drugs that you will administer.

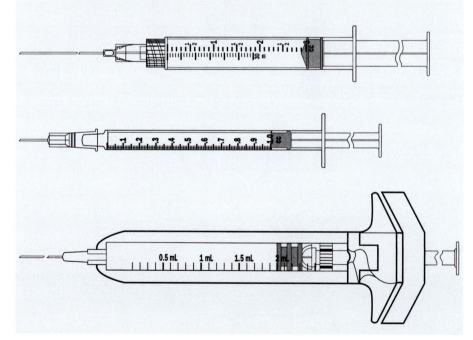

4. The patient is complaining of severe nausea. The Compazine vial is labeled 5 mg/mL. Draw a line on the appropriate syringe indicating the dose of Compazine to be administered in minims.

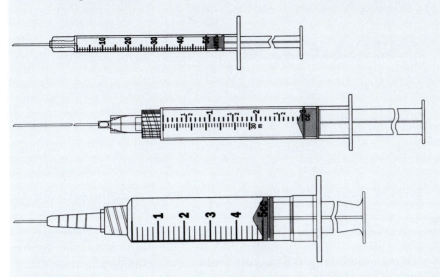

5. The information on the Mefoxin label states: add 10 mL of sterile water to the Mefoxin 1 g. Draw a line on the appropriate syringe indicating the amount of diluent that you will add to the vial.

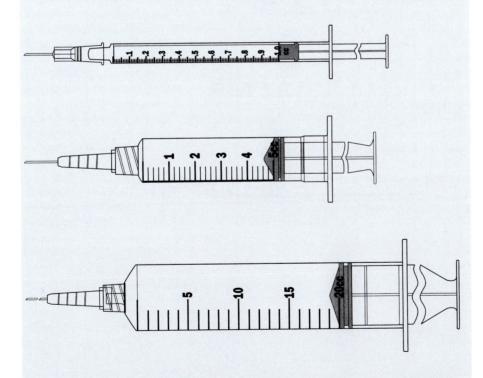

6. The patient is no longer NPO and the physician has ordered NPH insulin 15 units, and Regular insulin 8 units sc 30 minutes ac breakfast, and NPH insulin 6 units, Regular insulin 6 units, 30 minutes ac dinner.

a. Choose the syringe that you would use to administer the dose before dinner and draw a line on the syringe indicating the Regular insulin and then the NPH insulin.

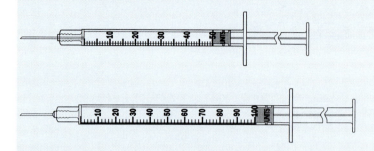

b. How many units of Regular insulin is she receiving each day?

7. The patient is being discharged on Lovenox 1 mg/kg sc q12h. The medication comes in 30 mg/0.3 mL; 40 mg/0.4 mL; 60 mg/0.6 mL; and 80 mg/0.8 mL and vials. Choose the appropriate vial and syringe to use and draw a line indicating the dose of Lovenox to be administered.

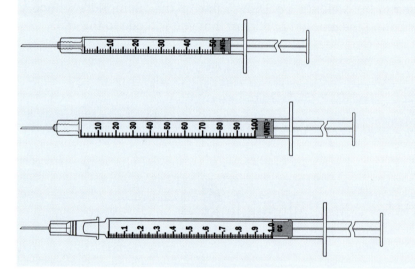

PRACTICE SETS

You will find the answers to *Try These for Practice, Exercises,* and *Cumulative Review Exercises* in Appendix A at the back of the book. The answers to the *Additional Exercises* can be found on the companion Website or ask your instructor.

Try These for Practice

Test your comprehension after reading the chapter.

In Problems 1 through 4, identify the type of syringe shown in the figure. Then, for each quantity, place an arrow at the appropriate level of measurement on the syringe.

1. _____ syringe; 0.7 cc

2. _____ syringe; 4.6 cc

3. _____ syringe; 34 units

4. _____ syringe; 78 units

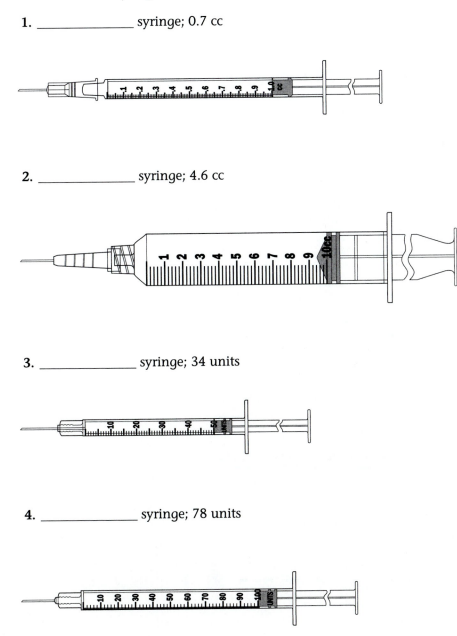

5. The prescriber ordered 5 mg of Adriamycin PFS IVPB. Read the label in Figure 7.26, do the calculation, and place an arrow at the appropriate level of measurement on the syringe below.

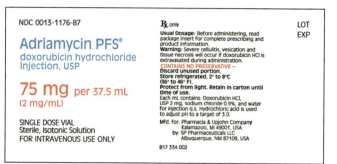

Figure 7.26 Drug Label For Adriamycin PFS.
(Courtesy of Pharmacia Corporation.)

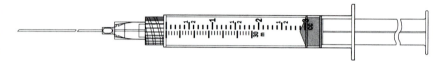

Exercises

Reinforce your understanding in class or at home.

In Problems 1 through 14, identify the type of syringe shown in the figure. Then, for each quantity, place an arrow at the appropriate level of measurement on the syringe.

1. _____ syringe; 42 units

2. _____ syringe; 14 units

3. _____ syringe; 2.6 cc

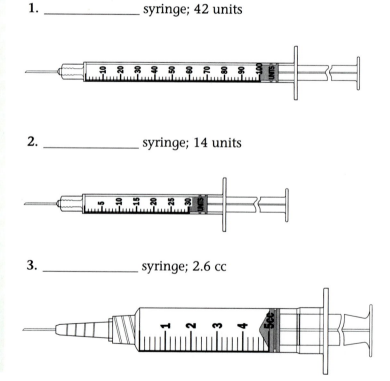

4. _____ syringe; 0.8 cc

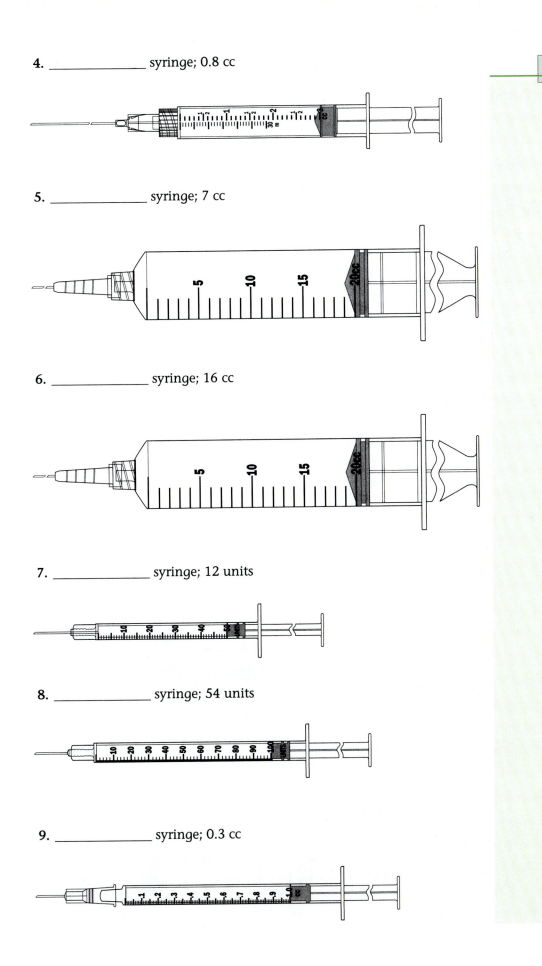

5. _____ syringe; 7 cc

6. _____ syringe; 16 cc

7. _____ syringe; 12 units

8. _____ syringe; 54 units

9. _____ syringe; 0.3 cc

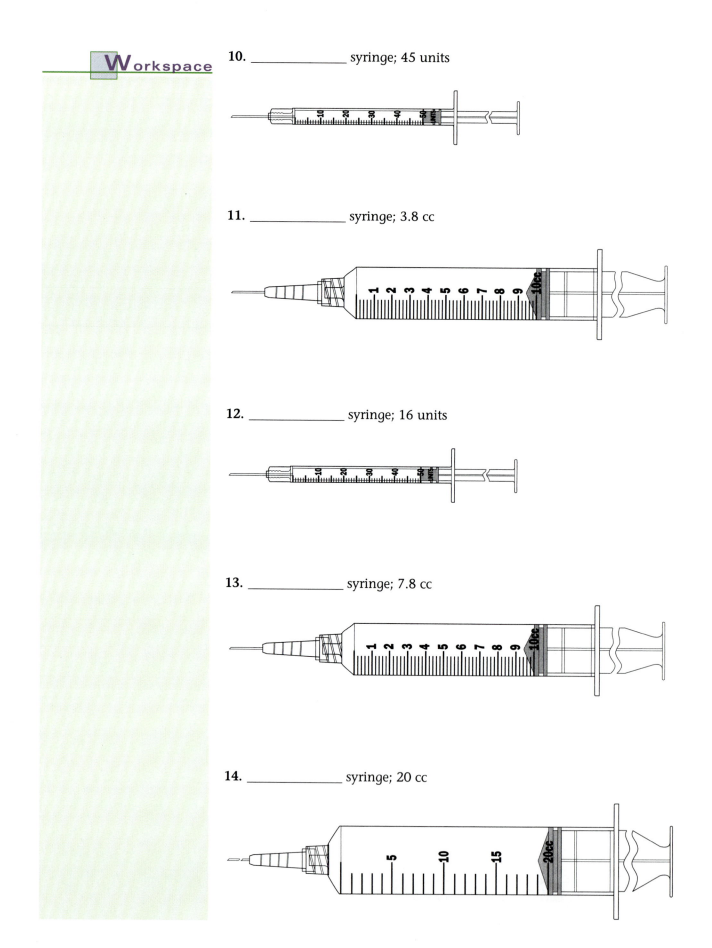

10. _____ syringe; 45 units

11. _____ syringe; 3.8 cc

12. _____ syringe; 16 units

13. _____ syringe; 7.8 cc

14. _____ syringe; 20 cc

In problems 15 through 20, read the order and use the appropriate label in Figure 7.27 (found *at the end of the Exercises*), calculate the dosage if necessary, and place an arrow at the appropriate level of measurement on the syringe.

15. Order: Dexamethasone 25 mg IV stat

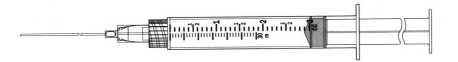

16. Order: 100 mg Lymphocyte immune globulin IV

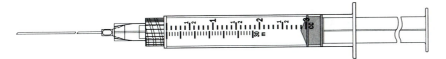

17. Order: Vancocin HCl 0.6 g IV

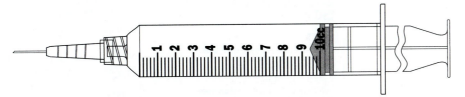

18. Order: Morphine Sulfate 4 mg IV

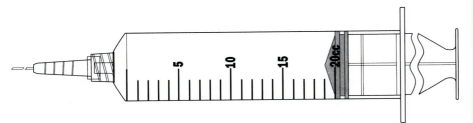

19. Order: Pancuronium 1.6 mg IV

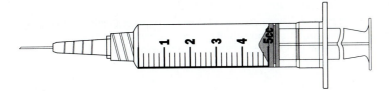

20. Order: Streptomycin 800 mg IM

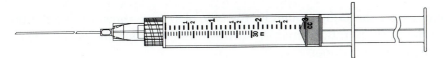

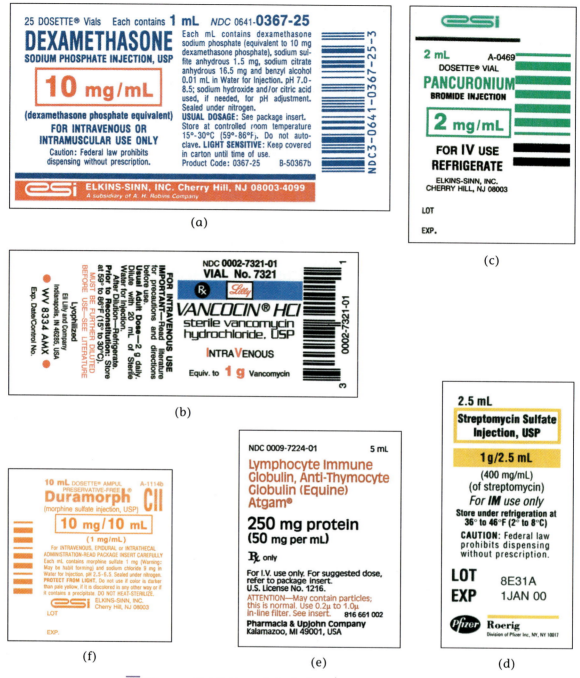

(a)

25 DOSETTE® Vials   Each contains **1 mL**   NDC 0641-**0367-25**

DEXAMETHASONE
SODIUM PHOSPHATE INJECTION, USP

10 mg/mL

(dexamethasone phosphate equivalent)

FOR INTRAVENOUS OR INTRAMUSCULAR USE ONLY
Caution: Federal law prohibits dispensing without prescription.

Each mL contains dexamethasone sodium phosphate (equivalent to 10 mg dexamethasone phosphate), sodium sulfite anhydrous 1.5 mg, sodium citrate anhydrous 16.5 mg and benzyl alcohol 0.01 mL in Water for Injection. pH 7.0-8.5; sodium hydroxide and/or citric acid used, if needed, for pH adjustment. Sealed under nitrogen.
USUAL DOSAGE: See package insert. Store at controlled room temperature 15°-30°C (59°-86°F). Do not autoclave. **LIGHT SENSITIVE:** Keep covered in carton until time of use.
Product Code: 0367-25   B-50367b

esi   ELKINS-SINN, INC. Cherry Hill, NJ 08003-4099
A subsidiary of A. H. Robins Company

NDC3-0641-0367-25-3

(c)

esi

2 mL   A-0469
DOSETTE® VIAL

PANCURONIUM
BROMIDE INJECTION

2 mg/mL

FOR IV USE
REFRIGERATE

ELKINS-SINN, INC.
CHERRY HILL, NJ 08003

LOT

EXP.

(b)

NDC 0002-7321-01
VIAL No. 7321

℞   Lilly

VANCOCIN® HCl
sterile vancomycin hydrochloride, USP

INTRAVENOUS

Equiv. to **1 g** Vancomycin

0002-7321-01

FOR INTRAVENOUS USE
IMPORTANT—Read literature for precautions and directions before use.
Usual Adult Dose—2 g daily.
Dilute with 20 mL of Sterile Water for Injection.
After Dilution—Refrigerate.
Prior to Reconstitution: Store at 59° to 86°F (15° to 30°C).

MUST BE FURTHER DILUTED BEFORE USE—SEE LITERATURE

Lyophilized
Eli Lilly and Company
Indianapolis, IN 46285, USA

WV 8334 AMX

Exp. Date/Control No.

(f)

10 mL DOSETTE® AMPUL   A-1114b
PRESERVATIVE-FREE®
Duramorph   **CII**
(morphine sulfate injection, USP)

10 mg/10 mL

(1 mg/mL)

For INTRAVENOUS, EPIDURAL or INTRATHECAL ADMINISTRATION-READ PACKAGE INSERT CAREFULLY
Each mL contains morphine sulfate 1 mg (Warning: May be habit forming) and sodium chloride 9 mg in Water for Injection, pH 2.5-6.5. Sealed under nitrogen.
PROTECT FROM LIGHT. Do not use if color is darker than pale yellow, if it is discolored in any other way or if it contains a precipitate. DO NOT HEAT-STERILIZE.

esi   ELKINS-SINN, INC.
Cherry Hill, NJ 08003

LOT

EXP.

(e)

NDC 0009-7224-01   5 mL

Lymphocyte Immune Globulin, Anti-Thymocyte Globulin (Equine) Atgam®

250 mg protein
(50 mg per mL)

℞ only

For I.V. use only. For suggested dose, refer to package insert.
U.S. License No. 1216.

ATTENTION—May contain particles; this is normal. Use 0.2μ to 1.0μ in-line filter. See insert.   **816 661 002**

Pharmacia & Upjohn Company
Kalamazoo, MI 49001, USA

(d)

2.5 mL

Streptomycin Sulfate Injection, USP

1g/2.5 mL

(400 mg/mL)
(of streptomycin)
*For **IM** use only*
Store under refrigeration at 36° to 46°F (2° to 8°C)

CAUTION: Federal law prohibits dispensing without prescription.

LOT   8E31A
EXP   1JAN 00

Pfizer **Roerig**
Division of Pfizer Inc, NY, NY 10017

Figure 7.27 Drug Labels for Exercises 15–20.

(a, c, f) Courtesy of ESI Lederle, a Business Unit of Wyeth Pharmaceuticals, Philadelphia, PA. (b) Courtesy of Eli Lilly and Company. (d) Registered Trademark of Pfizer Inc. Reproduced with permission. (e) Courtesy of Pharmacia & Upjohn Co.

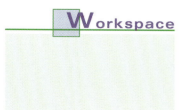

Workspace

Additional Exercises

Now, on your own, test yourself! The answers to the *Additional Exercises* can be found on the companion Website or ask your instructor.

In Problems 1 through 16, identify the type of syringe shown in the figure. Then, for each quantity, place an arrow at the appropriate level of measurement on the syringe.

1. _____ syringe; 9.8 cc

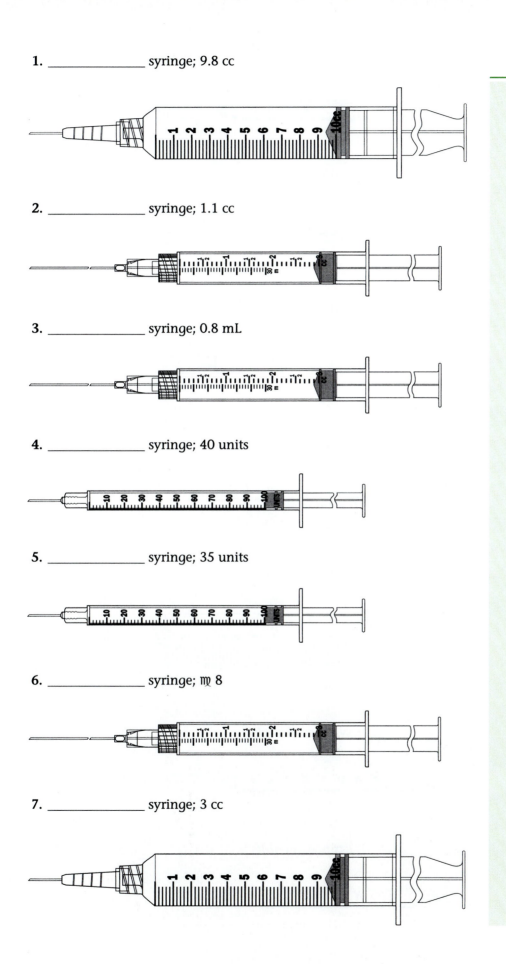

2. _____ syringe; 1.1 cc

3. _____ syringe; 0.8 mL

4. _____ syringe; 40 units

5. _____ syringe; 35 units

6. _____ syringe; ℳ 8

7. _____ syringe; 3 cc

8. _____ syringe; 90 units

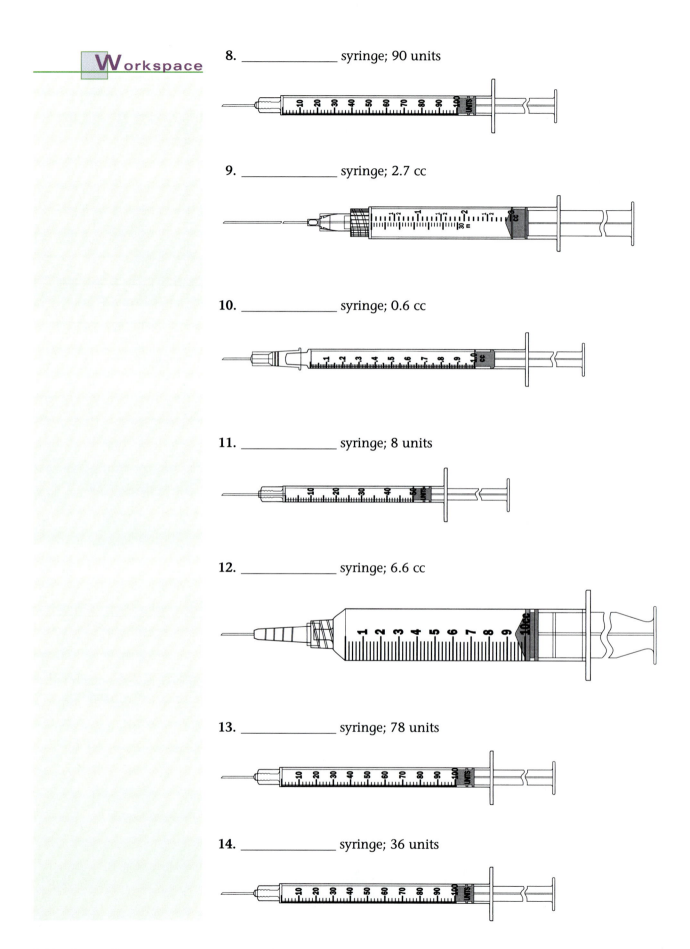

9. _____ syringe; 2.7 cc

10. _____ syringe; 0.6 cc

11. _____ syringe; 8 units

12. _____ syringe; 6.6 cc

13. _____ syringe; 78 units

14. _____ syringe; 36 units

15. _____ syringe; 3.4 cc

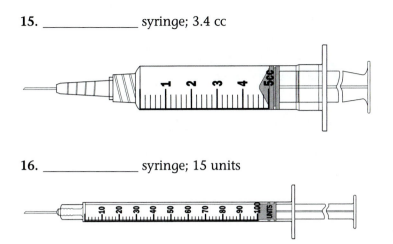

16. _____ syringe; 15 units

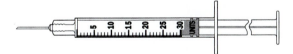

In problems 17 through 20, read the order and use the appropriate label in Figure 7.28 (found at the end of the *Additional Exercises*); calculate the dosage if necessary, and place an arrow at the appropriate level of measurement on the syringe.

17. Order: Fragmin 7500 units sc

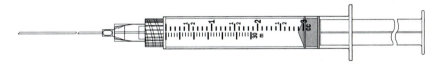

18. Order: Humulin R insulin 250 units IV

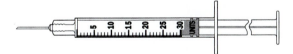

19. Order: Urokinase 125,000 units IV

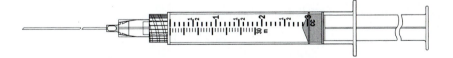

20. Order: Kefurox 750 mg IV

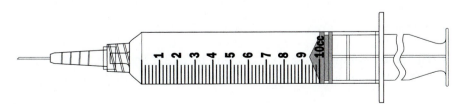

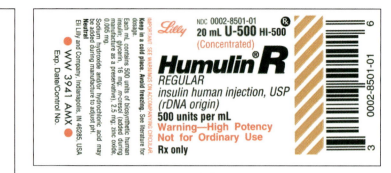

(a)

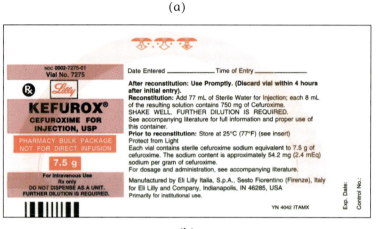

(b)

0.2 mL
Fragmin®
dalteparin sodium injection

**2500 IU
(anti-Xa)
per 0.2 mL**

Manufactured for:
Pharmacia & Upjohn
Company
132050198   KV0307-02

LOT
EXP

(d)

Figure 7.28 Drug labels for *Additional Exercises 17–20.*

(a, b) Courtesy of Eli Lilly and Company, (c) Reproduced with permission of Abbott Laboratories, (d) Reproduced with courtesy of Pharmacia & Upjohn Co.

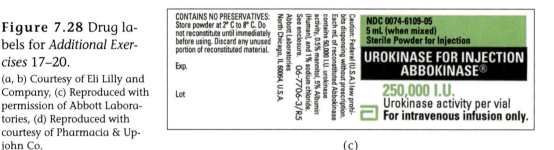

(c)

Workspace

CUMULATIVE REVIEW EXERCISES

Review your mastery of earlier chapters.

1. gr 20 = _____ mg   **2.** 1600 mL = _____ L

3. The prescriber ordered Prilosec 0.020 g po qd. Each capsule contains 20 milligrams. How many capsules will you administer to the patient? _____

4. The order reads: morphine sulfate gr $\frac{1}{8}$ IM q4h prn. Change grain $\frac{1}{8}$ to milligrams. _____

5. The prescriber ordered Biaxin 300 mg po q12h. The label reads 375 milligrams per 5 milliliters. How many milliliters will you administer to the patient? _____

6. Change grain $\dfrac{1}{500}$ to milligrams. _____

7. The prescriber ordered 120 mL H_2O po q2h for 10 h. How many ounces should the patient receive? _____

8. ℥ 24 = ℈ _____

9. 0.4 mg = gr _____

10. 0.004 g = gr _____

11. The prescriber ordered Cardura 4 mg po qd. Each tablet contains 0.002 g. How many tablets will you administer to the patient? _____

12. The prescriber ordered 0.3 milligram of clonidine hydrochloride. If each tablet contains 0.1 milligram, how many tablets will you administer to the patient? _____

13. Read the information on the label in Figure 7.29, and calculate the number of tablets equal to 0.001 gram. _____

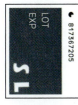
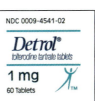

℞ only
See package insert for complete product information.
Dispense in tight container.
Store at controlled room temperature 20° to 25°C
(68° to 77°F) (see USP).

US Patent No. 5,382,600
Pharmacia & Upjohn Company
A subsidiary of Pharmacia Corporation
Kalamazoo, MI 49001, USA

NDC 0009-4541-02

Detrol®
tolterodine tartrate tablets

1 mg

60 Tablets

LOT
EXP
817367205
SL

Figure 7.29 Drug label for Detrol.
(Courtesy of Pharmacia and Upjohn Co.)

14. Read the label in Figure 7.30. How many milligrams of Trovan are contained in 35 mL? _____

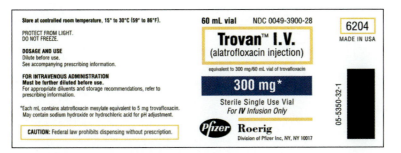

Store at controlled room temperature, 15° to 30°C (59° to 86°F).

PROTECT FROM LIGHT.
DO NOT FREEZE.

DOSAGE AND USE
Dilute before use.
See accompanying prescribing information.

FOR INTRAVENOUS ADMINISTRATION
Must be further diluted before use.
For appropriate diluents and storage recommendations, refer to prescribing information.

*Each mL contains alatrofloxacin mesylate equivalent to 5 mg trovafloxacin. May contain sodium hydroxide or hydrochloric acid for pH adjustment.

CAUTION: Federal law prohibits dispensing without prescription.

60 mL vial   NDC 0049-3900-28

Trovan™ I.V.
(alatrofloxacin injection)

equivalent to 300 mg/60 mL vial of trovafloxacin

300 mg*

Sterile Single Use Vial
For IV Infusion Only

Pfizer **Roerig**
Division of Pfizer Inc, NY, NY 10017

6204
MADE IN USA

05-5350-32-1

Figure 7.30 Drug label for Trovan.
(Reg. Trademark of Pfizer Inc. Reproduced with permission.)

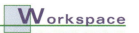

15. Read the label in Figure 7.31. How many milliliters equal
50 mg? _____

Figure 7.31 Drug label for Phenobarbital.
(Courtesy of ESI Lederle, a Business Unit of Wyeth Pharmaceuticals, Philadelphia PA.)

Additional questions, web links, matching exercises, fill-in-the-blanks, and glossary for this chapter
can be found on the companion Website at www.prenhall.com/olsen. Click on "Chapter 7" to
select the activities for this chapter.

CHAPTER EIGHT

Preparation of Solutions

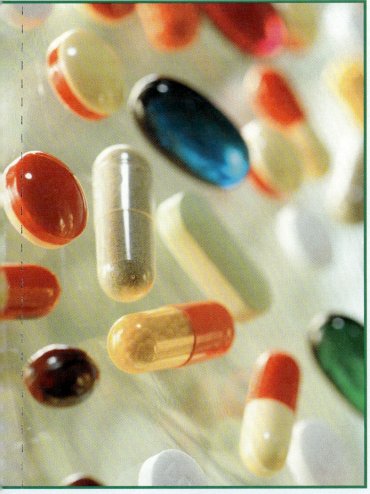

Objectives

After completing this chapter, you will be able to

- Use the strength of a solution, given in ratio form or percentage form, to calculate drug doses.

- Explain the relationships among the amount of solution, the strength of the solution, and the amount of pure drug that the solution contains.

- Do the calculations necessary to prepare solutions from pure drugs.

- Do the calculations necessary to prepare solutions by diluting stock solutions.

In this chapter you will learn about solutions. Although most solutions are prepared in the pharmacy by the pharmacist, nurses must understand the concepts involved and be able to prepare solutions, especially in home care situations.

Drugs are manufactured in both pure and diluted form. A pure drug contains only the drug and nothing else. A drug is frequently diluted by dissolving a quantity of pure drug in a liquid to form a solution. This solution is called a **stock solution**. The pure drug (either dry or liquid) is called the **solute**. The liquid added to the pure drug to form the solution is called the **solvent** or **diluent**. The solvents most commonly used are sterile water and normal saline solution.

Strength of Solutions

The strength of a solution can be stated as a **ratio** or a **percentage**.

- The ratio 1:2 (read "1 to 2") means that there is 1 part of the drug in 2 parts of solution. This solution is also referred to as a $\frac{1}{2}$ strength solution or a 50% solution.

- The ratio 1:10 (read "1 to 10") means that there is 1 part of the drug in 10 parts of solution. This solution is also referred to as a 10% solution.

- A 5% solution means that there are 5 parts of the drug in 100 parts of solution.

- A $2\frac{1}{2}$% solution means that there are $2\frac{1}{2}$ parts of the drug in 100 parts of solution.

Pure Drugs in Liquid Form

For a pure drug that is in liquid form, the ratio 1:40 means there is 1 milliliter of pure drug in every 40 milliliters of solution. So 40 milliliters of a 1:40 acetic acid solution means that 1 milliliter of pure acetic acid is diluted with water to make a total of 40 milliliters of solution. You would prepare this solution by placing 1 milliliter of pure acetic acid in a graduated cylinder and adding water until the level in the graduated cylinder reaches 40 milliliters. See Figure 8.1.

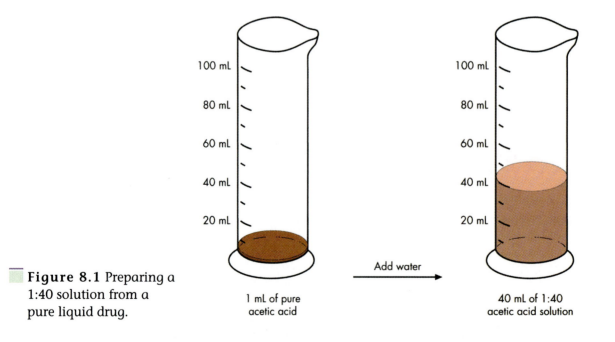

Figure 8.1 Preparing a 1:40 solution from a pure liquid drug.

100 mL   80 mL   60 mL   40 mL   20 mL

1 mL of pure acetic acid

Add water

100 mL   80 mL   60 mL   40 mL   20 mL

40 mL of 1:40 acetic acid solution

A 1% solution means that there is 1 part of the drug in 100 parts of solution. So you would prepare 100 milliliters of a 1% creosol solution by placing 1 milliliter of pure creosol in a graduated cylinder and adding water until the level in the graduated cylinder reaches 100 milliliters. See Figure 8.2.

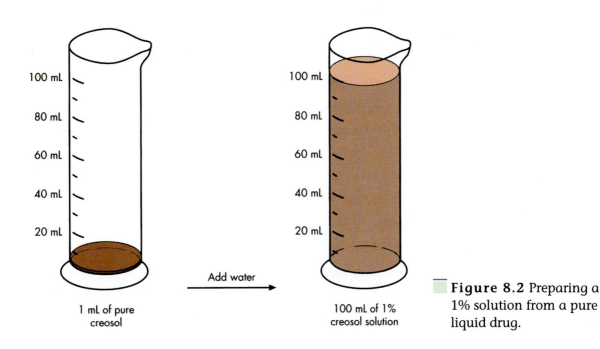

100 mL

80 mL

60 mL

40 mL

20 mL

1 mL of pure creosol

Add water

100 mL

80 mL

60 mL

40 mL

20 mL

100 mL of 1% creosol solution

Figure 8.2 Preparing a 1% solution from a pure liquid drug.

Pure Drugs in Dry Form

The ratio 1:20 means 1 part of the pure drug in 20 parts of solution, or 2 parts of the pure drug in 40 parts of solution, or 3 parts in 60, or 4 parts in 80, and so on. When a pure drug is in *dry* form, the ratio 1:20 means 1 *gram* of pure drug in every 20 *milliliters* of solution. So 100 milliliters of a 1:20 potassium permanganate solution means *5 grams* of pure potassium permanganate dissolved in water to make a total of *100 milliliters* of the solution. If each tablet is 5 grams, then you would prepare this solution by placing 1 tablet of the pure potassium permanganate in a graduated cylinder and adding water until the level in the graduated cylinder reaches 100 milliliters.

BY THE WAY

A 1:20 solution is the same as a 5% solution.

A 5% potassium permanganate solution means 5 grams of pure potassium permanganate in 100 milliliters of solution. So, the strength of a 5% potassium permanganate solution is written as $\dfrac{5\,g}{100\,mL}$ or $\dfrac{1\,g}{20\,mL}$. See Figure 8.3.

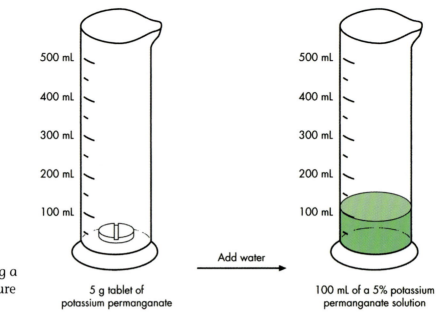

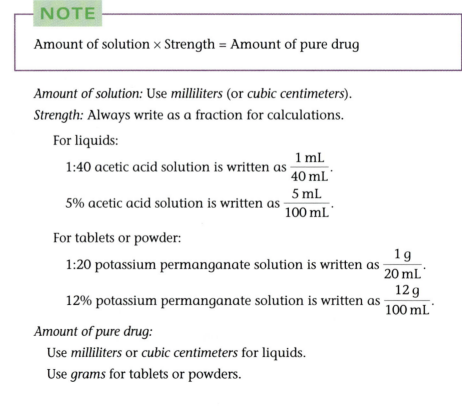

Figure 8.3 Preparing a 5% solution from a pure dry drug.

5 g tablet of potassium permanganate

Add water

100 mL of a 5% potassium permanganate solution

Preparing Solutions from Pure Drugs

The following formula shows the relationships among the amount of solution, the strength of the solution, and the amount of pure drug that the solution contains. You can use this formula to prepare a prescribed solution of a certain strength from a pure drug.

> **NOTE**
>
> Amount of solution × Strength = Amount of pure drug

Amount of solution: Use *milliliters* (or *cubic centimeters*).

Strength: Always write as a fraction for calculations.

For liquids:

1:40 acetic acid solution is written as $\dfrac{1\,mL}{40\,mL}$.

5% acetic acid solution is written as $\dfrac{5\,mL}{100\,mL}$.

For tablets or powder:

1:20 potassium permanganate solution is written as $\dfrac{1\,g}{20\,mL}$.

12% potassium permanganate solution is written as $\dfrac{12\,g}{100\,mL}$.

Amount of pure drug:

Use *milliliters* or *cubic centimeters* for liquids.

Use *grams* for tablets or powders.

Example 8.1

How many grams of sodium chloride would you need to prepare 100 milliliters of a 20% solution?

Because sodium chloride is in dry form, it is measured in grams. So, a 20% solution contains 20 grams of sodium chloride in 100 milliliters of solution.

Amount of solution is 100 milliliters.

Strength is 20% or $\dfrac{20}{100}$, so you use $\dfrac{20\,g}{100\,mL}$.

$$100\,mL \times \frac{20\,g}{100\,mL} = \text{Amount of pure drug}$$

$$\overset{1}{\cancel{100\,mL}} \times \frac{20\,g}{\underset{1}{\cancel{100\,mL}}} = 20\,g$$

So, you need 20 grams of sodium chloride to prepare 100 milliliters of a 20% solution.

Example 8.2

Read the label in Figure 8.4. How many grams of dextrose are contained in 30 mL of this solution?

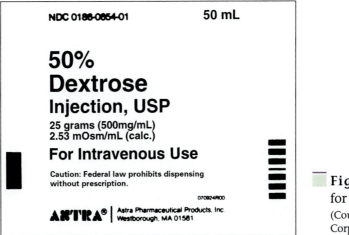

Figure 8.4 Drug label for 50% dextrose.
(Courtesy of Astra-Zeneca Corp.)

Amount of solution is 30 milliliters.

Strength is 50% or $\dfrac{50}{100}$, so you use $\dfrac{50\,g}{100\,mL}$.

$$30\,mL \times \frac{50\,g}{100\,mL} = \text{Amount of pure drug}$$

$$\cancel{30\,mL} \times \frac{50\,g}{\cancel{100\,mL}} = 15\,g$$

So, 15 grams of dextrose are contained in 30 milliliters of a 50% dextrose solution.

Example 8.3

How would you prepare 2000 milliliters of a 1:10 Clorox solution?

Because Clorox is a liquid, it is measured in milliliters. So, a 1:10 solution means 1 milliliter of Clorox in 10 milliliters of solution.

Amount of solution is 2000 milliliters.

Strength is 1:10 or $\frac{1}{10}$. You use $\frac{1\,\text{mL}}{10\,\text{mL}}$.

$$\overset{200}{\cancel{2000}}\,\cancel{\text{mL}} \times \frac{1\,\text{mL}}{\underset{1}{\cancel{10}\,\cancel{\text{mL}}}} = 200\,\text{mL}$$

So, you need 200 milliliters of Clorox to prepare 2000 milliliters of a 1:10 solution. This means that 200 milliliters of Clorox is diluted with water to 2000 milliliters of solution.

Example 8.4

How would you prepare 250 milliliters of a $\frac{1}{2}$% Lysol solution? Lysol is a liquid, so a $\frac{1}{2}$% solution means 0.5 milliliter of Lysol in 100 milliliters of solution. (*Remember:* $\frac{1}{2} = 0.5$)

Amount of solution is 250 milliliters.

Strength is $\frac{1}{2}$% or $\frac{0.5}{100}$, so you use $\frac{0.5\,\text{mL}}{100\,\text{mL}}$.

$$\overset{5}{\cancel{250}}\,\cancel{\text{mL}} \times \frac{0.5\,\text{mL}}{\underset{2}{\cancel{100}\,\cancel{\text{mL}}}} = 1.25\,\text{mL}$$

So, you need 1.25 milliliters of Lysol to prepare 250 milliliters of a $\frac{1}{2}$% Lysol solution. This means that 1.25 milliliters of Lysol is diluted with water to 250 milliliters of solution.

Example 8.5

How would you prepare 3 liters of a 1% urinary antiseptic solution using 5 g tablets of Neosporin?

Because the pure Neosporin is in dry form, it is measured in grams. So, a 1% solution means 1 gram of Neosporin in 100 milliliters of solution.

You must find the amount of pure drug necessary and convert to tablets.

Amount of solution is 3 liters.

Strength is 1% or $\dfrac{1}{100}$, so you use $\dfrac{1\,g}{100\,mL}$.

Because you are working in milliliters, change 3 liters to 3000 milliliters.

Because each tablet contains 5 grams, you use the fraction $\dfrac{1\,tab}{5\,g}$.

$$\overset{30}{\cancel{3000}}\ \cancel{mL} \times \dfrac{1\ \cancel{g}}{\underset{1}{\cancel{100}}\ \cancel{mL}} \times \dfrac{1\ tab}{5\ \cancel{g}} = 6\ tab$$

So, you dissolve 6 tablets of Neosporin in water and dilute to 3000 milliliters.

Diluting Stock Solutions

A stock solution is one in which a pure drug is already dissolved in a liquid. The strength of each stock solution is written on the label. If the order is for a stronger solution, you will need to prepare a new solution because you cannot strengthen a stock solution. However, if the order is for a weaker solution, you can dilute the stock solution to the prescribed strength. To find out how much stock solution to mix, use the following formula.

<table>
<tr><td>NOTE</td></tr>
<tr><td>$$\dfrac{\text{Amount prescribed} \times \text{Strength prescribed}}{\text{Strength of stock}} = \text{Amount of stock}$$</td></tr>
</table>

Example 8.6

How would you prepare 1 liter of a 25% solution from a 50% stock solution?

Amount prescribed is 1 liter, so you use 1000 milliliters.

Strength prescribed is 25%, so you use $\dfrac{25\,mL}{100\,mL}$.

Strength of stock is 50%, so you use $\dfrac{50\,mL}{100\,mL}$.

$$\dfrac{1000\ mL \times \dfrac{25\ \cancel{mL}}{100\ \cancel{mL}}}{\dfrac{50\ \cancel{mL}}{100\ \cancel{mL}}} = \text{Amount of stock}$$

$$1000\ mL \times \dfrac{25}{100} \div \dfrac{50}{100} =$$

$$1000\ mL \times \dfrac{\overset{1}{\cancel{25}}}{\underset{1}{\cancel{100}}} \times \dfrac{\overset{1}{\cancel{100}}}{\underset{2}{\cancel{50}}} = 500\ mL$$

So, you would take 500 milliliters of the 50% stock solution and add water to the level of 1000 milliliters.

Example 8.7

How would you prepare 2500 milliliters of a 1:10 boric acid solution from a 40% stock solution of this antiseptic?

Amount prescribed is 2500 milliliters.

Strength prescribed is 1:10, so you use $\dfrac{1\,\text{mL}}{10\,\text{mL}}$.

Strength of stock is 40%, so you use $\dfrac{40\,\text{mL}}{100\,\text{mL}}$.

$$\dfrac{2500\,\text{mL} \times \dfrac{1\,\text{mL}}{10\,\text{mL}}}{\dfrac{40\,\text{mL}}{100\,\text{mL}}} = \text{Amount of stock}$$

$$2500\,\text{mL} \times \dfrac{1}{10} \div \dfrac{40}{100} =$$

$$\overset{250}{\cancel{2500}}\,\text{mL} \times \dfrac{1}{\underset{1}{\cancel{10}}} \times \dfrac{100}{40} = 625\,\text{mL}$$

So, you would take 625 milliliters of the 40% stock solution of boric acid and add water to the level of 2500 milliliters.

Example 8.8

How would you prepare 500 milliliters of a 1:25 solution from a 1:4 stock solution of the antiseptic Argyrol?

Amount prescribed is 500 milliliters.

Strength prescribed is 1:25, so you use $\dfrac{1\,\text{mL}}{25\,\text{mL}}$.

Strength of stock is 1:4, so you use $\dfrac{1\,\text{mL}}{4\,\text{mL}}$.

$$\dfrac{500\,\text{mL} \times \dfrac{1\,\text{mL}}{25\,\text{mL}}}{\dfrac{1\,\text{mL}}{4\,\text{mL}}} = \text{Amount of stock}$$

$$500\,\text{mL} \times \dfrac{1}{25} \div \dfrac{1}{4} =$$

$$\overset{20}{\cancel{500}}\,\text{mL} \times \dfrac{1}{\underset{1}{\cancel{25}}} \times \dfrac{4}{1} = 80\,\text{mL}$$

So, you would take 80 milliliters of a 1:4 stock solution of Argyrol and add water to the level of 500 milliliters.

You have now learned how to prepare solutions by using formulas. In the following examples, you will use dimensional analysis to determine the amount of solution that contains a given amount of pure drug.

Example 8.9

How many milliliters of a 20% magnesium sulfate solution will contain 40 grams of the pure drug, magnesium sulfate?

You want to convert the 40 grams of pure drug to milliliters of solution.

$$40\,g = ?\,mL$$

You want to cancel the grams and obtain the equivalent amount in milliliters.

$$40\,g \times \frac{?\,mL}{?\,g} = ?\,mL$$

In a 20% solution there are 20 grams of pure drug per 100 mL of solution. So, the fraction is

$$\frac{100\,mL}{20\,g}$$

$$\overset{2}{\cancel{40}}\,\cancel{g} \times \frac{100\,mL}{\underset{1}{\cancel{20}\,\cancel{g}}} = 200\,mL$$

So, 200 milliliters of a 20% magnesium sulfate solution contains 40 grams of the pure drug, magnesium sulfate.

Example 8.10

How many milliliters of a 1:40 acetic acid solution will contain 25 milliliters of acetic acid?

You want to convert the 25 milliliters of pure acetic acid to milliliters of solution.

$$25\,mL\,(of\,pure\,drug) = ?\,mL\,(of\,solution)$$

There may be some confusion in the meaning of the previous line because there are milliliters on both sides of the equal sign. To aid your understanding, the parentheses are included to indicate whether "mL" refers to the amount of pure drug or to the amount of solution.

You want to cancel the milliliters of pure drug and obtain the equivalent amount in milliliters of solution.

$$25\,mL\,(of\,pure\,drug) \times \frac{?\,mL\,(of\,solution)}{?\,mL\,(of\,pure\,drug)} = ?\,mL\,(of\,solution)$$

In a 1:40 acetic acid solution there is 1 milliliter of pure acetic acid in 40 milliliters of solution. So, the fraction is

$$\frac{40\,mL\,(of\,solution)}{1\,mL\,(of\,pure\,drug)}$$

$$25\,\cancel{mL} \times \frac{40\,mL}{1\,\cancel{mL}} = 1000\,mL$$

So, 1000 milliliters of a 1:40 acetic acid solution contains 25 milliliters of pure acetic acid.

A 94-year-old female patient has a medical history of long-standing hypertension and diabetes mellitus type II. She is 5 feet tall and weighs 115 pounds. She makes an appointment with her primary physician. Her current medications are Inderal 20 mg tid, Isordil 20 mg tid, and one multivitamin per day.

Her physician examines her and finds the following symptoms: BP 220/132; P 110 irregular; R 32; T 100°F. She complains of urinary burning, has pedal edema + 3, and has gained 6 pounds. The physician orders 60 mg furosemide stat IV, a chest X ray, electrocardiogram, CBC, and SMA 18. Within 30 minutes she begins to diurese, and in 1 hour she is sent home with the following orders:

- Inderal 40 mg po tid

- Lasix 20 mg q12h po

- K-Lor 20 mEq q12h po

- Isordil 20 mg qid po

- multivitamin 1 qd po

- Zithromax 600 mg qd × 5 days po

- Glucotrol 0.01 g qd ac breakfast po

- hydroxyzine 0.05 g hs prn po
- trovafloxacin 0.1 g qd × 7 days po

1. How many tablets of Inderal will you administer to the patient if each tablet contains 0.04 g? _____

2. Calculate the number of grams of Lasix the patient will receive per day and per week. _____

3. Each packet of K-Lor contains 40 mEq. The directions state: Add packet to 4 oz of juice. How many milliliters equal the dose of potassium? _____

Read the labels found at the end of this case study in Figure 8.5 to answer questions 4 through 7.

4. How many tablets of azithromycin will you administer to this client? _____

5. How many tablets of trovafloxacin will you administer to the patient? _____

6. Determine how many tablets of glipizide you will administer ac breakfast. _____

7. Change the hydroxyzine order to milligrams, and determine the number of tablets you will administer. _____

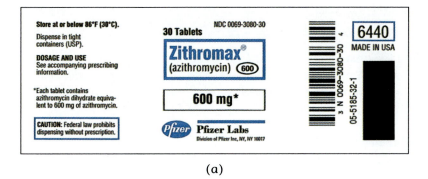

(a)

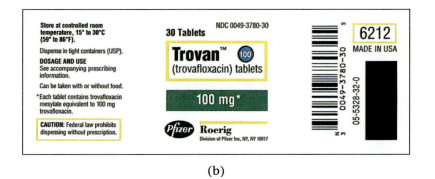

(b)

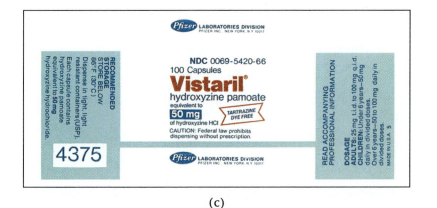

(c)

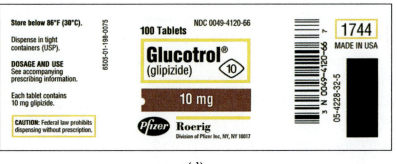

(d)

Figure 8.5 Drug labels for Case Study 8.1.

(Registered Trademark of Pfizer Inc. Reproduced with permission.)

PRACTICE SETS

You will find the answers to *Try These for Practice, Exercises,* and *Cumulative Review* in Appendix A at the back of the book. The answers to the *Additional Exercises* can be found on the companion Website or ask your instructor.

Try These for Practice

Test your comprehension after reading the chapter.

1. Describe how you would prepare 1000 milliliters of a 0.9% normal saline solution from the pure drug (sodium chloride). _____

2. How many grams of epsom salt crystals are required to make 500 milliliters of a 3% solution? _____

3. The prescriber has ordered 2 liters of a 1% neomycin solution for bladder irrigation. Calculate the amount needed from a 2% stock solution. _____

4. How would you prepare 300 mL of a 1:25 solution from a 1:5 solution? _____

5. How would you prepare 4000 milliliters of 5% potassium permanganate solution from 5 g tablets? _____

Exercises

Reinforce your understanding in class or at home.

1. Prepare 2 liters of a 1:50 solution of Lysol from a 100% solution.

2. Describe how you would prepare 500 mL of 0.5% Dakin's solution from a 10% solution.

3. Prepare 250 mL of a 3% hydrogen peroxide solution from a 15% solution.

4. Describe how you would prepare 240 mL of a $\frac{1}{2}$ strength solution of Ensure from pure drug Ensure (100%).

5. How many grams of amino acids are contained in 500 mL of an 8.5% amino acid solution?

6. A patient is receiving 250 mL of a 10% Intralipid solution. How many grams of lipids will this patient receive?

7. How many milliliters of a 20% solution of glucose will contain 50 g of a drug?

8. Physician's order:

   Magnesium sulfate 2 g in 10 mL D$_5$W IV push in 2 minutes

   The label on the vial reads 50% magnesium sulfate. How many milliliters will you prepare?

9. A patient has an order for 200 mL of a 2% lidocaine solution. How many milligrams of lidocaine are contained in this order?

10. A patient receives 4 mL of 1% lidocaine as a nerve block. How many grams of lidocaine did the patient receive?

11. Describe how you would prepare 100 mL of 0.9% normal saline from sodium chloride crystals.

12. How many grams of dextrose are contained in 4000 mL of a 25% dextrose solution?

13. Prepare a $\frac{1}{3}$ solution of Ensure from a can labeled 100% Ensure (240 mL). Explain how you would do this.

14. Describe how you would prepare 500 mL of a 0.25% solution from a 5% stock solution.

15. Use the information on the label in Figure 8.6 to determine the number of grams of calcium chloride in 2 mL of this solution.

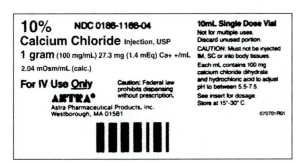

Figure 8.6 Drug label for calcium chloride.
(Courtesy of Astra-Zeneca Corp.)

16. Read the label in Figure 8.7. Determine how many milliliters of this solution will contain 0.001 g of Epinephrine.

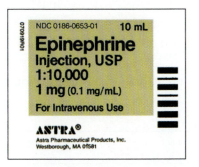

Figure 8.7 Drug label for Epinephrine.
(Courtesy of Astra-Zeneca Corp.)

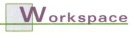
17. Read the label in Figure 8.8. How many grams of Mannitol are contained in 25 mL of this solution?

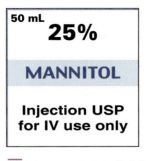

Figure 8.8 Label for Mannitol.

18. How many milliliters of a 1:30 acetic acid solution will contain 20 grams of acetic acid?

19. A client must have a foot soak. Prepare 4000 mL of a 4% solution of potassium permanganate solution from 5 gram tablets.

20. Describe how you would prepare 3500 mL of a 1:1000 aluminum acetate solution, an antiseptic, from 0.5 g tablets.

Additional Exercises

Now, on your own, test yourself! The answers to the *Additional Exercises* can be found on the companion Website or ask your instructor.

1. Describe how you would prepare 2000 milliliters of a 2% solution of formaldehyde, a disinfectant, from a 100% solution.

_____

_____

2. Explain how to prepare 500 milliliters of a 3% solution of Betadine from a 15% stock solution.

_____

_____

_____

3. How would you prepare 1000 milliliters of a 10% Weskodyne solution, a disinfectant, from pure drug?

_____

_____

_____

4. How would you prepare 250 milliliters of a 0.45% solution from sodium chloride crystals?

_____

_____

_____

5. Describe how you would prepare 2500 milliliters of a 1:1000 aluminum acetate solution, an antiseptic, from 0.5 g tablets.

_____

_____

_____

6. You must prepare 200 milliliters of a 2% boric acid solution, a mild antiseptic. How would you prepare this from boric acid crystals?

_____

_____

_____

7. Explain how to prepare a 1% ammonium chloride solution (1 liter) from 1 g tablets.

_____

_____

_____

8. Use the information found on the label in Figure 8.9 to determine the number of grams of calcium chloride contained in 5 milliliters of this solution.

_____

_____

_____

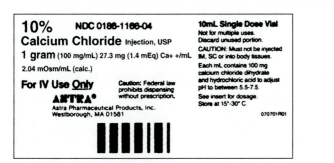

10% NDC 0186-1166-04
Calcium Chloride Injection, USP
1 gram (100 mg/mL) 27.3 mg (1.4 mEq) Ca+ +/mL
2.04 mOsm/mL (calc.)

For IV Use Only
ASTRA®
Astra Pharmaceutical Products, Inc.
Westborough, MA 01581

Caution: Federal law prohibits dispensing without prescription.

10mL Single Dose Vial
Not for multiple uses.
Discard unused portion.
CAUTION: Must not be injected IM, SC or into body tissues.
Each mL contains 100 mg calcium chloride dihydrate and hydrochloric acid to adjust pH to between 5.5-7.5.
See insert for dosage.
Store at 15°-30° C.

070701R01

Figure 8.9 Drug label for 10% calcium chloride.
(Courtesy of Astra-Zeneca Corp.)

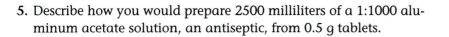

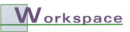

9. Describe how to prepare 600 milliliters of a 2.5% solution from a 3% solution of the antiseptic hydrogen peroxide.

_____

_____

_____

10. Read the label in Figure 8.10 and determine how many milliliters of this solution will contain 0.005 g epinephrine.

_____

_____

_____

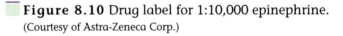

Figure 8.10 Drug label for 1:10,000 epinephrine.
(Courtesy of Astra-Zeneca Corp.)

11. Describe how to prepare 4000 milliliters of a 1:50 solution of the antiseptic potassium permanganate from 0.5 g tablets.

_____

_____

_____

12. How would you prepare 1000 milliliters of a 10% Lysol solution, a disinfectant, from a 25% stock solution?

_____

_____

_____

13. Using the information on the label in Figure 8.11, determine the number of grams of Mannitol contained in 40 milliliters of this solution.

_____

_____

_____

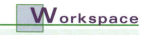

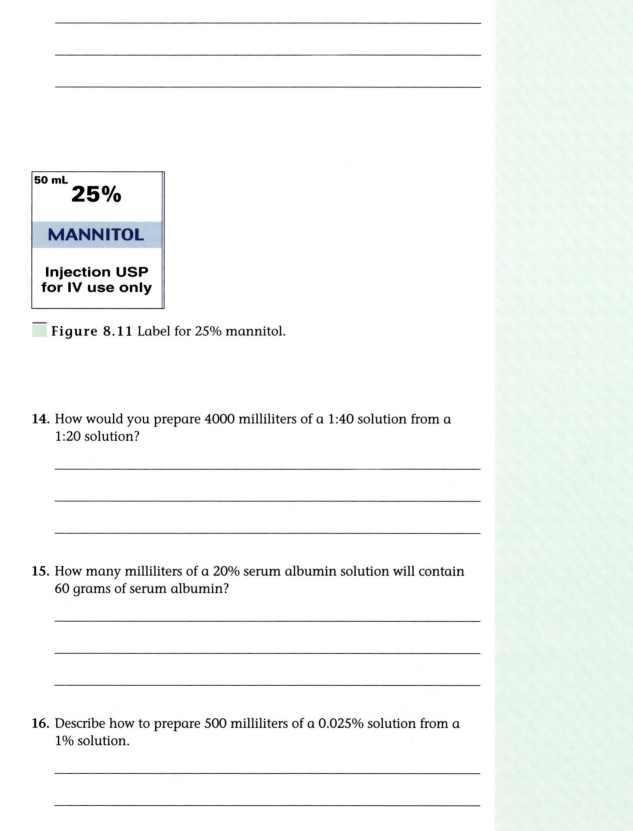

| 50 mL |
| **25%** |
| **MANNITOL** |
| **Injection USP for IV use only** |

Figure 8.11 Label for 25% mannitol.

14. How would you prepare 4000 milliliters of a 1:40 solution from a 1:20 solution?

_____

_____

_____

15. How many milliliters of a 20% serum albumin solution will contain 60 grams of serum albumin?

_____

_____

_____

16. Describe how to prepare 500 milliliters of a 0.025% solution from a 1% solution.

_____

_____

_____

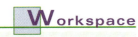

17. If 3 grams of pure drug are added to a container of sterile water and the total amount is now 1000 milliliters, what would be the strength of this solution?

_____

_____

_____

18. How would you prepare 1.25 liters of 10% aluminum acetate (Burow's) solution from 1 g tablets?

_____

_____

_____

19. The information found in the second order on the physician's order sheet in Figure 8.12 is, "Cleanse abdominal wound with 1:1000 normal saline solution q shift" (*q shift* means "every shift"). Describe how you would prepare 500 milliliters of this solution from a 2% solution.

_____

_____

_____

✚ GENERAL HOSPITAL ✚

PRESS HARD WITH BALLPOINT PEN. WRITE DATE & TIME AND SIGN EACH ORDER

DATE	TIME	A.M.
7/8/03	3	(P.M.)

1. *Apply flourocinonide 0.05% to affected skin qid*
2. *Cleanse abdominal wound with 1:1000 normal*
   saline q shift
3. *Tube feeding: 1/3 strength Meritine 240 mL q4h via*
   Gastrostomy tube

SIGNATURE
        L. Ablon   M.D.

IMPRINT
873667   7/8/03
Gene Martin   3/3/30
333Ocean Pkwy   Jewish
Huntington, NY   Aetna
41001
Dr. Leon Ablon

ORDERS NOTED
DATE _7/8/03_ TIME _3:10_ (A.M. / P.M.)
❑ MEDEX ❑ KARDEX
NURSE'S SIG. _A. Giangrasso RN_

FILLED BY   DATE

PHYSICIAN'S ORDERS

Figure 8.12 Physician's order sheet.

20. Read the information in the first order from the physician's order sheet in Figure 8.12. How would you prepare 250 milliliters of 0.05% fluorocinonide (Lidex) solution from a 1% solution?

_____

_____

_____

CUMULATIVE REVIEW EXERCISES

Review your mastery of earlier chapters.

Cumulative Exercises

1. Read the information on the label in Figure 8.13 and calculate the amount of dextrose in 25 milliliters.

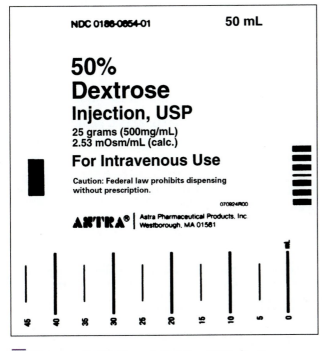

Figure 8.13 Drug label for 50% dextrose.
(Courtesy of Astra-Zeneca Corp.)

2. Physician's order:

   Add 0.06 g of Levophed to 1000 mL of normal saline.

   Each vial of Levophed is labeled 4 mL = 4 mg. How many milliliters of Levophed will you add to the normal saline?

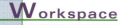

3. Your patient has an order for a tube feeding of 200 mL of $\frac{3}{4}$ strength Isocal, a nutritional supplement. Each can contains 200 mL of Isocal. How many milliliters of H_2O and how many milliliters of Isocal will you need to make a $\frac{3}{4}$ strength solution? (Hint: $\frac{3}{4}$ strength means 75% solution.)

4. gr $\frac{1}{240}$ = _____ mg

5. drams 4 = _____ ounces

6. 0.06 mg = gr _____

7. 0.0006 g = _____ mg

8. 100 mg = gr _____

9. gr $7\frac{1}{2}$ = _____ g

10. The order reads atropine sulfate 0.4 mg sc stat. How many grams will you administer?

11. The order is Digoxin 0.25 mg po qd. Convert this dose to micrograms.

12. You have 2 mL of Epinephrine 1:10,000. How many milligrams of Epinephrine are contained in this solution?

13. Physician's order:

    Zithromax 0.6 g bid for three days po

    How many grams of Zithromax will the patient receive in three days?

14. The antianxiety drug clorazepate (Tranxane) 0.0025 g po qd has been prescribed for a patient. The label reads 2.5 mg per tablet. How many tablets will you give your patient?

15. The order is Biaxin 600 mg po bid. The label reads 0.2 g in 5 mL. How many milliliters will you give your patient?

Additional questions, case studies, web links, matching exercises, fill-in-the-blanks, and glossary for this chapter can be found on the companion website at www.prenhall.com/olsen. Click on Chapter 8 to select the activities for this chapter.

CHAPTER NINE

Parenteral Medications

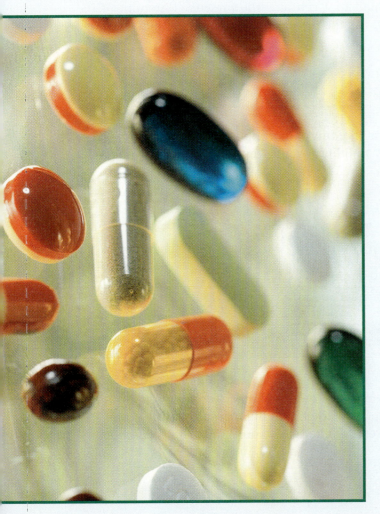

Objectives

After completing this chapter, you will be able to

- Do the calculations necessary to prepare medications for injection from drugs supplied in liquid form in vials and ampules.

- Do the calculations necessary to prepare medications for injection from drugs supplied in powdered form in vials.

- Do calculations involving units.

Parenteral medications are supplied in sterile liquid form in vials and ampules (Figure 9.1). They can also be supplied in powdered form in a sealed vial or ampule. Powdered drugs must be dissolved in sterile water or 0.9% sodium chloride (normal saline) prior to injection. This chapter introduces you to the calculations you will use to prepare and administer parenteral medications safely.

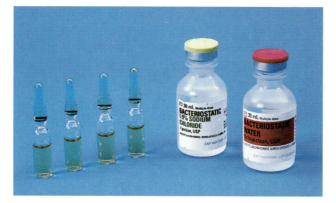

Figure 9.1 Ampules and vials.

(Photo by Al Dodge.)

Parenteral Medications Supplied as Liquids

When parenteral medications are supplied in liquid form, you need to calculate the volume of liquid that contains the prescribed amount of the drug. To do this, you will use the dimensional analysis method you have been using for all other calculations.

Example | 9.1

The prescriber ordered 9 milligrams of morphine sulfate sc. Study the label in Figure 9.2. How many milliliters would you administer to the patient?

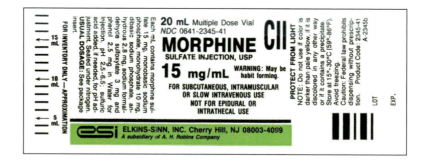

Figure 9.2 Drug label for morphine sulfate.

(Courtesy of ESI Lederle, a Business Unit of Wyeth Pharmaceuticals, Philadelphia, PA.)

Begin by finding out how many milliliters of the liquid in the vial contains the prescribed quantity of the drug (9 milligrams of morphine sulfate). That is, you want to convert 9 milligrams to an equivalent in milliliters.

$$9 \, \text{mg} = ? \, \text{mL}$$

You cancel the milligrams and obtain the equivalent quantity in milliliters.

$$9 \, \text{mg} \times \frac{? \, \text{mL}}{? \, \text{mg}} = ? \, \text{mL}$$

The label reads 15 milligrams per milliliter, which means 15 mg = 1 mL. So, the equivalent fraction is $\dfrac{1\,\text{mL}}{15\,\text{mg}}$.

$$\overset{3}{\cancel{9}}\,\text{mg} \times \dfrac{1\,\text{mL}}{\underset{5}{\cancel{15}}\,\text{mg}} = 0.6\,\text{mL}$$

So, 0.6 mL contains 9 milligrams of morphine sulfate, and you would administer 0.6 milliliter of the drug to your patient.

Example 9.2

The label on a drug vial reads 2500 milligrams per minims 150. How many minims would you administer if the medication order reads 750 milligrams IM of the drug? You want to convert the order (1500 milligrams) to its equivalent in minims.

$$750\,\text{mg} = \text{m}\!\!\!\!/\,?$$

You cancel the milligrams and obtain the equivalent amount in minims.

$$1500\,\text{mg} \times \dfrac{\text{m}\!\!\!\!/\,?}{?\,\text{mg}} = \text{m}\!\!\!\!/\,?$$

The label reads 2500 milligrams per minims 150. So, the equivalent fraction is $\dfrac{\text{m}\!\!\!\!/\,150}{2500\,\text{mg}}$.

$$\overset{3}{\cancel{750}}\,\text{mg} \times \dfrac{\text{m}\!\!\!\!/\,150}{\underset{10}{\cancel{2500}}\,\text{mg}} = \text{m}\!\!\!\!/\,45$$

So, minims 45 contain 750 milligrams, and you would administer minims 45 IM of the drug to your patient.

Example 9.3

The prescriber ordered 0.005 gram of Compazine (prochlorperazine) IM. Read the label in Figure 9.3, and calculate how many milliliters of this anti-emetic drug you would administer.

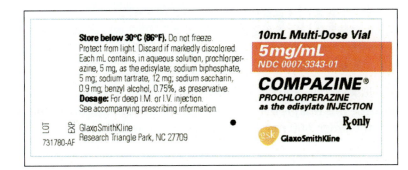

Figure 9.3 Drug label for Compazine.
(Reproduced with permission of GlaxoSmithKline.)

The label shows Compazine in milligrams per milliliter, so you want to convert 0.005 gram to its equivalent in milligrams and then change milligrams to milliliters.

$$0.005\,g \longrightarrow mg \longrightarrow mL$$

Do this on one line as follows:

$$0.005\,g \times \frac{?\,mg}{?\,g} \times \frac{?\,mL}{?\,mg} = ?\,mL$$

The first equivalent fraction is $\dfrac{1000\,mg}{1\,g}$.

The label reads 5 milligrams per milliliter which means 5 mg = 1 mL. So, the second fraction is $\dfrac{1\,mL}{5\,mg}$.

$$0.005\,\cancel{g} \times \frac{\overset{200}{\cancel{1000}}\,\cancel{mg}}{1\,\cancel{g}} \times \frac{1\,mL}{\underset{1}{\cancel{5}}\,\cancel{mg}} = 1\,mL$$

You would administer 1 milliliter of Compazine IM which would contain 0.005 gram of Compazine.

Example 9.4

The medication order reads 660 milligrams of cefazolin (Kefzol) IM. Read the label in Figure 9.4, and calculate how much of this antibiotic you would administer.

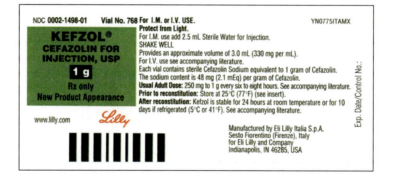

Figure 9.4 Drug label for Kefzol.
(Courtesy of Eli Lilly and Company.)

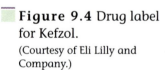

The label reads: add 2.5 mL of sterile water to the vial and 1 mL = 330 mg. Because this drug is available in milligrams per milliliter, you want to convert the order, 660 mg, to its equivalent in milliliters.

$$660\,mg = ?\,mL$$

You cancel the milligrams and obtain the equivalent amount in milliliters.

$$660\,\text{mg} \times \frac{?\,\text{mL}}{?\,\text{mg}}$$

Because the label reads 330 milligram per milliliter, you use the equivalent fraction $\dfrac{1\,\text{mL}}{330\,\text{mg}}$.

$$\overset{2}{\cancel{660}}\,\text{mg} \times \frac{1\,\text{mL}}{\underset{1}{\cancel{330}}\,\text{mg}} = 2\,\text{mL}$$

So, 2 mL of Kefzol contain 660 milligrams and you would administer 2 milliliters IM to your patient.

Example 9.5

Mr. Jones is to receive grain $\dfrac{1}{600}$ of atropine sulfate sc. The ampule of liquid is labeled grain $\dfrac{1}{150}$ per minims 15. How many minims of this anticholinergic drug should be administered to the patient?

You want to convert the order of grain $\dfrac{1}{600}$ to its equivalent in minims.

$$\text{gr}\,\frac{1}{600} = \text{m} \,?$$

You cancel the grains and obtain the equivalent amount in minims.

$$\text{gr}\,\frac{1}{600} \times \frac{\text{m}\,?}{\text{gr}\,?} = \text{m}\,?$$

Because the label on the ampule reads grain $\dfrac{1}{150}$ per minims 15, the equivalent fraction is $\dfrac{\text{m}\,15}{\text{gr}\,\dfrac{1}{150}}$.

$$\cancel{\text{gr}}\,\frac{1}{600} \times \frac{\text{m}\,15}{\cancel{\text{gr}}\,\dfrac{1}{150}} = \text{m}\,\frac{1 \times 15}{\dfrac{600}{150}} = \text{m}\,\frac{15}{4} = \text{m}\,3\frac{3}{4}$$

So, minims $3\dfrac{3}{4}$ of this solution contains grain $\dfrac{1}{600}$ of atropine sulfate. Normally, you would give the patient minims 4, since three-fourths of a minim is too small to measure into the syringe. See Figure 9.5.

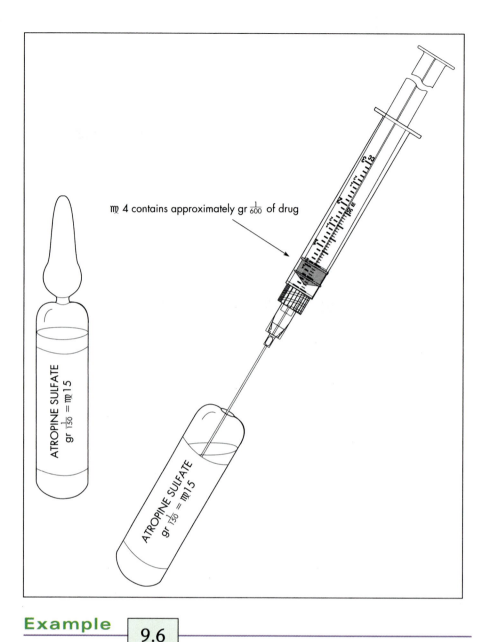

$\mathfrak{m}$ 4 contains approximately gr $\frac{1}{600}$ of drug

ATROPINE SULFATE
gr $\frac{1}{150}$ = $\mathfrak{m}$ 15

ATROPINE SULFATE
gr $\frac{1}{150}$ = $\mathfrak{m}$ 15

Figure 9.5 Preparing atropine sulfate gr $\dfrac{1}{600}$ from an ampule.

Example 9.6

The prescriber ordered: Chlorpromazine 0.075 g IM. Read the information on the label in Figure 9.6, and explain how to prepare the medication for administration to the patient.

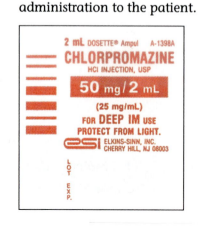

2 mL DOSETTE® Ampul   A-1398A
CHLORPROMAZINE
HCl INJECTION, USP
50 mg / 2 mL
(25 mg/mL)
FOR **DEEP IM** USE
PROTECT FROM LIGHT.
ELKINS-SINN, INC.
CHERRY HILL, NJ 08003

L O T
E X P.

Figure 9.6 Drug label for Chlorpromazine.
(Courtesy of ESI Lederle, a Business Unit of Wyeth Pharmaceuticals, Philadelphia, PA.)

Because the vial contains medication measured in milligrams per milliliter, you want to convert 0.075 gram to milligrams and then find the amount in milliliters.

$$0.075\,g \longrightarrow ?\,mg \longrightarrow ?\,mL$$

$$0.075\,g \times \frac{?\,mg}{?\,g} \times \frac{?\,mL}{?\,mg} = ?\,mL$$

The first equivalent fraction is $\dfrac{1000\,mg}{1\,g}$.

The label reads 50 milligrams per 2 milliliters, so the second equivalent fraction is $\dfrac{2\,mL}{50\,mg}$.

$$0.075\,\cancel{g} \times \frac{1000\,\cancel{mg}}{1\,\cancel{g}} \times \frac{2\,mL}{50\,\cancel{mg}} = \frac{150}{50}\,mL = 3\,mL$$

So, 3 milliliters contains 0.075 gram of Chlorpromazine, and you would administer 3 milliliters IM to your patient.

Example 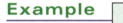 9.7

Examine the label in Figure 9.7, and determine the quantity of solution to be withdrawn from the vial if the medication order reads 80 micrograms of Sufentanil IV push.

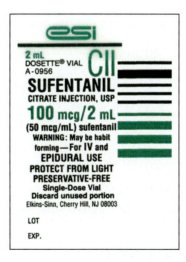

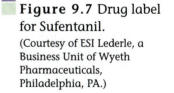

Figure 9.7 Drug label for Sufentanil.

(Courtesy of ESI Lederle, a Business Unit of Wyeth Pharmaceuticals, Philadelphia, PA.)

You want to convert micrograms to milliliters.

$$80\,mcg \longrightarrow ?\,mL$$

$$80\,mcg \times \frac{?\,mL}{?\,mcg} = ?\,mL$$

The label reads 100 mcg/2 mL, which means 100 mcg of Sufentanil are in 2 mL. So, the equivalent fraction is $\dfrac{2\,mL}{100\,mcg}$.

$$\overset{4}{\cancel{80}} \text{ mcg} \times \frac{2 \text{ mL}}{\underset{5}{\cancel{100}} \text{ mcg}} = 1.6 \text{ mL}$$

So you would withdraw 1.6 mL from the vial.

Example 9.8

The prescriber ordered 40 units of NPH insulin (NPH Iletin II) sc for a patient, and you must use a standard syringe because no insulin syringe is available. What would the dose be in milliliters? The label on the vial is shown in Figure 9.8.

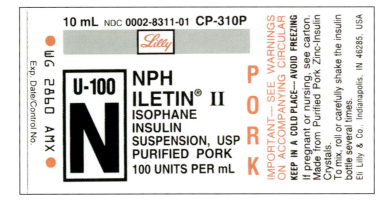

Figure 9.8 Drug label for NPH Iletin II.

(Courtesy of Eli Lilly and Company.)

You want to convert 40 units to milliliters.

40 units = ? mL

You cancel the units and obtain the equivalent amount in milliliters.

$$40 \text{ units} \times \frac{? \text{ mL}}{? \text{ units}} = ? \text{ mL}$$

The label reads 100 units per milliliter, which means 100 units = 1 mL. So, the equivalent fraction is $\frac{1 \text{ mL}}{100 \text{ units}}$.

$$\overset{4}{\cancel{40}} \text{ units} \times \frac{1 \text{ mL}}{\underset{10}{\cancel{100}} \text{ units}} = 0.4 \text{ mL}$$

So, 40 units would be contained in 0.4 milliliter, and you would draw 0.4 milliliter into a tuberculin syringe.

Heparin

Heparin is an anticoagulant (clot-preventing) medication that can be administered to a patient by subcutaneous injection, intermittent intravenous injection, and by continuous intravenous infusion or to flush a "hep-lock" device or a central intravenous line. Like insulin, penicillin, and some other medications, heparin is supplied in *USP units*, which are often shortened (as noted in Chapter 7) to *units*. The heparin concentration used to flush a hep-lock device or a central intravenous line is 10 units in 1 mL or 100 units in 1 mL. Heparin is prepared by the manufacturer in a variety of strengths. **Some** examples of heparin preparations are shown in Table 9.1.

Table 9.1

USP Unit Potencies of Heparin

Supplied Form	Strength
Vials	1000 units in 1 mL
	2000 units in 1 mL
	2500 units in 1 mL
	5000 units in 1 mL
	7500 units in 1 mL
	10,000 units in 1 mL
	20,000 units in 1 mL
	40,000 units in 1 mL
Ampules	1000 units in 1 mL
	5000 units in 1 mL
	10,000 units in 1 mL
Premixed Intravenous Solutions	1000 units in 500 mL of 0.9% NaCl
	2000 units in 1000 mL of 0.9% NaCl
	12,500 units in 250 mL of 0.45% NaCl
	25,000 units in 250 mL of 0.45% NaCl
	25,000 units in 500 mL of 0.45% NaCl
	10,000 units in 100 mL of D_5W
	12,500 units in 250 mL of D_5W
	25,000 units in 250 mL of D_5W
	25,000 units in 500 mL of D_5W
	20,000 units in 500 mL of D_5W

In order to administer a premixed parenteral solution, you must convert the physician's order to the volume of solution that contains the amount of heparin ordered. As a safety factor, the strength of the heparin concentration is usually noted in the intravenous solutions in red.

Example 9.9

The prescriber ordered:

Heparin 2000 units sc q12h

The label on the vial (Figure 9.9) reads 1000 units per milliliter. How many milliliters will you administer to the patient?

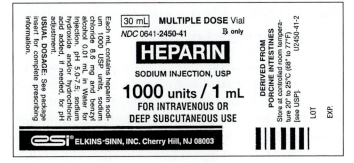

Figure 9.9 Drug label for Heparin.

(Courtesy of ESI Lederle, a Business Unit of Wyeth Pharmaceuticals, Philadelphia, PA.)

You want to convert units to milliliters.

$$2000 \text{ units} = ? \text{ mL}$$

You cancel the units and obtain the equivalent amount in milliliters.

$$2000 \text{ units} \times \frac{? \text{ mL}}{? \text{ units}} = ? \text{ mL}$$

The label on the vial reads 1000 units per milliliter, so the equivalent fraction is $\dfrac{1 \text{ mL}}{1000 \text{ units}}$.

$$\overset{2}{\cancel{2000}} \text{ } \cancel{\text{units}} \times \frac{1 \text{ mL}}{\cancel{1000} \text{ } \cancel{\text{units}}} = 2 \text{ mL}$$

So, 2 milliliters contain 2000 units of heparin, and you would administer 2 milliliters of heparin to the patient sc.

Example 9.10

The prescriber ordered:

heparin 8000 units sc q8h

The label on the drug vial reads 10,000 units per milliliter, how many minims would equal 8000 units?

You want to convert 8000 units to minims.

$$8000 \text{ units} = ℥ \text{ } ?$$

You cancel the units and obtain the equivalent amount in minims.

$$8000 \text{ units} \times \frac{℥ \text{ } ?}{? \text{ units}} = ℥ \text{ } ?$$

The label on the vial reads 10,000 units per mL, so the fraction is $\dfrac{1 \text{ mL}}{10,000 \text{ units}}$. The second fraction is $\dfrac{℥ \text{ } 15}{\text{mL}}$.

$$\overset{8}{\cancel{8000}} \text{ } \cancel{\text{units}} \times \frac{1 \text{ } \cancel{\text{mL}}}{\underset{10}{\cancel{10,000}} \text{ } \cancel{\text{units}}} \times \frac{℥ \text{ } 15}{1 \text{ } \cancel{\text{mL}}} = ℥ \text{ } 12$$

So, minims 12 contain 8000 units of heparin, and you would administer minims 12 sc to your patient.

Parenteral Medications Supplied in Powdered Form

Some parenteral medications are supplied in powdered form in sealed vials (Figure 9.10). The powder cannot be removed from these vials. You must add a diluent, sterile water or saline to the vial and dissolve the powder to form a solution. This is referred to as reconstituting the drug. Sterile technique must be used during this process. You then inject the liquid volume of prepared solution that contains the proper amount of the drug.

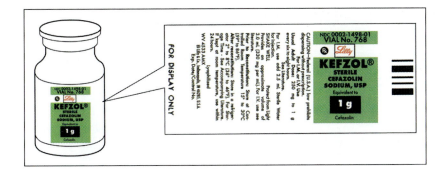

Figure 9.10a A sealed vial of Kefzol in powdered form with label detail.
(Courtesy of Eli Lilly and Company.)

The pharmaceutical manufacturer provides instructions that specify the amount of diluent that must be injected into the vial of powder to make a solution of a given strength. After preparing the solution, you need to calculate the volume that contains the prescribed amount of the drug.

Example 9.11

The prescriber ordered 165 milligrams of cefazolin (Kefzol) IV. Read the label shown in Figure 9.10. How would you prepare this dose?

First prepare the solution. Inject 2.5 milliliters of sterile water into the vial. Now the vial contains a solution in which

$$1 \text{ mL} = 330 \text{ mg}$$

To calculate the amount of this solution, you need to convert milligrams to milliliters.

$$165 \text{ mg} \times \frac{? \text{ mL}}{? \text{ mg}} = ? \text{ mL}$$

The vial now contains 330 milligrams per 1 milliliter, so the equivalent fraction is $\frac{1 \text{ mL}}{330 \text{ mg}}$.

$$165 \text{ mg} \times \frac{1 \text{ mL}}{330 \text{ mg}} = 0.5 \text{ mL}$$

So, you would add 2.5 mL of sterile water to the vial, then withdraw 0.5 milliliters from the vial and administer it to the patient.

Example 9.12

The prescriber has ordered 0.2 gram IVPB of the antibiotic, alatrofloxacin (Trovan). Read the label in Figure 9.11. How would you prepare this dose?

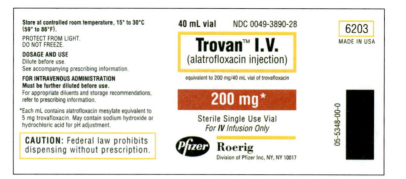

Figure 9.11 Drug label for Trovan.

(Registered Trademark of Pfizer Inc. Reproduced with permission.)

The directions tell you to add the 40 mL of Trovan to 60 mL D5W. Now, you have a solution that contains 200 mg of Trovan in 100 mL.

$$100 \, mL = 200 \, mg$$

To calculate the amount of solution, you must convert grams to milliliters. This is a two step procedure.

$$0.2 \, g \longrightarrow ? \, mg \longrightarrow ? \, mL$$

$$0.2 \, g \times \frac{? \, mg}{? \, g} \times \frac{? \, mL}{? \, mg} = ? \, mL$$

The first equivalent fraction is $\dfrac{1000 \, mg}{1 \, g}$. Because the prepared solution is $100 \, mL = 200 \, mg$, the second fraction is $\dfrac{100 \, mL}{200 \, mg}$.

$$0.2 \, \cancel{g} \times \frac{\overset{5}{\cancel{1000}} \, \cancel{mg}}{1 \, \cancel{g}} \times \frac{100 \, mL}{\underset{1}{\cancel{200}} \, \cancel{mg}} = 100 \, mL$$

So 100 mL of the Trovan solution contains 0.2 g.

Example 9.13

The prescriber ordered: cefoxitin sodium 0.75 g IM q12h. The vial of cefoxitin sodium, an antibiotic, contains 5 grams of powder. The instructions are as follows: Add 13.2 mL of sterile water to the vial, 3 mL = 1 g. How many milliliters of the solution would contain the prescribed dose?

You want to change 0.75 gram to milliliters.

$$0.75 \, g \times \frac{? \, mL}{? \, g} = ? \, mL$$

Because the prepared solution is $3 \, mL = 1 \, g$, the equivalent fraction is $\dfrac{3 \, mL}{1 \, g}$.

$$0.75 \, \cancel{g} \times \frac{3 \, mL}{1 \, \cancel{g}} = 2.25 \, mL$$

So, 2.25 milliliters of the prepared solution contains 0.75 gram of cefoxitin sodium.

A 34-year-old man is admitted to the emergency room with a chief complaint of pain in the throat. He reports a medical history of recently completing chemotherapy for cancer of the lung. He also has diabetes mellitus and is allergic to fish and penicillin. He is admitted with the diagnosis of febrile neutropenia and upper respiratory infection. His vital signs are: T 101.4°F; BP 110/60; P 80; R 18. The admitting orders are as follows:

- Regular diet as tolerated
- V/S q4h
- CBC q am
- Blood culture
- Urine analysis, C/S
- Chest X ray, PA & Lateral
- NPH 30 units sc $\frac{1}{2}$ h ac breakfast
- Neupogen 300 mcg sc stat
- Maxipime (cefepime HCl) 2 g IM q12h
- Gentamicin 240 mg in 50 mL D_5W IVPB q8h; infuse over 1 h
- Fentanyl 50 mcg IM q2h prn
- IV D_5N/S 1 liter q 8 hr

Refer to labels in Figure 9.12 when necessary to answer the following questions.

1. The Maxipime is supplied in 500 mg and 1000 mg vials. Which vial would you choose and how many will you need for the prescribed dose?

2. The label on the vial of Gentamicin reads 0.04 gram/mL. How many mL of this antibiotic will you prepare for one dose?

3. The label on the vial of Neupogen reads 300 µg/mL. How many milliliters will you administer?

4. The order for Maxipime was changed to Unasyn 1500 mg IM q6h. How many vials will you use to prepare one dose?

5. The patient became very restless and the physician ordered Phenobarbital grains 2 IM stat. How many milliliters will you give the patient?

6. The patient's blood pressure increased to 190/110. The physician ordered Atenolol 0.025 g daily. How many tablets will you give the patient?

7. How many milliliters of Fentanyl will you prepare for your patient?

8. Order: Humalog insulin 6 units sc before dinner. Place an arrow at the correct measurement on the most appropriate syringe.

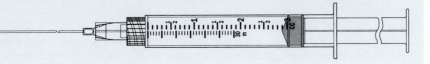

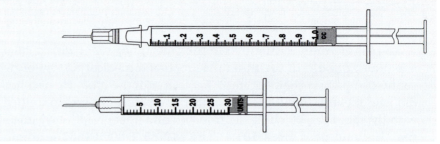

9. Neupogen 5 mcg/kg sc daily has been ordered. The patient weighs 110 pounds. The label on the vial reads 300 mcg/mL. How many milliliters will you prepare?

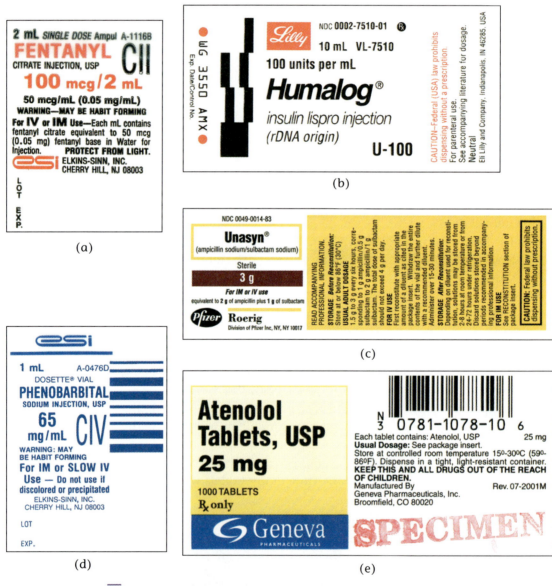

Figure 9.12 Drug Labels for Case Study 9.

(a, d) Courtesy of ESI Lederle, a Business Unit of Wyeth Pharmaceuticals, Philadelphia, PA. (b) Courtesy of Eli Lilly and Company. (c) Reg. Trademark of Pfizer Inc. Reproduced with permission. (e) Courtesy of Genova Pharmaceuticals.

The answers to *Try These for Practice, Exercises,* and *Cumulative Review* appear in Appendix A at the back of the book. The answers to the *Additional Exercises* can be found on the companion Website or ask your instructor.

Try These for Practice

Test your comprehension after reading the chapter.

1. The prescriber ordered cefazolin sodium 0.66 g IM q8h. The directions on the package insert state: Add 2.5 mL of sterile water to a vial labeled 1 g and 1 mL = 330 mg. How many milliliters equal 0.66 gram?_____

2. The prescriber ordered insulin 0.54 units/kg sc qd. The label on the vial reads 100 units per milliliter. How many milliliters will you give your patient, who weighs 65 kilograms?_____

3. Your patient is to receive grain $\dfrac{1}{400}$ of atropine sulfate sc. The label on the vial reads 0.1 milligram per milliliter. How many milliliters equal grain $\dfrac{1}{400}$?_____

4. An ampule of Digoxin is labeled 0.125 milligram per milliliter. How many milliliters equal 0.5 milligram?_____

5. If your patient's medication order is for 5000 units of heparin sc and the vial is labeled 10,000 units per milliliter, how many minims equal 5000 units?_____

Exercises

Reinforce your understanding in class or at home.

1. The prescriber ordered cefuroxime (Kefurox) 0.75 g IV, an anti-infective drug. Read the information on the label in Figure 9.13. How many milliliters would you prepare for the patient?

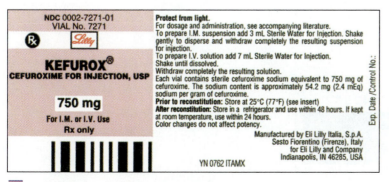

Figure 9.13 Drug label for Kefurox.
(Courtesy of Eli Lilly and Company.)

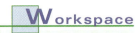

2. The medication order is Streptomycin 500 mg IM daily for thirty days. Read the label in Figure 9.14 and calculate how much antibiotic you would administer to your patient?

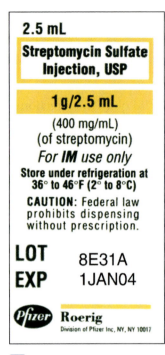

Figure 9.14 Drug label for Streptomycin.
(Registered Trademark of Pfizer Inc. Reproduced with permission.)

3. A vial of medication is labeled 250 mg = 15 minims. How many minims would you prepare if the medication order for this drug reads 700 mg IM of this drug?

4. The prescriber ordered Digoxin 0.2 mg IM. Read the label in Figure 9.15 and calculate how many milliliters of this cardiovascular drug you would administer.

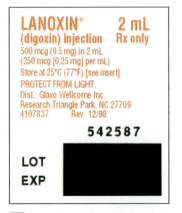

Figure 9.15 Drug label for Digoxin.
(Reproduced with permission of GlaxoSmithKline.)

5. Mr. Petagra is to receive gr $\frac{1}{400}$ of atropine sulfate sc. The vial is labeled gr $\frac{1}{150}$ per minims 15. How many minims would you prepare for this patient?

6. The antiviral opthalmic drug, fomivirsen sodium (Vitravene), has been ordered by the physician, 330 mcg. The vial is labeled 6.6 mg/mL. How many milliliters contain the prescribed dose?

7. The physician ordered 0.725 mg of droperidol (Inapsine) IV stat. The vial reads 2.5 mg in 2 mL. Calculate the amount of drug you will administer to this patient in milliliters.

8. Physicians's order: ciprofloxacin (Cipro) 400 mg IVPB q12h. The vial reads 20 mg/mL. How many milliliters contain the dose?

9. Order: Add 30 mg of morphine sulfate to 250 mL D5W IVPB. The vial reads 10 mg/mL. How many milliliters of morphine will you prepare?

10. The prescriber ordered 175,000 units of Urokinase IVPB. The vial directions read: Add 4.2 mL to vial and each mL contains 50,000 units. How many milliliters will you prepare?

11. Order: Vancomycin (Vancocin) 0.45 g IV daily. Read the label in Figure 9.16. How many milliliters equal the prescribed dose?

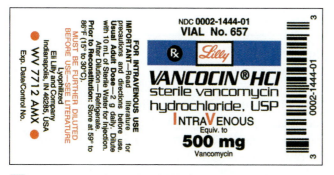

Figure 9.16 Drug label for Vancocin.
(Courtesy of Eli Lilly and Company.)

12. Order: Cleocin 600 mg IM q12h. The label reads: Add 4.8 mL of sterile water to vial, 0.4 g = 1 mL. How many milliliters contain the prescribed dose?

13. Prepare a 10 g vial of cefazolin (Kefzol). Read the label in Figure 9.17. If you add 45 mL of diluent to the vial, how many milliliters contain 500 mg?

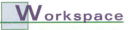

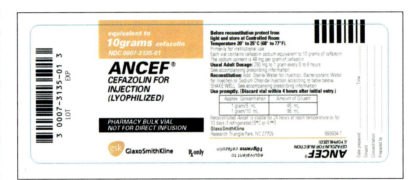

Figure 9.17 Drug label for Kefzol.
(Courtesy of Eli Lilly and Company.)

14. The order is Ancef 10.7 mg/kg IV daily. Read the information on the label in Figure 9.18. Calculate the amount of drug you will administer to your patient in milliliters. The patient weighs 70 kg.

Figure 9.18 Drug label for Ancef.
(Reproduced with permission of GlaxoSmithKline.)

15. Order: cidofovir (Vistide) IVPB, an antiviral medication used for the treatment of CMV retinitis in patients with AIDS. The order is 5 mg/kg. Weight: 55 kg. Vial reads 75 mg/mL in a 5 mL vial. How many milliliters will contain the required dose?

16. Foscarnet (Foscavir) is an antiviral drug used in the treatment of CMV retinitis in clients with AIDS. The order for this drug is 2000 mg/m² IVPB. BSA is 1.8 m². The drug is available in 250 mL bottles with 24 mg/mL of foscarnet. How many milliliters contain the prescribed dose?

17. Order: Pentamidine isethionate (Pentam) 3 mg/kg IM qid. The label reads: Add 3 mL of sterile water to each 300 mg vial. How many milliliters of Pentam contain the prescribed dose for the patient who weighs 90 pounds?

18. The antifungal medication Amphotericin B IVPB has been ordered for a patient who weighs 60 kg , 0.25 mg/kg. The vial reads 50 mg/10 mL. How many milliliters contain the dose?

19. Cefoxitin sodium (Mefoxin) 1.5 g IM stat has been ordered. The label on the vial reads: Add 4 mL of 0.5% Lidocaine to the vial containing 2 g of Mefoxin. How many milliliters contain the prescribed dose?

20. Order: Ampicillin 0.3 g IM 30 minutes prior to dental surgery. The vial is labeled 2 g. If you add 6 mL to the vial, how many milliliters contain the prescribed dose?

Additional Exercises

Now, on your own, test yourself! Answers to the *Additional Exercises* are in the *Instructor's Guide* and on the companion Website.

1. A patient is to receive 25 units of the hormonal drug vasopressin (Pitressin) IM. If the label reads 50 units per 2 milliliters, how many milliliters will you administer to the patient? _____

2. The order reads: calcitonin 2.5 units/kg sc daily. The label reads: 100 units per milliliter. How many milliliters will you administer to a patient who weighs 62 kilograms? _____

3. The order reads: amitriptyline 0.025 g IM tid. If the drug vial is labeled 10 milligrams per milliliter, how many milliliters will you prepare for the patient? _____

4. The prescriber ordered clindamycin 200 mg IM q6h. The label reads: 1 mL = 150 mg. How many milliliters will equal 200 milligrams?

_____

5. Read the first medication order in Figure 9.19. The vial of furosemide is labeled 10 milligrams per milliliter. How many milliliters would you prepare for a patient who weighs 45 kilograms? _____

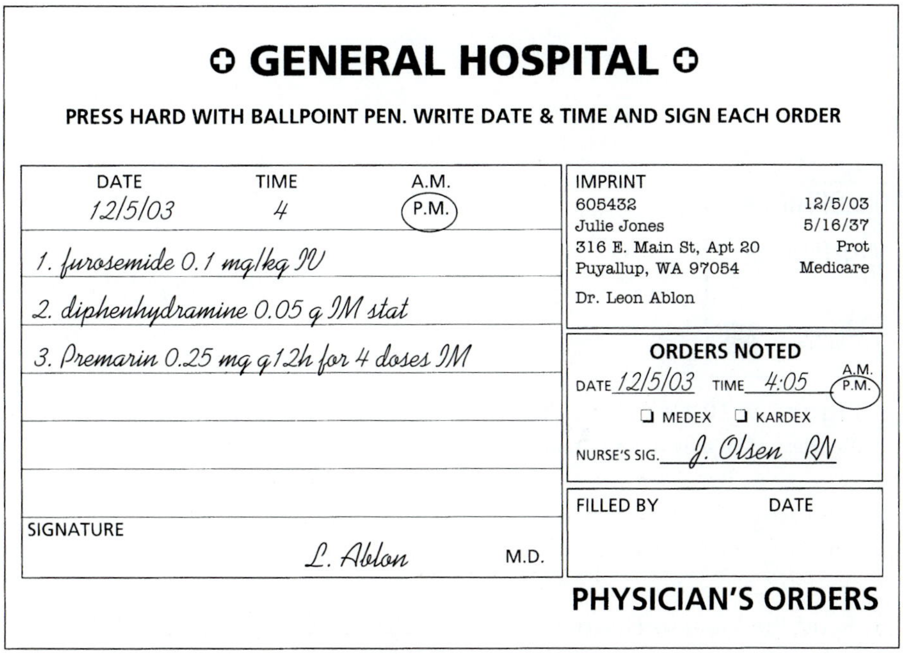

✛ **GENERAL HOSPITAL** ✛

PRESS HARD WITH BALLPOINT PEN. WRITE DATE & TIME AND SIGN EACH ORDER

DATE	TIME	A.M.
12/5/03	4	(P.M.)

1. *furosemide 0.1 mg/kg IV*
2. *diphenhydramine 0.05 g IM stat*
3. *Premarin 0.25 mg q12h for 4 doses IM*

IMPRINT
605432   12/5/03
Julie Jones   5/16/37
316 E. Main St, Apt 20   Prot
Puyallup, WA 97054   Medicare

Dr. Leon Ablon

ORDERS NOTED
DATE 12/5/03   TIME 4:05 A.M. (P.M.)

❏ MEDEX ❏ KARDEX

NURSE'S SIG. *J. Olsen RN*

FILLED BY   DATE

SIGNATURE
L. Ablon   M.D.

PHYSICIAN'S ORDERS

Figure 9.19 Physician's order sheet.

6. In the second medication order in Figure 9.19, the patient must receive 0.05 gram of the antihistamine diphenhydramine (Benadryl) IM stat. The vial is labeled 50 milligrams per milliliter. How many milliliters will you administer to this patient? _____

7. Read the information in the third medication order in Figure 9.19. If the vial of Premarin is labeled 0.025 gram per 5 milliliters, how many milliliters equal the prescribed single dose? _____

8. Prescriber's order Dobutamine (Dobutrex) 100 micrograms per kilogram IVPB. If a patient weighs 75 kilograms and the vial is labeled 12.5 milligrams per milliliter, how many milliliters would you prepare? _____

9. The order reads: nitroglycerine 0.3 mg IV once only. The vial is labeled 50 milligrams per 10 milliliters. Calculate the amount in milliliters required for this dose. _____

10. The label on the vial of verapamil HCl reads: 10 milligrams per 4 milliliters. If the medication order is 2.5 milligrams IVPB, calculate the amount in milliliters you would prepare for this patient. _____

11. The label on a vial reads: penicillin G 1,000,000 units. The instructions are as follows: Add 19.6 mL of sterile diluent to vial, 1 mL = 50,000 units. How many milliliters contain 100,000 units? _____

12. The prescriber ordered: Dolophine HCl 0.015 g IM q4h prn. Read the label in Figure 9.20. How many milliliters will you prepare for this patient? _____

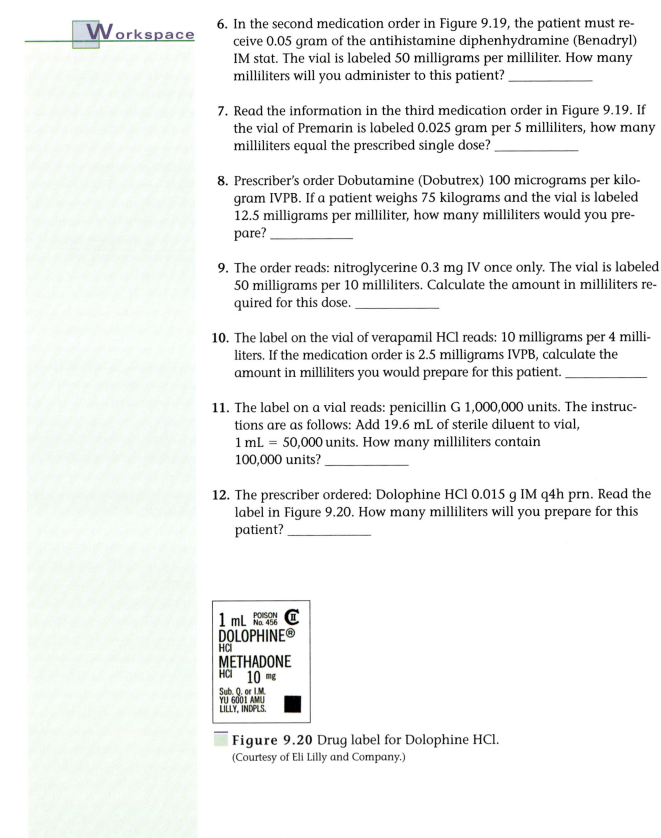

1 mL	POISON No. 456 **Ⓒ**

DOLOPHINE®
HCl

METHADONE
HCl 10 mg

Sub. Q. or I.M.
YU 6001 AMU
LILLY, INDPLS.

Figure 9.20 Drug label for Dolophine HCl.
(Courtesy of Eli Lilly and Company.)

13. Read the label in Figure 9.21. Calculate how many milliliters of insulin you will prepare if the order reads: Lente insulin 40 units sc at breakfast. _____

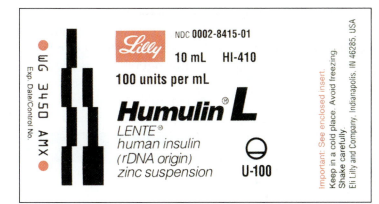

Figure 9.21 Drug label for Humulin L.
(Courtesy of Eli Lilly and Company.)

14. The order reads: Terramycin 10 mg/kg IM q12h. Read the label in Figure 9.22. How many milliliters will you prepare for a patient who weighs 25 kilograms? _____

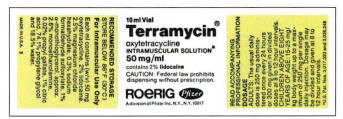

Figure 9.22 Drug label for Terramycin.
(Registered Trademark of Pfizer Inc. Reproduced with permission.)

15. The patient must receive 190 milligrams of ceftizoxime (Cefizox) IM. The 1 g vial has the following directions: Add 10 mL of sterile water, 1 mL = 95 mg. How many minims of this antibiotic will you administer to the patient? _____

16. Your patient is to receive 75 milligrams of dexamethasone (Dalalone), injected into a joint by the physician. If the vial is labeled 20 milligrams per milliliters, how many milliliters will you prepare? _____

17. The order reads: phenytoin 0.2 g IM stat. The drug label reads 200 milligrams per 2 milliliters. How many milliliters of this anticonvulsant will you administer to your patient? _____

18. Your patient has been prescribed 1.3 milliliters of the antineoplastic drug methotrexate sodium (Folex) IM per day. The recommended dose is 3.3 milligrams per square meter per day. The label on the vial reads 25 milligrams per milliliter. If this patient's body surface area (BSA) is 1.42 square meters, is this an appropriate dose? _____

19. Prepare 1550 milligrams of ticarcillin (Ticar) from a vial that has the following directions: Add 13 mL of sterile water to the vial, 200 mg = 1 mL. How many milliliters contain this dose? _____

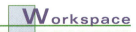

20. The order reads: methylergonovine maleate (Methergine) 0.0002 g IM q4h for three doses. The drug label reads 0.2 milligram per milliliter. a. How many milliliters will you administer in one dose? b. What is the total number of milligrams this patient will receive in three doses of this oxytocic drug?_____

CUMULATIVE REVIEW EXERCISES

Review your mastery of earlier chapters.

1. The medication order is 10 milligrams/kilogram of Zithromax. Read the label in Figure 9.23. How many tablets contain this dose for a patient who weighs 61 Kg?

Store at or below 86°F (30°C).

Dispense in tight containers (USP).

DOSAGE AND USE
See accompanying prescribing information.

*Each tablet contains azithromycin dihydrate equivalent to 600 mg of azithromycin.

CAUTION: Federal law prohibits dispensing without prescription.

NDC 0069-3080-30

30 Tablets

Zithromax®
(azithromycin) (600)

600 mg*

Pfizer **Pfizer Labs**
Division of Pfizer Inc, NY, NY 10017

6440
MADE IN USA

3 N 0069-3080-30
05-5185-32-1

Figure 9.23 Drug label for Zithromax.
(Registered Trademark of Pfizer Inc. Reproduced with permission.)

2. The medication order is grain $\frac{1}{3}$ po of dicyclomine HCl (Bentyl), an antispasmodic drug. The tablets on hand are 10 milligrams. How many tablets would you administer?

3. The medication order reads 0.12 gram po qd of propranolol (Inderal SL), an antihypertensive drug. Each capsule contains 60 milligrams. How many capsules would you administer?

4. The medication order reads: Viagra 0.05 g po. How many tablets would you administer if each tablet contains 50 mg?

5. A vial is labeled meperidine HCl (Demerol), 50 milligrams per milliliter. The prescriber orders 12.5 milligrams IM. How many minims of this analgesic narcotic would you administer?

6. The order is for K-Lor 60 mEq po stat. Each packet contains 20 mEq. How many packets of K-Lor will you need?

7. The prescriber ordered: norfloxacin 0.4 g po. The drug label reads 1 tab = 400 mg. How many tablets of this oral antibiotic would you administer?

8. The medication order is for 0.3 gram of cimetidine (Tagamet) po bid, an anti-ulcer agent. The drug label reads 300 milligrams per 2 milliliters. How many milliliters would you administer to the patient?

9. The medication order is 0.6 g po q.d. of rifabutin (Mycobutin), an antibiotic. Each capsule contains 150 mg. How many capsules would you administer to the patient?

10. The drug vial contains 1,000,000 units of Penicillin G. The label directions state: Add 2.3 mL of sterile water to the vial, 1.2 mL = 500,000 units. How many milliliters equal 200,000 units?

11. gr $\dfrac{1}{200}$ = _____ g

12. 0.003 g = _____ mg

13. 90 mg = gr _____

14. $2\dfrac{1}{2}$ t = _____ gtt

15. 0.06 mg = gr _____

Additional questions, case studies, web links, matching exercises, fill-in-the-blanks, and glossary for this chapter can be found on the companion website at www.prenhall.com/olsen. Click on Chapter 9 to select the activities for this chapter.

UNIT FOUR

Specialized Medication Preparations

CHAPTER TEN

Calculating Flow Rates for Enteral Solutions and Intravenous Infusions

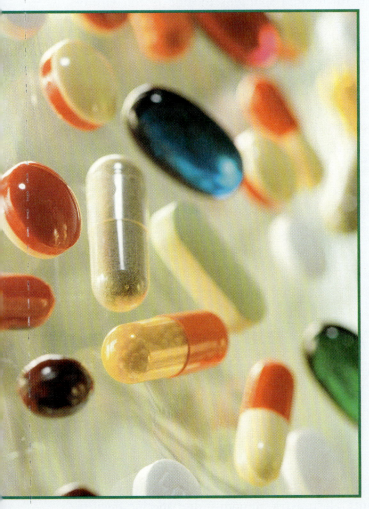

Objectives

*After completing this chapter,
you will be able to*

- Describe the basic concepts and standard equipment involved in the delivery of intravenous (IV) and enteral infusions.

- Calculate the flow rate of IV solutions.

- Calculate the flow rate of enteral solutions.

This chapter introduces the basic concepts and standard equipment involved in intravenous and enteral therapy. You will also learn how to use dimensional analysis to calculate flow rates for these infusions.

Introduction to Intravenous and Enteral Solutions

Fluids can be given to a patient slowly over a period of time through a vein (***intravenous***) or through a tube inserted into the alimentary tract (***enteral***).

Enteral Solutions

When a patient needs nutrients, fluid, or medications and cannot swallow, the prescriber may write an order for an enteral feeding. Enteral feedings provide nutrients by way of a tube into the alimentary tract.

There are various methods for tube feeding. The feeding tube is inserted into the stomach either indirectly (through the nares and esophagus) or directly (through an incision in the abdomen and the stomach).

A tube inserted directly into the stomach and sutured in place is called a ***gastrostomy tube***. The ***percutaneous endoscopic gastrostomy (PEG)*** tube is another type of feeding tube inserted directly into the stomach.

Currently available enteral feeding solutions include Isocal, Ensure, and Sustacal.

An enteral solution order might read:

Isocal 50 mL/hr via nasogastric tube

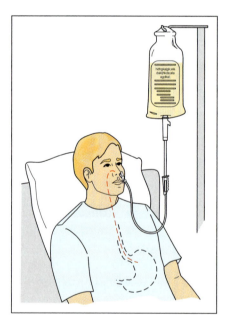

Figure 10.1 Using a calibrated plastic bag to administer a tube feeding.

Intravenous Fluids

Intravenous means through the veins. Fluids are administered intravenously to provide fluid, nutrients, electrolytes, minerals, and specific medications to the patient.

Intravenous Solutions

The most commonly prescribed intravenous solutions are listed in Table 10.1.

Table 10.1

Intravenous Solutions

Name of Solution	Common Abbreviation
0.45% sodium chloride injection USP	0.45% NS
0.9% sodium chloride injection USP	0.9% NS
5% dextrose in 0.22% sodium chloride injection USP	5% D/0.22% NS
5% dextrose injection USP	5% D/W, D/5/W
5% dextrose in 0.45% sodium chloride injection USP	5% D/0.45% NS or D/5/0.45% NS
5% dextrose in 0.9% sodium chloride injection USP	5% D/0.9% NS or D/5/0.9% NS
Lactated Ringer's injection USP	LR, RL, or RLS
Lactated Ringer's and 5% dextrose injection USP	5% D/RL, or D/5/RL

Intravenous fluids generally contain dextrose, sodium chloride, and/or electrolytes:

- D/5/W (or 5% D/W) is a 5% dextrose solution, which means that 5 milliliters or 5 grams of dextrose are dissolved in water to make each 100 milliliters of this solution. See Figure 10.2a and b.

- 0.9% NS stands for a solution in which each 100 milliliters contains 0.9 gram of sodium chloride. See Figure 10.2c and d.

- 5% D/0.45% NS stands for a solution containing 5 milliliters or 5 grams of dextrose in each 100 milliliters of 0.45% normal saline solution. See Figure 10.3b

- Ringer's lactate (RL), also called lactated Ringer's solution (LRS), is a solution containing electrolytes. See Figure 10.3c.

Additional information on IV fluids can be found in nursing and pharmacology textbooks.

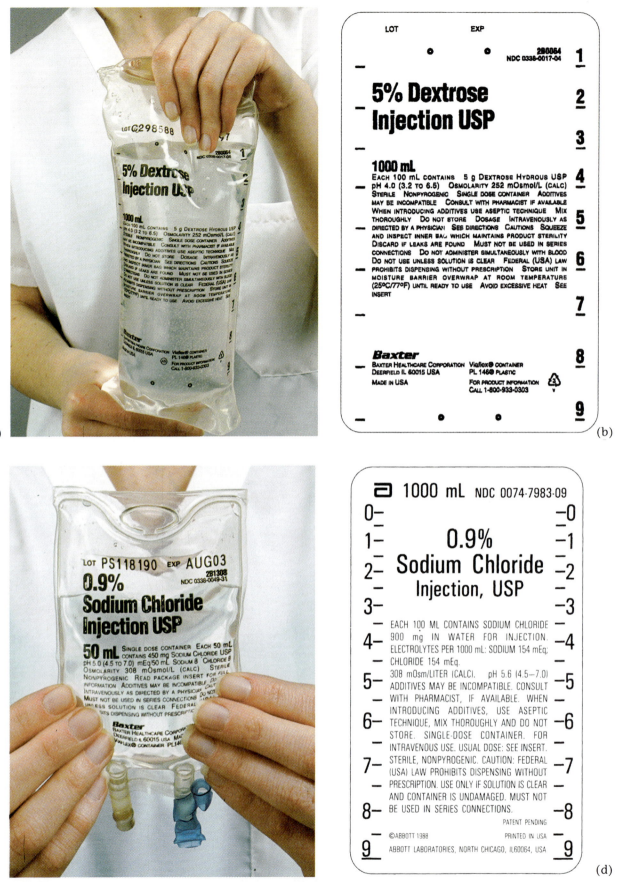

(a)

(b)

(c)

(d)

Figure 10.2 IV bag and label from 0.9% Sodium Chloride 1000 mL bag.

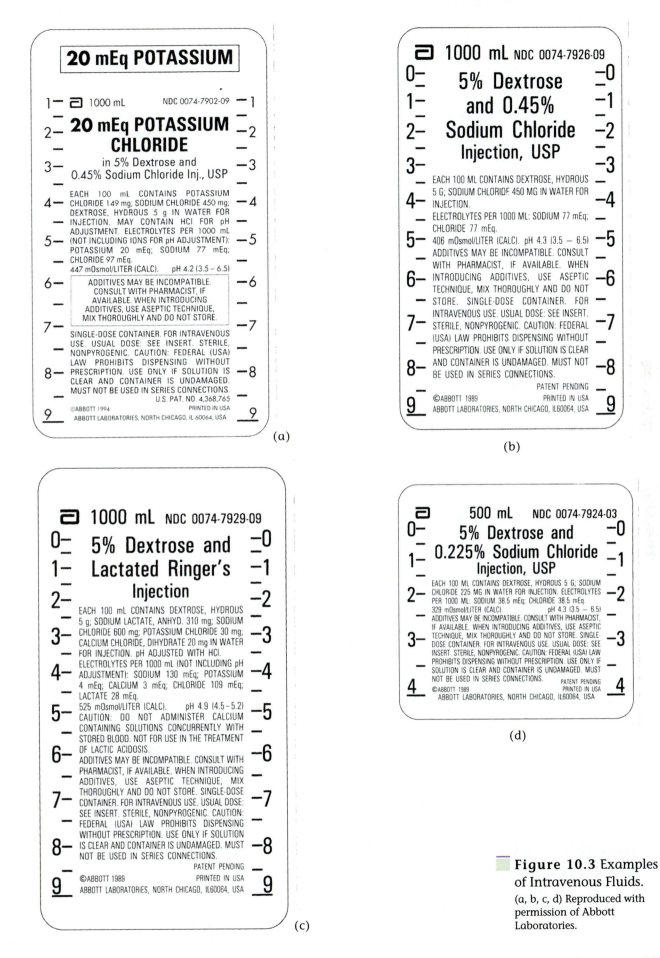

(a)

20 mEq POTASSIUM

🔲 1000 mL   NDC 0074-7902-09

20 mEq POTASSIUM CHLORIDE

in 5% Dextrose and 0.45% Sodium Chloride Inj., USP

EACH 100 mL CONTAINS POTASSIUM CHLORIDE 149 mg; SODIUM CHLORIDE 450 mg; DEXTROSE, HYDROUS 5 g IN WATER FOR INJECTION. MAY CONTAIN HCl FOR pH ADJUSTMENT. ELECTROLYTES PER 1000 mL (NOT INCLUDING IONS FOR pH ADJUSTMENT): POTASSIUM 20 mEq; SODIUM 77 mEq; CHLORIDE 97 mEq.
447 mOsmol/LITER (CALC).   pH 4.2 (3.5 – 6.5)

ADDITIVES MAY BE INCOMPATIBLE. CONSULT WITH PHARMACIST, IF AVAILABLE. WHEN INTRODUCING ADDITIVES, USE ASEPTIC TECHNIQUE, MIX THOROUGHLY AND DO NOT STORE.

SINGLE-DOSE CONTAINER. FOR INTRAVENOUS USE. USUAL DOSE: SEE INSERT. STERILE, NONPYROGENIC. CAUTION: FEDERAL (USA) LAW PROHIBITS DISPENSING WITHOUT PRESCRIPTION. USE ONLY IF SOLUTION IS CLEAR AND CONTAINER IS UNDAMAGED. MUST NOT BE USED IN SERIES CONNECTIONS.
U.S. PAT. NO. 4,368,765
©ABBOTT 1994   PRINTED IN USA
ABBOTT LABORATORIES, NORTH CHICAGO, IL 60064, USA

(b)

🔲 1000 mL NDC 0074-7926-09

5% Dextrose and 0.45% Sodium Chloride

Injection, USP

EACH 100 ML CONTAINS DEXTROSE, HYDROUS 5 G; SODIUM CHLORIDE 450 MG IN WATER FOR INJECTION.
ELECTROLYTES PER 1000 ML: SODIUM 77 mEq; CHLORIDE 77 mEq.
406 mOsmol/LITER (CALC).   pH 4.3 (3.5 – 6.5)
ADDITIVES MAY BE INCOMPATIBLE. CONSULT WITH PHARMACIST, IF AVAILABLE. WHEN INTRODUCING ADDITIVES, USE ASEPTIC TECHNIQUE, MIX THOROUGHLY AND DO NOT STORE. SINGLE-DOSE CONTAINER. FOR INTRAVENOUS USE. USUAL DOSE: SEE INSERT. STERILE, NONPYROGENIC. CAUTION: FEDERAL (USA) LAW PROHIBITS DISPENSING WITHOUT PRESCRIPTION. USE ONLY IF SOLUTION IS CLEAR AND CONTAINER IS UNDAMAGED. MUST NOT BE USED IN SERIES CONNECTIONS.
PATENT PENDING
©ABBOTT 1989   PRINTED IN USA
ABBOTT LABORATORIES, NORTH CHICAGO, IL60064, USA

(c)

🔲 1000 mL NDC 0074-7929-09

5% Dextrose and Lactated Ringer's

Injection

EACH 100 mL CONTAINS DEXTROSE, HYDROUS 5 g; SODIUM LACTATE, ANHYD. 310 mg; SODIUM CHLORIDE 600 mg; POTASSIUM CHLORIDE 30 mg; CALCIUM CHLORIDE, DIHYDRATE 20 mg IN WATER FOR INJECTION. pH ADJUSTED WITH HCl.
ELECTROLYTES PER 1000 mL (NOT INCLUDING pH ADJUSTMENT): SODIUM 130 mEq; POTASSIUM 4 mEq; CALCIUM 3 mEq; CHLORIDE 109 mEq; LACTATE 28 mEq.
525 mOsmol/LITER (CALC).   pH 4.9 (4.5 – 5.2)
CAUTION: DO NOT ADMINISTER CALCIUM CONTAINING SOLUTIONS CONCURRENTLY WITH STORED BLOOD. NOT FOR USE IN THE TREATMENT OF LACTIC ACIDOSIS.
ADDITIVES MAY BE INCOMPATIBLE. CONSULT WITH PHARMACIST, IF AVAILABLE. WHEN INTRODUCING ADDITIVES, USE ASEPTIC TECHNIQUE, MIX THOROUGHLY AND DO NOT STORE. SINGLE-DOSE CONTAINER. FOR INTRAVENOUS USE. USUAL DOSE: SEE INSERT. STERILE, NONPYROGENIC. CAUTION: FEDERAL (USA) LAW PROHIBITS DISPENSING WITHOUT PRESCRIPTION. USE ONLY IF SOLUTION IS CLEAR AND CONTAINER IS UNDAMAGED. MUST NOT BE USED IN SERIES CONNECTIONS.
PATENT PENDING
©ABBOTT 1989   PRINTED IN USA
ABBOTT LABORATORIES, NORTH CHICAGO, IL60064, USA

(d)

🔲 500 mL   NDC 0074-7924-03

5% Dextrose and 0.225% Sodium Chloride

Injection, USP

EACH 100 ML CONTAINS DEXTROSE, HYDROUS 5 G; SODIUM CHLORIDE 225 MG IN WATER FOR INJECTION. ELECTROLYTES PER 1000 ML: SODIUM 38.5 mEq; CHLORIDE 38.5 mEq.
329 mOsmol/LITER (CALC).   pH 4.3 (3.5 – 6.5)
ADDITIVES MAY BE INCOMPATIBLE. CONSULT WITH PHARMACIST, IF AVAILABLE. WHEN INTRODUCING ADDITIVES, USE ASEPTIC TECHNIQUE, MIX THOROUGHLY AND DO NOT STORE. SINGLE-DOSE CONTAINER. FOR INTRAVENOUS USE. USUAL DOSE: SEE INSERT. STERILE, NONPYROGENIC. CAUTION: FEDERAL (USA) LAW PROHIBITS DISPENSING WITHOUT PRESCRIPTION. USE ONLY IF SOLUTION IS CLEAR AND CONTAINER IS UNDAMAGED. MUST NOT BE USED IN SERIES CONNECTIONS.
PATENT PENDING
©ABBOTT 1989   PRINTED IN USA
ABBOTT LABORATORIES, NORTH CHICAGO, IL60064, USA

Figure 10.3 Examples of Intravenous Fluids.
(a, b, c, d) Reproduced with permission of Abbott Laboratories.

An order for intravenous fluids must include the name of the solution, medication (if required), and the length of time the solution is to infuse. For example, an intravenous order might read:

1000 mL 5% D/W IV for 8 hr

The registered professional nurse, vocational nurse, or licensed practical nurse must perform the necessary calculations to determine the correct rate at which the enteral or intravenous solutions will enter the body (***flow rate***). The flow rate will be measured in drops per minute, milliliters per minute, or milliliters per hour.

Equipment for IV Infusions

The equipment that must be used for the administration of IV infusions includes the IV solution, the package of tubing, and the drop chamber (Figure 10.4).

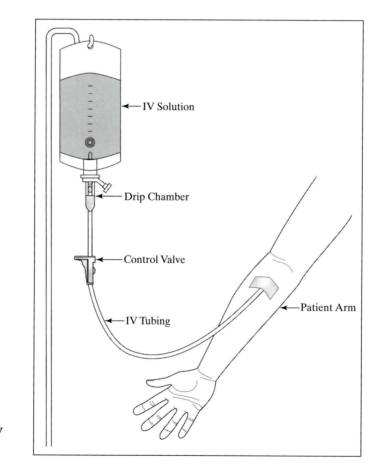

IV Solution

Drip Chamber

Control Valve

Patient Arm

IV Tubing

Figure 10.4 Primary intravenous line.

Figure 10.5 shows packaging of IV tubing.

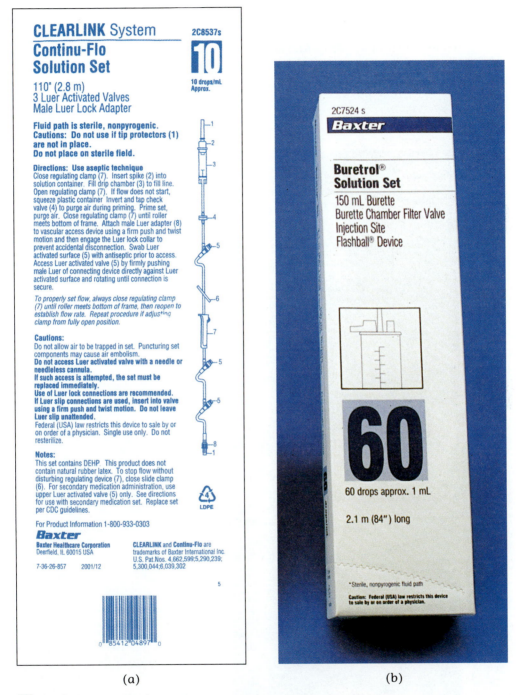

(a)

(b)

Figure 10.5 Samples of IV tubing with various drop factors.

[(a, b) Courtesy of Baxter Healthcare Corporations. All rights reserved. Photos by Al Dodge.]

The drip chamber (Figure 10.6) is located at the site of the entrance of the tubing into the container of intravenous solution. It allows you to count the number of drops per minute that the client is receiving (flow rate).

A roll valve clamp or clip (Figure 10.6) is connected to the tubing and can be manipulated to increase or decrease the flow rate.

The size of the drop that IV tubing delivers is not standard; it depends on the way the tubing is designed. Manufacturers specify the number of drops that equal 1 milliliter for their particular tubing. This equivalent is called the tubing's **drop factor**; see Table 10.2. You must know the tubing's drop factor when calculating the flow rate of solutions in drops per minute (gtt/min) or microdrops per minute (μgtt/min).

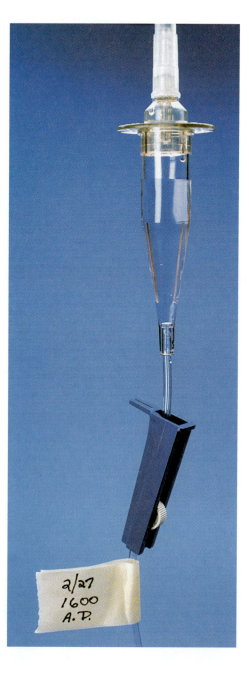

Figure 10.6 Tubing with drip chamber and roll valve clamp.
(Photo by Al Dodge.)

Table 10.2

Table 10.2

Common Drop Factors

10 gtt	=	1 mL
12 gtt	=	1 mL
15 gtt	=	1 mL
20 gtt	=	1 mL
60 μgtt	=	1 mL

Note: 60 microdrops = 1 milliliter is a universal equivalent for IV tubing calibrated in microdrops.

Intravenous infusions can also be controlled by electronic infusion devices. These devices are operated by electricity or by battery and can be set to deliver the IV solution in either milliliters per minute or milliliters per hour. There are many different types of infusion devices. These include syringe pumps, controllers, and volumetric pumps (See Figures 10.7 and 10.8).

The burette is generally used for smaller amounts of solution and is not electronic.

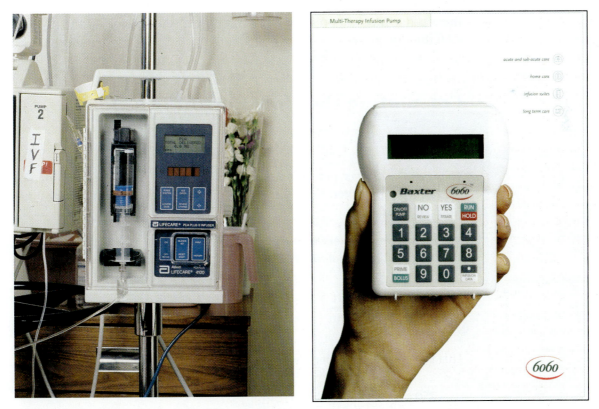

(a)   (b)

Figure 10.7 Volumetric infusion pumps: (a) Typical hospital infusion pump (Kozier, *Fundamentals of Nursing*, Figure 48.30, page 1345.) (b) Portable infusion pump.
(Courtesy of Baxter Healthcare Corporation. All rights reserved.)

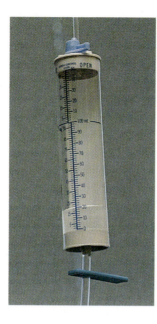

Figure 10.8 A Volume-control set (Burette) below the drip chamber of an intravenous solution.

Pumps have many advantages over traditional tubing. Pumps allow for a precise amount of drug solution to be administered within a specified period of time. On the newer pumps, the amount of fluid, the amount of medication, and the flow rate can easily be coded on the pump panel. If there is an interruption in the flow, an alarm sounds to alert the nursing staff and the patient.

Calculating the Flow Rate of Infusions

Example | 10.1 |

The order is 1250 cc per 12 hours of D/5/W IV. The tubing is calibrated at 10 drops per milliliter. Calculate the number of drops per minute that you would administer.

1250 cubic centimeters in a 12-hour period means $\dfrac{1250\,cc}{12\,hr}$. You want to convert cubic centimeters per hour to drops per minute.

$$\frac{1250\,cc}{12\,hr} \longrightarrow \frac{?\,gtt}{?\,min}$$

This is a two-step problem, which you do in one line as follows:

$$\frac{1250\,cc}{12\,hr} \times \frac{?\,gtt}{?\,cc} \times \frac{?\,hr}{?\,min} = ?\,\frac{gtt}{min}$$

Because 10 gtt = 1 cc, the first equivalent fraction is $\dfrac{10\,gtt}{1\,cc}$. Because 60 min = 1 hr, the second equivalent fraction is $\dfrac{1\,hr}{60\,min}$.

$$\frac{1250 \text{ cc}}{12 \text{ h}} \times \frac{10 \text{ gtt}}{1 \text{ cc}} \times \frac{1 \text{ h}}{\underset{6}{60} \text{ min}} = \frac{1250 \text{ gtt}}{72 \text{ min}} \text{ or } 17.4 \text{ gtt/min}$$

So, 1250 cubic centimeters given over a 12-hour period would be administered at the rate of 17 drops per minute.

Example 10.2

The medication order reads:

250 mL 0.9% NS in 4 h IV

The drop factor is 60 microdrops per milliliter. How many microdrops per minute would you administer?

"250 milliliters in a 4-hour period" means $\frac{250 \text{ mL}}{4 \text{ hr}}$. You want to convert milliliters per hour to microdrops per minute:

$$\frac{250 \text{ mL}}{4 \text{ hr}} \longrightarrow \frac{? \, \mu \text{gtt}}{? \text{ min}}$$

This is a two-step problem, which you do on one line, as follows:

$$\frac{250 \text{ mL}}{4 \text{ hr}} \times \frac{? \, \mu \text{gtt}}{? \text{ mL}} \times \frac{? \text{ hr}}{? \text{ min}} = ? \frac{\text{gtt}}{\text{min}}$$

Because 60 μgtt = 1 mL, the first equivalent fraction is $\frac{60 \, \mu \text{gtt}}{1 \text{ mL}}$. Because 60 min = 1 hr, the second equivalent fraction is $\frac{1 \text{ hr}}{60 \text{ min}}$.

$$\frac{250 \text{ mL}}{4 \text{ hr}} \times \frac{\overset{1}{60} \, \mu \text{gtt}}{1 \text{ mL}} \times \frac{1 \text{ hr}}{\underset{1}{60} \text{ min}} = \frac{250 \, \mu \text{gtt}}{4 \text{ min}} = 62.5 \frac{\mu \text{gtt}}{\text{min}}$$

So, 63 microdrops per minute would be administered.

Example 10.3

The prescriber ordered:

850 mL of 0.225% NS IV in 8 hr

The label on the box containing the intravenous set to be used for this infusion is shown in Figure 10.9. Calculate the flow rate in drops per minute.

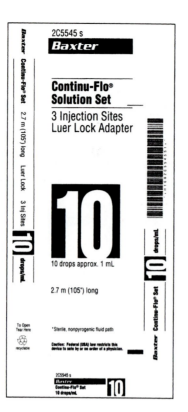

Figure 10.9 Continu-Flo Solution Set box label.

(Courtesy of Baxter Healthcare Corporation. All rights reserved.)

You want to convert the flow rate from milliliters per hour to drops per minute.

$$\frac{850 \text{ mL}}{8 \text{ hr}} \longrightarrow ?\frac{\text{gtt}}{\text{min}}$$

Do this on one line as follows:

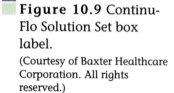

$$\frac{850 \text{ mL}}{8 \text{ hr}} \times \frac{1 \text{ hr}}{\underset{6}{60} \text{ min}} \times \frac{\overset{1}{10} \text{ gtt}}{1 \text{ mL}} = \frac{850 \text{ gtt}}{48 \text{ min}} = 17.7\frac{\text{gtt}}{\text{min}}$$

So, the flow rate is 18 drops per minute.

Sometimes, the infusion flow rate can change for a variety of reasons. A change will affect the prescribed duration of time in which the solution will be administered. Therefore, the nurse must assess the flow rate periodically and make any necessary adjustments.

Example 10.4

The order is 500 milliliters of 5% D/W to infuse IV in 5 hours. Calculate the flow rate in drops per minute if the drop factor is 15 drops per milliliter. To calculate the flow rate, you want to convert milliliters per hour to drops per minute.

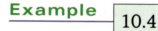

$$\frac{500 \text{ mL}}{5 \text{ hr}} \longrightarrow \frac{?\text{ gtt}}{\text{min}}$$

You can do this in one line as follows:

$$\frac{\overset{100}{\cancel{500}} \text{ mL}}{\cancel{5} \text{ hr}} \times \frac{\cancel{15} \text{ gtt}}{1 \cancel{\text{ mL}}} \times \frac{1 \cancel{\text{ h}}}{\cancel{60} \text{ min}} = \frac{100 \text{ gtt}}{4 \text{ min}} = 25 \text{ gtt/min}$$

So, the original flow rate was 25 gtt/min.

When the nurse later checks the infusion, 400 milliliters remain to be absorbed in 3 hours. Now you must recalculate the flow rate for the remaining 400 milliliters.

You want to convert milliliters per hour to drops per minute.

$$\frac{400 \text{ mL}}{3 \text{ hr}} \longrightarrow ?\frac{\text{gtt}}{\text{min}}$$

Do this on one line as follows:

$$\frac{400 \text{ mL}}{3 \text{ hr}} \times \frac{? \text{ gtt}}{? \text{ mL}} \times \frac{? \text{ hr}}{? \text{ min}}$$

Because 15 gtt = 1 mL, the first equivalent fraction is $\dfrac{15 \text{ gtt}}{1 \text{ mL}}$. Because 60 min = 1 hr, the second equivalent fraction is $\dfrac{1 \text{ hr}}{60 \text{ min}}$.

$$\frac{400 \cancel{\text{ mL}}}{3 \cancel{\text{ hr}}} \times \frac{\overset{1}{\cancel{15}} \text{ gtt}}{1 \cancel{\text{ mL}}} \times \frac{1 \cancel{\text{ hr}}}{\underset{4}{\cancel{60}} \text{ min}} = \frac{400 \text{ gtt}}{12 \text{ min}} = 33.3 \frac{\text{gtt}}{\text{min}}$$

So, the new flow rate is 33 drops per minute.

Example 10.5

The order is 875 mL of 5% D/W in 6 hours. The flow rate was set at 29 drops per minute. You assess the infusion flow 3 hours later, and the patient has received 500 mL IV with 375 mL remaining to be infused. Recalculate the flow rate with a drop factor of 10 drops per milliliter.

You want to convert milliliters per hour to drops per minute.

$$\frac{375 \text{ mL}}{3 \text{ hr}} \longrightarrow \frac{? \text{ gtt}}{\text{min}}$$

Do this on one line as follows:

$$\frac{375 \text{ mL}}{3 \text{ hr}} \times \frac{? \text{ gtt}}{? \text{ mL}} \times \frac{? \text{ hr}}{\text{min}}$$

Because 10 gtt = 1 mL, the first equivalent fraction is $\dfrac{10 \text{ gtt}}{1 \text{ mL}}$. Because 60 min = 1 hr, the second equivalent fraction is $\dfrac{1 \text{ hr}}{60 \text{ min}}$.

$$\frac{375 \cancel{\text{ mL}}}{3 \cancel{\text{ hr}}} \times \frac{\overset{1}{\cancel{10}} \text{ gtt}}{\cancel{\text{ mL}}} \times \frac{1 \cancel{\text{ hr}}}{\underset{6}{\cancel{60}} \text{ min}} = \frac{375 \text{ gtt}}{18 \text{ min}} = 20.8 \text{ or } 21 \frac{\text{gtt}}{\text{min}}$$

So, the new flow rate would be 21 drops per minute.

Notice that if you had realized that 3 hours is equivalent to 180 minutes, Example 10.5 could have been done more simply as follows:

$$\frac{375 \, \overline{mL}}{\underset{18}{\cancel{180} \, min}} \times \frac{\overset{1}{\cancel{10} \, gtt}}{\overline{mL}} = 20.8 \text{ or } 21 \frac{gtt}{min}$$

Example 10.6

The prescriber ordered 500 milliliters of 0.45% N/S IV. It has been calculated that the flow rate is 31 drops per minute. The drop factor is 10 drops per mL. What is the flow rate in milliliters per hour?

You want to convert drops per minute to milliliters per hour.

$$\frac{31 \, gtt}{1 \, min} \longrightarrow ? \frac{mL}{hr}$$

Do this on one line as follows:

$$\frac{31 \, gtt}{1 \, min} \times \frac{? \, mL}{? \, gtt} \times \frac{? \, min}{? \, hr} = ? \frac{mL}{hr}$$

Because 10 gtt = 1 mL and 60 min = 1 hr, the two equivalent fractions are $\frac{1 \, mL}{10 \, gtt}$ and $\frac{60 \, min}{1 \, hr}$.

$$\frac{31 \, \cancel{gtt}}{1 \, \overline{min}} \times \frac{1 \, mL}{\cancel{10} \, \underset{1}{\cancel{gtt}}} \times \frac{\overset{6}{\cancel{60} \, \overline{min}}}{1 \, hr} = 186 \frac{mL}{hr}$$

So, the patient would receive 186 milliliters per hour.

Example 10.7

The prescribers ordered 850 mL of D/5/.45% NS IV to infuse at 21 drops per minute. If the drop factor is 20 drops per milliliter, how many milliliters per hour will the patient receive?

You want to convert drops per minute to milliliters per hour.

$$\frac{21 \, gtt}{1 \, min} \longrightarrow \frac{mL}{hr}$$

Do this on one line as follows:

$$\frac{21 \, gtt}{1 \, min} \times \frac{? \, mL}{? \, gtt} \times \frac{? \, min}{? \, hr} = \frac{? \, mL}{? \, hr}$$

Because 20 gtt = 1 mL and 60 min = 1 hr, the two equivalent fractions are $\frac{1 \, mL}{20 \, gtt}$ and $\frac{60 \, min}{1 \, hr}$.

$$\frac{21 \, \cancel{gtt}}{1 \, \overline{min}} \times \frac{1 \, mL}{\cancel{20} \, \underset{1}{\cancel{gtt}}} \times \frac{\overset{3}{\cancel{60} \, \overline{min}}}{1 \, hr} = \frac{63 \, mL}{hr}$$

So, the patient would receive 63 milliliters per hour.

Example 10.8

The order reads:

125 mL 5% D/W IV in 1 hour

The drop factor is 60 microdrops per milliliter. What is the flow rate in microdrops per minute?

You want to change the flow rate from milliliters per hour to microdrops per minute.

$$\frac{125\,mL}{1\,hr} = \frac{?\,\mu gtt}{?\,min}$$

Do this in one line as follows:

$$\frac{125\,\cancel{mL}}{1\,\cancel{hr}} \times \frac{1\,\cancel{hr}}{60\,min} \times \frac{60\,\mu gtt}{1\,\cancel{mL}} = \frac{125\,\mu gtt}{min}$$

So, you would administer 125 microdrops per minute.

> **NOTE**
>
> In Example 10.8, it was shown that 125 milliliters per hour is the same flow rate as 125 microdrops per minute. Therefore, the flow rates of milliliters per hour and microdrops per minute are equivalent. So, for example, calculations are not necessary to change 137 mL/hr to 137 μgtt/min.

Calculating the Flow Rate of Enteral Solutions

Example 10.9

A patient must receive a tube-feeding of Ensure, 240 milliliters in 60 minutes. The calibration of the tubing is 20 drops per milliliter. Calculate the flow rate in drops per minute.

You want to convert milliliters per minute to drops per minute.

$$\frac{240\,mL}{60\,min} \longrightarrow ?\,\frac{gtt}{min}$$

Do this on one line as follows:

$$\frac{\overset{4}{\cancel{240}}\,\cancel{mL}}{\underset{1}{\cancel{60}}\,min} \times \frac{20\,gtt}{1\,\cancel{mL}} = 80\,\frac{gtt}{min}$$

So, the flow rate is 80 drops per minute.

Example 10.10

A patient has an order for Sustacal 240 milliliters in 2 hours via a feeding tube. Calculate the rate of flow in milliliters per minute.

You want to convert the milliliters per hour into milliliters per minute.

$$\frac{240\,mL}{2\,hr} \longrightarrow \frac{?\,mL}{?\,min}$$

Do this in one line as follows

$$\frac{\overset{4}{\cancel{240}}\,mL}{2\,\cancel{hr}} \times \frac{1\,\cancel{h}}{\underset{1}{\cancel{60}}\,min} = 2\,\frac{mL}{min}$$

So, the patient would receive 2 mL per minute.

Case Study 10.1

An 82-year-old female is seen in the emergency room complaining of neck pain for three days, and weakness, fever, chills, and cough. She is admitted with a diagnosis of sepsis, hypertension, congestive heart failure, and osteoarthritis. She has no known drug allergies and her vital signs are: T 99.2°; BP 120/70; P 86; R 20. She is 5 feet, 5 inches tall and weighs 180 pounds. The orders are as follows:

- 2 g Na Diet
- CBC qd in am
- Chest X ray stat
- IV: N/S @ 83 cc/h
- Cefuroxime 750 mg IVPB q8h
- Zithromax 500 mg IVPB qd
- Accupril 10 mg po qd
- Lopressor 50 mg po bid
- Heparin 5000 units sc q12h

1. Calculate the flow rate for the IV infusion. The drop factor is 10 gtts/mL.

2. How many mL of N/S will the patient receive in 24 h?

Read the Cefuroxime label in Figure 10.10 to answer Question 3.

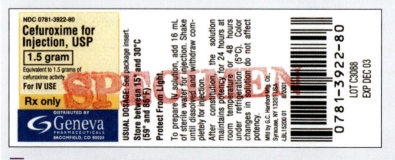

Figure 10.10 Drug label for Cefuroxime.
(Courtesy of Geneva Pharmaceuticals.)

3. a. What type and how much diluent will you add to the cefuroxime vial to reconstitute the solution?

  b. Calculate the number of milliliters you will withdraw from the cefuroxime vial to administer the prescribed dose?

  c. You then add the Cefuroxime to a 50 mL bag of N/S and infuse over 30 minutes. The drop factor is 15 gtts/mL. Calculate the flow rate.

4. Heparin is available in a vial labeled 20,000 units/mL. How many milliliters will you administer to the patient?

5. Place an arrow at the correct measurement on the most appropriate syringe to indicate the amount of Heparin to be administered.

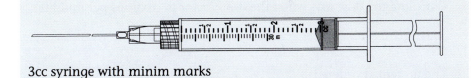

3cc syringe with minim marks

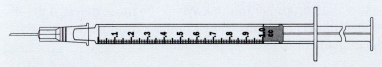

tuberculin syringe

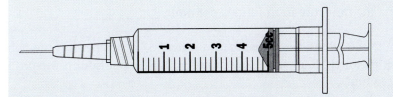

5cc syringe

6. How many units of Heparin is the patient receiving each day?

7. You have a 250 mL IV bag of D/5/W with 500 mg of zithromax. Infuse in 60 minutes via infusion pump. At what flow rate (mL/h) will you set the infusion pump?

8. The Accupril is supplied in 5 mg tablets and 20 mg tablets. Which tablets will you administer and how many?

9. State the dose of Accupril in micrograms.

10. The drug, Lopressor, is labeled as a 0.05 g tablet. How many tablets will you administer?

PRACTICE SETS

The answers to *Try These for Practice, Exercises,* and *Cumulative Review* appear in Appendix A at the back of the book. The answers to the *Additional Exercises* can be found on the companion Website or ask your instructor.

Try These for Practice

Test your comprehension after reading the chapter.

1. The prescriber ordered:

> *250 mL 5% D/W in 4 hr IV*

Calculate the flow rate when the drop factor is 10 drops per milliliter.

_____

2. The prescriber ordered:

> *1000 mL 0.9% NS in 8 hr IV*

The flow rate is 31 drops per minute. When the nurse assessed the infusion, 400 milliliters had infused in 4 hours. Calculate the new flow rate if the drop factor is 15 drops per milliliter. _____

3. The prescriber ordered:

> *850 mL 5% D/W IV in 8 hr*

Calculate the flow rate in milliliters per hour. _____

4. An IV of D/5/0.45% NS is infusing at a rate of 37 drops per minute. The drop factor is 15 gtt/mL. How many milliliters per hour is the patient receiving? _____

5. An IV solution is infusing at the rate of 60 milliliters per hour. How many microdrops per minute is this flow rate? _____

Exercises

1. The physician ordered 3000 milliliters of 5% Dextrose and Lactated Ringer's solution IV q24h. Calculate the flow rate in drops per minute. The drop factor is 10 gtt = 1 mL.

_____

2. The order reads:

> *D5W 250 cc per 8 hours IV*

Calculate the flow rate in microdrops per minute. _____

3. The patient is to receive 1000 mL of 0.9% NS in 8 hours. Set the rate on the infusion pump in milliliters per hour.

_____

4. The physician ordered the enteral solution, Ensure, via feeding tube 75 milliliters per hour. The drop factor is 18 drops per milliliter. Calculate the flow rate in drops per minute. _____

5. A patient is to receive 100 milliliters D/5/0.45% NS IV in 60 minutes. Calculate the flow rate in microdrops per minute. _____

6. The order reads:

   650 mL D5W q 8 h IV

   Set the flow rate on the infusion pump in milliliters per hour. _____

7. The medication order is 300 mL D/5/W IV in 3 hours. Calculate the flow rate in drops per minute. The drop factor is 12 gtt/mL. _____

8. A patient is receiving 10% D/W via a peripheral line at a rate of 55 milliliters per hour. How many microdrops per minute is the patient receiving? _____

9. A patient has an order for total parenteral nutrition (TPN) solution 2500 mL of 20% D/W in 24 hours. Set the rate on the infusion pump in milliliters per hour. _____

10. The order reads:

    850 mL D/5/0.45% NS q6h IV

    The drop factor is 15 gtt/mL. Calculate the flow rate in drops per minute. _____

11. The physician ordered 500 mL 0.9% saline as a fluid replacement IV in 3 hours. The rate of flow was 167 microdrops per minute. How many milliliters per hour was the patient receiving? _____

12. An intravenous solution is infusing at a rate of 17 drops per minute. The drop factor is 10 drops per milliliter. How many milliliters per hour is the patient receiving?

_____

13. The order reads:

    250 cc of 2 1/2% D/W IV. Infuse over a 24 h period

    Set the flow rate on the infusion pump in milliliters per hour. _____

14. An IV solution is infusing at a rate of 50 microdrops per minute.

    a. How many milliliters per hour is the patient receiving? _____
    b. How many milliliters will the patient receive in 24 h? _____

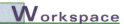

15. The order reads:

> *8 am: 1000 mL D/5/W IV in 8 h*

The infusion pump is set at 125 mL/hr. The IV was stopped for one hour with 625 mL remaining. Calculate the new flow rate. _____

16. The flow rate for an intravenous solution of 750 mL in 5 hours is 150 microdrops per minute. The new flow rate ordered by the physician is 125 microdrops per minute. Recalculate the flow rate in mL/h. _____

17. The patient has an order for 1250 mL D/5/0.45% NS in 15 hours IV. The drop factor is 10 gtt/mL and the flow rate is 14 drops per minute. Five hours later 700 milliliters remained in the IV bag. If you have to recalculate the flow rate, what will be the new flow rate in milliliters per hour? _____

18. A patient must have a continuous tube feeding of 1000 mL Ensure for 10 hours. The drop factor is 20 gtt/mL.

    a. Calculate the setting for the pump in drops per minute. _____

    b. If each can of Ensure contains 200 mL, how many cans of Ensure will you need? _____

19. An IV is infusing at a rate of 31 drops per minute. The drop factor is 15 gtt/mL. Calculate the flow rate in milliliters per hour. _____

20. An IV solution is infusing at 40 microdrops per minute. How many milliliters of this solution will the patient receive in 18 hours? _____

Additional Exercises

Now, on your own, test yourself! The answers to the *Additional Exercises* can be found on the companion Website or ask your instructor.

    1. The prescriber ordered 1800 milliliters of 5% D/W in 24 hours IV. The patient was receiving 75 microdrops per minute. After 12 hours, the patient had received 1240 milliliters. Recalculate the flow rate.

        _____

    2. An intravenous solution of 5% D/W is infusing at a flow rate of 42 drops per minute. The drop factor was 10 drops per milliliter. How many milliliters per hour will the patient receive? _____

    3. The flow rate of an intravenous solution is 16 drops per minute. The drop factor is 15 drops per milliliter. How many milliliters per hour is the patient receiving? _____

    4. The prescriber ordered 500 milliliters of 5% D/W to infuse in 10 hours. After 4 hours, 400 milliliters of the infusion remained to be infused. Recalculate the flow rate. The drop factor is 10 drops per milliliter.

        _____

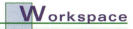

5. An infusion of 5% D/W has a flow rate of 36 drops per minute. The drop factor is 15 drops per milliliter. What is the flow rate in milliliters per hour? _____

6. An infusion of 1000 milliliters of 5% D/W is infusing at a rate of 31 drops per minute. The drop factor is 20 drops per milliliter. How many milliliters per hour is the patient receiving? _____

7. A patient is receiving 10% D/W via a peripheral line at a rate of 40 milliliters per hour. How many microdrops per minute is this?

_____

8. The prescriber ordered:

   250 mL 5% D/W IV in 2.5 hr

   Calculate the flow rate when the drop factor is 15 drops per minute.

_____

9. The physician ordered tube feedings of Ensure 240 milliliters per 4 hours. Calculate the flow rate in milliliters per hour. _____

10. The prescriber ordered a tube feeding of Sustacal 480 milliliters in 2 hours. The drop factor is 20 drops per milliliter. Calculate the flow rate.

_____

11. A patient has an order for total parenteral nutrition (TPN), 3000 milliliters of 20% D/W in 24 hours. Calculate the flow rate in milliliters per hour. _____

12. The prescriber ordered:

   2500 mL 5% D/W in 24 hr IV

   The drop factor is 10 drops per milliliter. Calculate the flow rate.

_____

13. 125 μgtt/min = ? mL/hr _____

14. The physician's order reads:

   400 mL Ensure via PEG in 4.4 hr

   Calculate the flow rate in milliliters per hour. _____

15. The patient has PEG. What is the meaning of this - abbreviation? _____

16. The order is 1250 milliliters of 5% D/W IV in 12 hours. The flow rate is 25 drops per minute; the drop factor is 15 drops per milliliter. How many milliliters per hour is the patient receiving? _____

17. An infusion of 20% D/0.225% NS has been prepared for a patient. The flow rate is 26 drops per minute. The drop factor is 15 drops per milliliter. How many milliliters per hour is this patient receiving IV?

_____

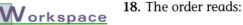

18. The order reads:

> *900 mL 5% D/0.45% NS IV 5 hr*

Calculate the flow rate when the drop factor is 10 drops per milliliter.

_____

19. Calculate the flow rate in milliliters per hour for the order in the previous problem. _____

20. Recalculate the flow rate for an intravenous infusion of 500 milliliters of 5% D/W that is infusing at 100 microdrops per minute in 5 hours. The new flow rate ordered by the physician is 80 microdrops per minute. How many milliliters per hour will this patient receive? _____

CUMULATIVE REVIEW EXERCISES

Review your mastery of earlier chapters.

1. An intravenous solution is infusing at 80 microdrops per minute. How many milliliters per hour is the patient receiving? _____

2. The order reads:

> *1500 mL lactated Ringer's solution IV for 24 hr.*

How many milliliters per hour will the patient receive? _____

3. The prescriber orders TPN, 2500 milliliters of 20% D/W to infuse in 16 hours. Set the rate on the infusion pump at milliliters per hour. _____

4. An infusion of 1000 milliliters of 5% D/W was to infuse at a rate of 30 drops per minute for 10 hours. After 4 hours the patient had received 600 milliliters. The drop factor is 15 drops per milliliter. Recalculate the flow rate. _____

5. A patient has an order for $gr\frac{1}{500}$ of atropine sulfate sc. Convert $gr\frac{1}{500}$ to mg. _____

6. The patient has a BSA of 1.6 m². The medication order is 0.8 mg/m². The capsule is labeled 1.2 mg. How many capsules will you prepare? _____

7. You have a sodium chloride solution with a concentration of 0.45%. How many milligrams of sodium chloride are in 1 milliliter? _____

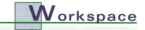

8. You are to prepare 0.75 g of Cefuroxime IM for your patient. The label reads 250 mg/mL. How many milliliters will you prepare for your patient? _____

9. Your patient weighs 101 pounds. The prescriber has ordered 6.6 milligrams per kilogram of lithium po. You have lithium capsules labeled 300 milligrams each. How many capsules will you prepare? _____

10. The order reads:

Levalbuterol (Xopenex) 0.32 mg by inhalation

The label reads 0.31 mg/3 mL. How many milliliters will you prepare of this drug? _____

11. 4 T = ? tsp _____

12. 6 mg = gr ? _____

13. 10 mL = ? gtt _____

14. gr $\dfrac{1}{100}$ = ? g _____

15. 1 oz = ? mL _____

Additional questions, web links, matching exercises, fill-in-the-blanks, and glossary for this chapter can be found on the companion Website at www.prenhall.com/olsen. Click on Chapter 10 to select the activities for this chapter.

CHAPTER ELEVEN

Calculating Flow Rates for Intravenous Medications and Duration of Flow

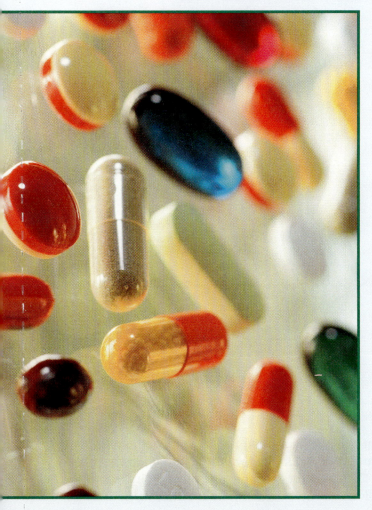

Objectives

After completing this chapter, you will be able to

- Describe intravenous piggyback medication administration.

- Calculate the rate of flow of intravenous piggyback medications.

- Calculate the flow rate of intravenous solutions based on the amount of drug per minute or per hour.

- Determine the amount of drug a patient will receive IV per minute or per hour.

- Calculate IV flow rates based on weight.

- Calculate IV flow rates based on body surface area.

- Calculate the infusion time of an IV solution.

This chapter extends the discussion of intravenous infusions to include intravenous piggyback (IVPB) infusions. You will also learn how to calculate the infusion time of an IV as well as how to determine flow rates for IVs based on weight or BSA.

Intravenous Piggyback Infusions

Patients can receive a drug through a port in an existing IV line. This is called **intravenous piggyback (IVPB)**; see Figure 11.1. IVPB tubing can be used to administer small amounts of medication along with the IV solution. The IVPB tubing that delivers the medication is called the **secondary set**.

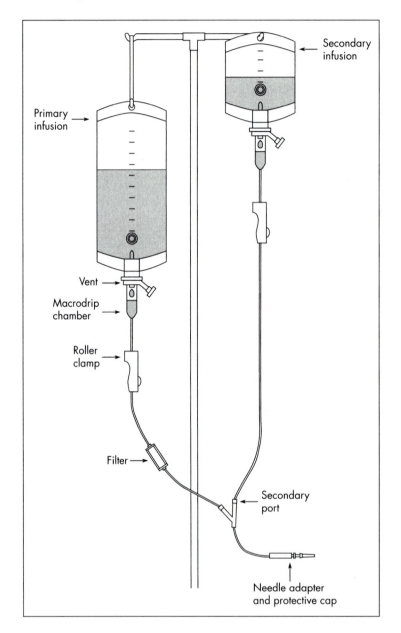

Figure 11.1 Primary and secondary (IVPB) infusion setup.

Notice in Figure 11.1 that the secondary bag is higher than the primary bag so that the pressure in the secondary line will be greater than the pressure in the primary line. Therefore, the secondary medication infuses first. Once the secondary infusion is completed, the primary line begins to flow. Remember to maintain the patency of both systems. If you close the primary line, when the secondary IVPB is completed the primary line will not flow into the vein.

The box in Figure 11.2 is an example of a secondary medication set.

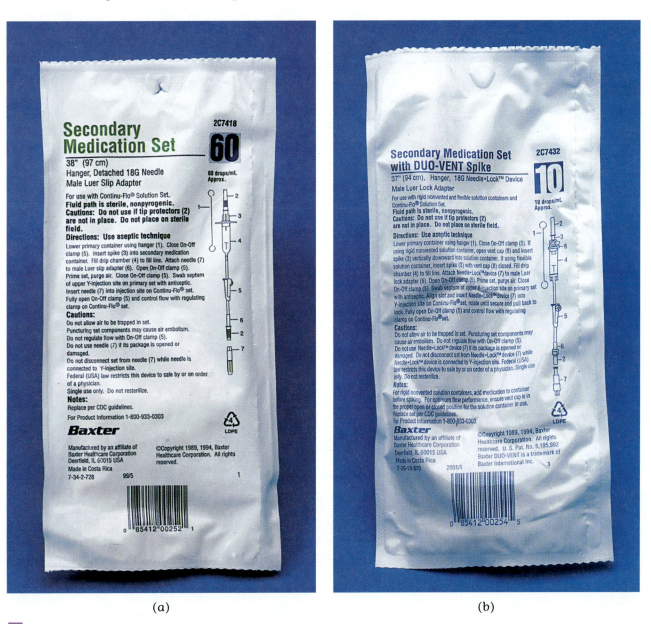

Figure 11.2 Package of secondary IV tubing.
(Courtesy of Baxter Healthcare Corporation. All rights reserved. Photos by Al Dodge.)

Let's look at some examples involving IVPB or secondary IV medications. Keep in mind that some medications for intermittent infusion are premixed by the manufacturer in 50 milliliters or 100 milliliters of D/5/W or 0.9% NS.

Intravenous Piggyback Medications

A patient who is already receiving 5% D/W via an IV line is to receive 1 gram of cefazolin (Ancef) every 4 hours. The prescriber's order reads:

Ancef 1 g IVPB q4h

This indicates that the patient will receive 1 gram of Ancef in solution via a secondary IV line that is attached to a port (piggyback) on the primary line.

Example 11.1

The prescriber ordered:

Ancef 1 g IVPB q4h

The package insert information is as follows: Add 50 mL sterile water to the bag of Ancef 1 g and infuse in 30 min. The tubing is labeled 20 drops per milliliter. Calculate the flow rate for this antibiotic.

You want to change the flow rate from milliliters per minute to drops per minute.

$$\frac{50 \, \text{mL}}{30 \, \text{min}} \longrightarrow ? \, \frac{\text{gtt}}{\text{min}}$$

Do this on one line as follows:

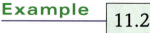

$$\frac{\overset{5}{\cancel{50 \, \text{mL}}}}{\underset{3}{\cancel{30 \, \text{min}}}} \times \frac{20 \, \text{gtt}}{1 \, \cancel{\text{mL}}} = \frac{100 \, \text{gtt}}{3 \, \text{min}} = 33.3 \, \frac{\text{gtt}}{\text{min}}$$

So, the flow rate is 33 drops per minute.

Example 11.2

The prescriber ordered:

Cefuroxime 1500 mg IVPB q12h

Read the information for this antibiotic medication in Figure 11.3. Follow the directions on the label, and infuse in 1 hour. The tubing is labeled 60 microdrops per milliliter. Calculate the flow rate. Add the required amount of Cefuroxime to 100 mL D/5/W.

Figure 11.3 Drug label for Cefuroxime.
(Courtesy of Geneva Pharmaceuticals.)

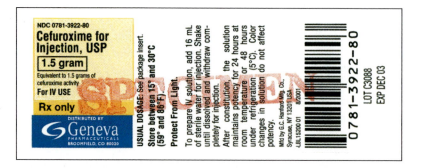

The label says to "add 16 mL of sterile water" to the vial, which contains 1.5 g (1500 mg) of Cefuroxime. The reconstituted solution has 1500 mg in 16 mL. This entire solution is added to the 100 mL of D/5/W. So, 116 mL (100 mL + 16 mL) must be infused in 1 hour.

Because 1 hour equals 60 minutes, you want to change the flow rate from milliliters per minute to microdrops per minute.

$$\frac{116 \text{ mL}}{60 \text{ min}} \longrightarrow ? \frac{\mu\text{gtt}}{\text{min}}$$

Do this on one line as follows:

$$\frac{116 \text{ mL}}{60 \text{ min}} \times \frac{60 \text{ }\mu\text{gtt}}{1 \text{ mL}} = 116 \frac{\mu\text{gtt}}{\text{min}}$$

So, the flow rate is 116 microdrops per minute.
Note: Remember that 116 μgtt/min is the same as 116 mL/h.

Example 11.3

The medication order reads:

1000 mL 5% D/W with 1000 mg lidocaine at 1 mg/min

Calculate the flow rate if the drop factor is 15 drops per milliliter. In this example, the prescriber has specified the solution (1000 milliliters of 5% D/W containing 1000 milligrams of the drug lidocaine) and also the amount of lidocaine per minute (1 milligram per minute) that the patient is to receive.

You want to change the flow rate from milligrams per minute to drops per minute.

$$1 \frac{\text{mg}}{\text{min}} \longrightarrow ? \frac{\text{gtt}}{\text{min}}$$

Do this on one line as follows:

$$\frac{1 \text{ mg}}{1 \text{ min}} \times \frac{? \text{ mL}}{? \text{ mg}} \times ? \frac{\text{gtt}}{\text{mL}} = ? \frac{\text{gtt}}{\text{min}}$$

Because 1000 milliliters contain 1000 milligrams and because 15 gtt = 1 mL, the equivalent fractions are

$$\frac{1 \text{ mg}}{1 \text{ min}} \times \frac{1000 \text{ mL}}{1000 \text{ mg}} \times \frac{15 \text{ gtt}}{1 \text{ mL}} = 15 \frac{\text{gtt}}{\text{min}}$$

So, you would administer 15 drops per minute.

Example 11.4

The prescriber writes an order for 1000 milliliters of 5% D/W with 10 units of synthetic oxytocin (Pitocin). Your patient must receive 30 milliunits of this drug per minute. The drop factor is 60 microdrops per milliliter. Calculate the flow rate in microdrops per minute.

You want to change the flow rate from milliunits per minute to microdrops per minute.

$$30\,\frac{mU}{min} \longrightarrow ?\,\frac{\mu gtt}{min}$$

NOTE

1000 milliunits (mU) = 1 unit (u)

Do this on one line as follows:

$$\frac{30\,mU}{1\,min} \times \frac{?\,unit}{?\,mU} \times \frac{?\,mL}{?\,unit} \times \frac{?\,\mu gtt}{?\,mL} = ?\,\frac{\mu gtt}{min}$$

Because $1000\,mU = 1\,unit$, $1000\,mL = 10\,units$, and $60\,\mu gtt = 1\,mL$, the equivalent fractions are

$$\frac{30\,\cancel{mU}}{1\,min} \times \frac{1\,\cancel{unit}}{1000\,\cancel{mU}} \times \frac{1000\,\cancel{mL}}{10\,\cancel{units}} \times \frac{60\,\mu gtt}{1\,\cancel{mL}} = 180\,\frac{\mu gtt}{min}$$

So, you will administer 180 microdrops per minute.

Example 11.5

Calculate the flow rate in milliliters per hour if the medication order reads: Add 10,000 units of heparin to 1000 mL 5% D/W IV. Your patient is to receive 1250 units of this anticoagulant per hour via an infusion pump.

You want to change the flow rate from units per hour to milliliters per hour.

$$\frac{1250\,units}{1\,hr} \longrightarrow ?\,\frac{mL}{hr}$$

Do this on one line as follows:

$$\frac{1250\,\cancel{units}}{1\,hr} \times \frac{\overset{1}{\cancel{1000}}\,mL}{\underset{10}{\cancel{10,000}}\,\cancel{units}} = \frac{1250\,mL}{10\,hr} = 125\,\frac{mL}{hr}$$

So, your patient will receive 125 milliliters per hour.

In Examples 11.6, 11.7, and 11.8, you are given the flow rate in milliliters per hour, and you need to determine the amount of medication the patient will receive per hour.

Example 11.6

Calculate the amount of Regular insulin a patient is receiving per hour if the order is 500 mL NS with 300 units of Regular insulin and it is infusing at the rate of 12.5 mL per hour on the pump.

You want to convert the flow rate from mL per hour to units per hour.

$$\frac{12.5 \text{ mL}}{h} \longrightarrow ?\frac{\text{units}}{h}$$

Do this in one line as follows:

$$\frac{12.5 \text{ mL}}{h} \times \frac{300 \text{ units}}{500 \text{ mL}} = \frac{37.5 \text{ units}}{5 \text{ h}} \quad \text{or} \quad 7.5 \frac{\text{units}}{\text{hour}}$$

So, the patient is receiving 7.5 units per hour.

Example 11.7

The medication order reads:

500 mL 5% D/W with 50,000 units of heparin IV. Infuse at rate of 10 milliliters per hour

How many units is your patient receiving per hour?

You want to convert the flow rate from milliliters per hour to units per hour.

$$\frac{10 \text{ mL}}{1 \text{ hr}} \longrightarrow ?\frac{\text{units}}{\text{hr}}$$

Do this on one line as follows:

$$\frac{10 \text{ mL}}{1 \text{ hr}} \times \frac{50,000 \text{ units}}{500 \text{ mL}} = 1000 \text{ units/hr}$$

So, your patient is receiving 1000 units of heparin per hour.

Example 11.8

Your patient is receiving an IV of 1000 milliliters of 0.9% NS with 1000 milligrams of the bronchodilator aminophylline (somophyllin). The flow rate is 50 milliliters per hour. How many milligrams per hour is your patient receiving?

You want to convert the flow rate from milliliters per hour to milligrams per hour.

$$\frac{50 \text{ mL}}{1 \text{ hr}} \longrightarrow ?\frac{\text{mg}}{\text{hr}}$$

Do this on one line as follows:

$$\frac{50 \text{ mL}}{1 \text{ hr}} \times \frac{\overset{1}{1000} \text{ mg}}{\underset{1}{1000} \text{ mL}} = 50 \frac{\text{mg}}{\text{hr}}$$

So your patient is receiving 50 milligrams of aminophylline per hour.

Calculating Flow Rates Based on Body Weight

Some IV and enteral medications are prescribed based on your patient's weight. For example, the medication order might read:

0.001 mg/kg/min

This means that each minute, your patient is to receive 0.001 milligram of the drug for every kilogram of body weight. This can also be written as $\dfrac{0.001 \text{ mg}}{\text{kg} \times \text{min}}$.

Example 11.9

The prescriber ordered:

250 mL 5% D/W with 60 mg Aredia, 0.006 mg/kg/min IV.

The patient weighs 75 kilograms, and the drop factor is 20 drops per milliliter. Calculate the flow rate for this antihypercalcemic drug in drops per minute.

Because the amount of drug ordered is based on the weight of the patient (kilograms), the weight will determine the flow rate (drops per minute). You want to convert kilograms to drops per minute. You have the following information:

The patient weighs 75 kg

The order is 0.006 mg/kg/min

60 mg = 250 mL

20 gtt = 1 mL

Do this problem on one line as follows:

$$75 \text{ kg} \times \frac{0.006 \text{ mg}}{\text{kg} \times \text{min}} \times \frac{250 \text{ mL}}{60 \text{ mg}} \times \frac{20 \text{ gtt}}{1 \text{ mL}} = 37.5 \frac{\text{gtt}}{\text{min}}$$

So, the flow rate is 38 drops per minute.

Example 11.10

The medication order reads:

Vibramycin 0.012 mg/kg/min in 200 mL 5% D/W IV.

The directions on the label read: "To prepare: add 20 mL of sterile water to the 300 mg vial and further dilute with 200 mL of D/5/W." How many milliliters will you add to the vial? The patient weighs 60 kilograms. How many milliliters per hour will your patient receive?

If 20 mL of sterile water are added to the vial, and this drug is then added to the 200 mL of 5% D/W, the total infusion will be 220 mL. You have the following information:

The patient weighs 60 kg

The order is 0.012 mg/kg/min

220 mL = 200 mg

Do this problem on one line as follows:

$$60 \text{ kg} \times \frac{0.012 \text{ mg}}{\text{kg} \times \text{min}} \times \frac{220 \text{ mL}}{200 \text{ mg}} \times \frac{60 \text{ min}}{1 \text{ hr}} = 47.5 \frac{\text{mL}}{\text{hr}}$$

So, your patient will receive 47.5 milliliters per hour.

Calculating Flow Rates Based on Body Surface Area

As you know, certain medications are ordered based on body surface area (BSA). Chapter 6 discusses how to determine BSA, and you will find a nomogram, in Appendix G.

The following examples show how to calculate flow rates for this type of medication order.

Example 11.11

The prescriber ordered 1 gram of vancomycin (Vancocin), an antibiotic drug, in 250 milliliters 0.9% NS to be infused at a rate of 500 milligrams per square meter per hour (see the label in Figure 11.4 for drug information). Your patient's BSA is 1.5 square meters. How many milliliters per hour should your patient receive?

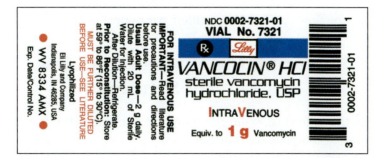

Figure 11.4 Drug label for Vancocin.
(Courtesy of Eli Lilly and Company.)

Because the medication order is based on the BSA of the patient, the BSA will determine the flow rate (milliliters per hour). You have the following information:

The BSA of the patient is 1.5 m²

The order is 500 mg/m²/hr

250 mL = 1 g of Vancocin

Do this problem on one line as follows:

$$1.5 \; \text{m}^2 \times \frac{\overset{1}{\cancel{500 \; \text{mg}}}}{\text{m}^2 \times \text{h}} \times \frac{250 \; \text{mL}}{\underset{2}{\cancel{1000 \; \text{mg}}}} = 187.5 \; \frac{\text{mL}}{\text{h}}$$

So, your patient should receive 187.5 milliliters per hour.

Example 11.12

The prescriber ordered:

Cefobid 1000 mg/m²/h IVPB q12h

Read the label in Figure 11.5 and use 20 milliliters per 2 grams for reconstitution, add to 100 mL of D/5/W. Calculate the flow rate in milliliters per hour if the patient's BSA is 1.7 square meters.

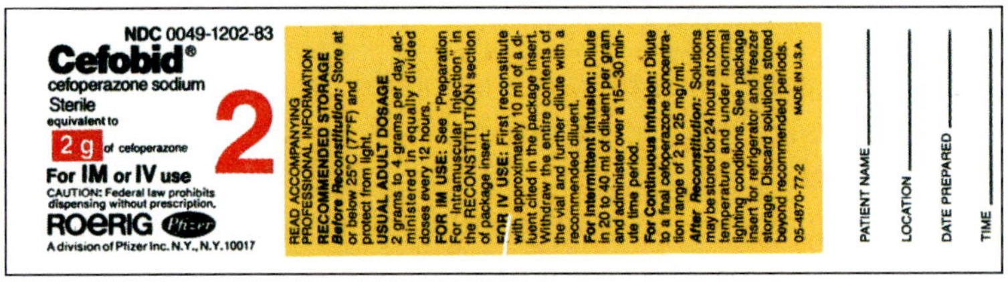

Figure 11.5 Cefobid 2 g.

(Registered Trademark of Pfizer Inc. Reproduced with permission.)

You have the following information:

The BSA of the patient is 1.7 m²

The order is 1000 mg/m²/h

Because 2 g = 20 mL, 2000 mg = 20 mL

If 20 mL of sterile water is added to the vial, and the reconstituted solution is then added to the 100 mL of D/5/W, the total infusion will be 120 mL. Do this problem on one line as follows:

$$1.7 \; \text{m}^2 \times \frac{\overset{1}{\cancel{1000 \; \text{mg}}}}{\text{m}^2 \times \text{hr}} \times \frac{120 \; \text{mL}}{\underset{2}{\cancel{2000 \; \text{mg}}}} = 102 \; \frac{\text{mL}}{\text{hr}}$$

So, the flow rate is 102 milliliters per hour.

Calculating the Duration of Flow for IV and Enteral Solutions

In the following examples, you will determine the length of time it will take to complete an infusion.

Example 11.13

An infusion of 5% D/W has solution remaining in the bag (Figure 11.6). It is infusing at a rate of 20 drops per minute. If the drop factor is 12 drops per milliliter, how many hours will it take for the remaining solution in the bag to infuse?

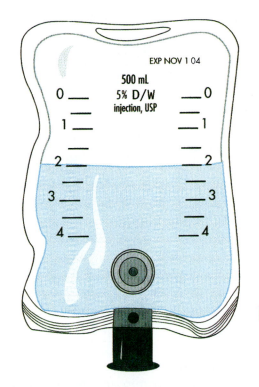

Figure 11.6 5% D/W intravenous solution (300 mL remaining in bag).

You can see that 500 milliliters of solution were originally in the bag and that the patient has received 200 milliliters. Therefore, 300 milliliters remain to be infused.

You want to convert milliliters to hours.

$$300 \, \text{mL} \longrightarrow ? \, \text{gtt} \longrightarrow ? \, \text{min} \longrightarrow ? \, \text{hr}$$

Do this on one line as follows:

$$300 \, \text{mL} \times \frac{? \, \text{gtt}}{? \, \text{mL}} \times \frac{? \, \text{min}}{? \, \text{gtt}} \times \frac{? \, \text{hr}}{? \, \text{min}} = ? \, \text{hr}$$

Because 12 gtt = 1 mL, 20 gtt = 1 min, and 60 min = 1 hr, these become the equivalent fractions.

$$\overset{15}{\cancel{300}} \, \text{mL} \times \frac{\overset{1}{\cancel{12}} \, \text{gtt}}{1 \, \text{mL}} \times \frac{1 \, \text{min}}{\underset{1}{\cancel{20}} \, \text{gtt}} \times \frac{1 \, \text{hr}}{\underset{5}{\cancel{60}} \, \text{min}} = 3 \, \text{hr}$$

So, it will take 3 hours to infuse this solution.

Example 11.14

A patient is receiving an IV of 500 milliliters of 5% D/W. The flow rate is 27 drops per minute. If the drop factor is 15 drops per milliliter, how many hours will it take for this infusion to finish?

You want to convert milliliters to hours.

$$500 \, \text{mL} \longrightarrow ? \, \text{gtt} \longrightarrow ? \, \text{min} \longrightarrow ? \, \text{hr}$$

Do this on one line as follows:

$$500\,\text{mL} \times \frac{?\,\text{gtt}}{?\,\text{mL}} \times \frac{?\,\text{min}}{?\,\text{gtt}} \times \frac{?\,\text{hr}}{?\,\text{min}} = ?\,\text{hr}$$

Because 15 gtt = 1 mL, 27 gtt = 1 min, and 60 min = 1 hr, these become the equivalent fractions.

$$500\,\cancel{\text{mL}} \times \frac{\overset{1}{\cancel{15}}\,\cancel{\text{gtt}}}{1\,\cancel{\text{mL}}} \times \frac{1\,\cancel{\text{min}}}{27\,\cancel{\text{gtt}}} \times \frac{1\,\text{hr}}{\underset{4}{\cancel{60}}\,\cancel{\text{min}}} = 4.63\,\text{hr}$$

Convert the portion of an hour to minutes—that is, convert 0.63 hour to minutes.

$$0.63\,\cancel{\text{hr}} \times \frac{60\,\text{min}}{1\,\cancel{\text{hr}}} = 37.8\,\text{min}$$

So, the infusion will take 4 hours and 38 minutes.

Example 11.15

An IV of 1000 milliliters of 5% D/0.9% NS is started at 8 P.M. The flow rate is 38 drops per minute, and the drop factor is 10 drops per milliliter. At what time will this infusion finish?

You want to convert milliliters to hours.

$$1000\,\text{mL} \longrightarrow ?\,\text{gtt} \longrightarrow ?\,\text{min} \longrightarrow ?\,\text{hr}$$

Do this on one line as follows:

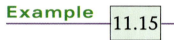

$$1000\,\text{mL} \times \frac{?\,\text{gtt}}{?\,\text{mL}} \times \frac{?\,\text{min}}{?\,\text{gtt}} \times \frac{?\,\text{hr}}{?\,\text{min}} = ?\,\text{hr}$$

Because 10 gtt = 1 mL, 38 gtt = 1 min, and 60 min = 1 hr, these become the equivalent fractions.

$$1000\,\cancel{\text{mL}} \times \frac{\overset{1}{\cancel{10}}\,\cancel{\text{gtt}}}{1\,\cancel{\text{mL}}} \times \frac{1\,\cancel{\text{min}}}{38\,\cancel{\text{gtt}}} \times \frac{1\,\text{hr}}{\underset{6}{\cancel{60}}\,\cancel{\text{min}}} = 4.4\,\text{hr}$$

You then convert 0.4 hour to minutes.

$$0.4\,\cancel{\text{hr}} \times \frac{60\,\text{min}}{1\,\cancel{\text{hr}}} = 24\,\text{min}$$

So, the IV will infuse for 4 hours and 24 minutes. Because the infusion started at 8 P.M., it will finish at 12:24 A.M. on the following day.

Example 11.16

An IV of 2000 milliliters of 20% D/W is to infuse at a rate of 100 μgtt/min. The drop factor is 60 μgtt/mL. If this IV solution begins to infuse at 10:15 A.M., at what time will it finish?

You want to convert milliliters to hours.

$$2000 \, \text{mL} \longrightarrow ? \, \text{gtt} \longrightarrow ? \, \text{min} \longrightarrow ? \, \text{hr}$$

Do this on one line as follows:

$$2000 \, \text{mL} \times \frac{? \, \text{gtt}}{? \, \text{mL}} \times \frac{? \, \text{min}}{? \, \text{gtt}} \times \frac{? \, \text{hr}}{? \, \text{min}} = ? \, \text{hr}$$

Because $60 \, \mu\text{gtt} = 1 \, \text{mL}$, $100 \, \mu\text{gtt} = 1 \, \text{min}$, and $60 \, \text{min} = 1 \, \text{hr}$, these become the equivalent fractions.

$$2000 \, \cancel{\text{mL}} \times \frac{60 \, \cancel{\mu\text{gtt}}}{\cancel{\text{mL}}} \times \frac{1 \, \cancel{\text{min}}}{100 \, \cancel{\mu\text{gtt}}} \times \frac{1 \, \text{h}}{60 \, \cancel{\text{min}}} = 20 \, \text{h}$$

So, the IV will infuse for 20 hours. Because the infusion started at 10:15 A.M., it will finish at 6:15 A.M. on the following day.

Example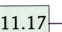

The prescriber ordered Vancomycin 1.5 g in 200 mL of D/5/W. Infuse in 60 minutes, the label reads: 1.5 g of Vancomycin. The vial available is used with a reconstitution device similar to that shown in Figure 11.7. The tubing is labeled 15 drops per milliliter. Calculate the flow rate in drops per minute.

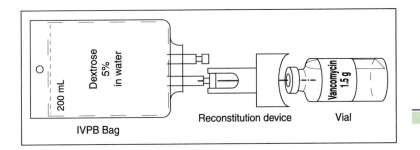

Figure 11.7
Reconstitution system.

You want to change the flow rate from milliliters per minute to drops per minute.

$$\frac{200 \, \text{mL}}{60 \, \text{min}} \longrightarrow \frac{? \, \text{drops}}{\text{min}}$$

Do this in one line as follows:

$$\frac{200 \, \cancel{\text{mL}}}{60 \, \text{min}} \times \frac{15 \, \text{gtt}}{\cancel{\text{mL}}} = 50 \, \text{gtt/min}$$

So, the flow rate is 50 drops per minute.

There are reconstitution systems that now enable the nurse to reconstitute a powdered drug and place it into an IVPB bag without using a syringe. One such device is shown in Figure 11.7. With this device, when the IVPB bag is squeezed, fluid is forced into the vial, dissolving the powder. The system is then placed in a vertical configuration with the vial on top and the IVPB bag on the bottom. The IVPB bag is then squeezed and released, thereby creating a negative pressure, which allows the newly reconstituted drug to flow into the IVPB bag.

Case Study 11.1

A 46-year-old male has been hospitalized for 3 weeks following a motor vehicle accident and head injury. During this time he has had a feeding tube and foley catheter inserted. Recently he has developed pneumonia and a decrease in his urinary output. He has no known drug allergies. His orders include:

- Clindamycin (Cleocin) 150 mg via feeding tube q6h
- Zantac (ranitidine) 150 mg via feeding tube bid
- Dilantin (phenytoin) 100 mg IVPB in 50 cc NS q8h, infuse over 30 min
- Ensure 480 mL q6h, followed by 50 mL of sterile water via feeding tube
- Mannitol (osmitrol) 100 g IVPB over 3 h, administer via infusion pump

1. The label on the Cleocin reads 75 mg/5 mL. How many milliliters are needed to administer the prescribed dose?

2. The label on the vial of Zantac reads 15 mg/mL. How many milliliters will you prepare?

3. How many milligrams of Zantac will the patient receive each day?

4. The vial of Dilantin is labeled 50 mg/mL. How many milliliters will you prepare?

5. Calculate the flow rate for the IVPB Dilantin. The drop factor is 15 gtt/mL.

6. Calculate the flow rate of the Ensure. The drop factor is 18 gtt/mL.

7. You have a 20% solution of Mannitol available. How many milliliters per hour will you set the infusion pump?

8. The patient's antibiotic has been changed to Kefzol 750 mg IVPB q8h; infuse in 100 mL of D_5W over 30 minutes. At what rate will you set the infusion pump (mL/h)?

9. Flagyl (metronidazole) has been added to the patient's regimen. The order is for 7.5 mg/kg q6h, to be infused in 100 cc over 1 h for 7 days. The patient weighs 178 pounds. How many milligrams will he receive per dose?

10. Calculate the flow rate needed to administer the Flagyl as noted in Question 9. The drop factor is 15 gtt/mL.

11. Calculate the total amount of enteral fluid this patient will receive in 24 hours.

12. The physician has now ordered the diuretic furosemide (Lasix) 60 mg oral suspension via feeding tube qd. The label reads 0.08 g = 30 mL. How may milliliters will you administer to the patient? _____

PRACTICE SETS

The answers to the *Try These for Practice, Exercises*, and *Cumulative Review Exercises* appear in Appendix A at the back of the book. The answers to the *Additional Exercises* can be found on the companion Website or ask your instructor.

Try These for Practice

Test your comprehension after reading the chapter.

1. The patient must receive 3 grams of cefuroxime IVPB in 200 ml D/5/W. Infuse in 120 minutes at 6:00 A.M. Read the label in Figure 11.8.

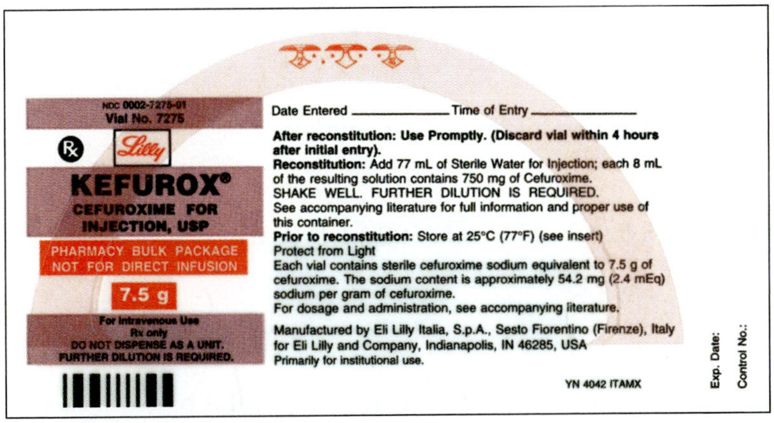

NDC 0002-7275-01
Vial No. 7275
Lilly
KEFUROX®
CEFUROXIME FOR INJECTION, USP
PHARMACY BULK PACKAGE
NOT FOR DIRECT INFUSION
7.5 g
For Intravenous Use
Rx only
DO NOT DISPENSE AS A UNIT.
FURTHER DILUTION IS REQUIRED.
Date Entered ____ Time of Entry ____
After reconstitution: Use Promptly. (Discard vial within 4 hours after initial entry).
Reconstitution: Add 77 mL of Sterile Water for Injection; each 8 mL of the resulting solution contains 750 mg of Cefuroxime.
SHAKE WELL. FURTHER DILUTION IS REQUIRED.
See accompanying literature for full information and proper use of this container.
Prior to reconstitution: Store at 25°C (77°F) (see insert)
Protect from Light
Each vial contains sterile cefuroxime sodium equivalent to 7.5 g of cefuroxime. The sodium content is approximately 54.2 mg (2.4 mEq) sodium per gram of cefuroxime.
For dosage and administration, see accompanying literature.
Manufactured by Eli Lilly Italia, S.p.A., Sesto Fiorentino (Firenze), Italy for Eli Lilly and Company, Indianapolis, IN 46285, USA
Primarily for institutional use.
YN 4042 ITAMX
Exp. Date:
Control No.:

Figure 11.8 Drug label for cefuroxime.
(Courtesy of Eli Lilly and Company.)

   a. How many milliliters of cefuroxime will you add to the 200 mL of D/5/W? ____________

   b. The drop factor is 60 microdrops per milliliter. Calculate the flow rate. ____________

2. The order reads:

   Pitocin 10 units in 1000 mL of 0.9% NS IV. Infuse at a rate of 20 milliunits/min.

   Calculate the flow rate in mL/h. ____________

3. The patient is to receive 1400 units of heparin qh IV. The order is 500 milliliters of 5% D/W with 25,000 units of heparin. How many milliliters per hour will the patient receive of this drug? See Figure 11.9. ____________

See literature for dosage. Each ml contains 10,000 USP Heparin units, derived from porcine intestinal mucosa, sodium chloride 0.1%. Preservative—1% benzyl alcohol added during manufacture. Sodium hydroxide and/or hydrochloric acid may have been added during manufacture to adjust pH. Store at 59° to 86°F.
NDC 0002-7217-01
5 ml
VIAL No. 520
Lilly
HEPARIN SODIUM
INJECTION, USP
10,000 USP
Units per ml
Multiple Dose
YD 1380 AMX
ELI LILLY AND COMPANY
Indianapolis, IN 46285, U.S.A.
Exp. Date/Control No.

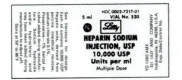

Figure 11.9 Drug label for Heparin.
(Courtesy of ESI Lederle, a Business Unit of Wyeth Pharmaceuticals, Philadelphia, Pa.)

Workspace

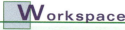

4. A patient has an IV of 250 milliliters of 5% D/W. The flow rate is 19 microdrops per minute. If the drop factor is 60 microdrops per milliliter, how many hours will it take for this infusion to finish?_____

5. Order:

Clindamycin phosphate 600 mg IVPB q6h × 5 days

The label for this drug reads: 900 mg/2 mL.

a. How many milliliters of clindamycin phosphate would you add to a 50 mL bag of 5% D/W? _____

b. Calculate the infusion rate in microdrops per minute when the total time of this infusion is 1 hour. _____

Exercises

Reinforce your understanding in class or at home.

1. Physician's Order:

Dobutamine (Dobutrex) 500 mg in 500 mL D₅W, 6 mcg/kg/min IVPB. Weight 145 lb.

a. Set the flow rate on the infusion pump in milliliters per hour. _____

b. If the above infusion begins at 6 A.M., when will it be completed? _____

2. Order: Amiodarone 160 mg in 20 mL D₅W IVPB; infuse over 10 minutes. The label reads 50 mg/mL. The drop factor is 60 µgtt/mL. Calculate the flow rate. _____

3. The dose of amiodarone (Cordarone) in Question 2 is increased to 720 mg in 24 hours in 500 mL D₅W. Set the rate on the infusion pump in milliliters per hour. _____

4. Pamidronate disodium (Aredia), an antihypercalcemic drug, 0.09 gram IV has been prescribed. The label reads: Add 10 mL to a 90 mg vial.

a. How many milliliters contain the prescribed dose? _____

b. Add the correct amount of Aredia to 1000 mL of 0.45% NS and infuse in 24 hours. Set the flow rate on the infusion pump in milliliters per hour. _____

5. Lidocaine HCl 2% 0.75 mg/kg has been ordered IVPB in 500 milliliters of D₅W. Weight is 150 pounds.

a. How many milliliters of the lidocaine contain this dose? _____

b. Calculate the flow rate in milliliters per hour so that the patient receives 5 mg/h _____

6. Order: Diltiazem (Cardizem) 0.25 mg/kg IV push over 2 minutes. The label on the vial reads 5 mg/mL. The patient weighs 210 pounds.

   a. How many milligrams of Cardizem will the patient receive? _____

   b. How many milliliters contain the dose of medication? _____

7. Physician's order:

   Phenytoin (Dilantin) 500 mg IV push over 10 min

   The label on the vial reads 50 mg/mL.

   a. How many milliliters will you prepare? _____

   b. Calculate the flow rate in microdrops per minute. _____

8. The loading dose of digoxin is 0.25 mg IV push q6h for 4 doses. The label on the ampule reads 0.5 mg/mL. How many milliliters contain this dose? _____

9. The prescriber ordered cefuroxime, an antibiotic drug, 18 mg/kg IV in 200 mL NS. Infuse in 1.5 hours. The patient weighs 80 kg. Read the label in Figure 11.10.

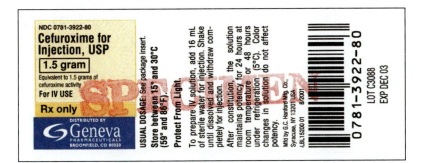

Figure 11.10 Drug label for cefuroxime.
(Courtesy of Geneva Pharmaceuticals.)

   a. How many milligrams of cefuroxime will the patient receive? _____

   b. How many milliliters of cefuroxime will you add to the 200 mL of NS? _____

   c. Calculate the flow rate in milliliters per hour. _____

10. Adenocor, an antiarrhythmic drug used in the treatment of PSVT (premature supraventricular tachycardia), 6 mg IV push over 1–2 seconds has been prescribed for your patient. The label on the vial reads 3 mg/mL. How many milliliters will you prepare? _____

11. The order for cefuroxime is 500 mg in 100 mL D$_5$W IVPB q8h; infuse in 20 minutes. Read the label in Figure 11.11.

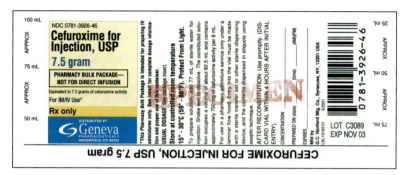

Figure 11.11 Drug label for cefuroxime.
(Courtesy of Geneva Pharmaceuticals.)

a. How many milliliters of cefuroxime contain this dose? _____

b. Calculate the flow rate in milliliters per minute. _____

12. Your patient has developed bradycardia and Atropine gr $\frac{1}{60}$ IV push stat is ordered. The label reads 0.5 mg/mL. How many milliliters will you administer? _____

13. Ritodrine HCL (Yutopar) 150 mg added to 500 mL D$_5$W has been ordered for a patient who is having premature uterine contractions.

a. Calculate the flow rate in microdrops per minute over a 15 hour period. _____

b. Change the flow rate to milliliters per hour. _____

14. A patient has been admitted to the ER with a diagnosis of lead poisoning. The physician orders edetate calcium disodium (calcium EDTA) 1.5 g/m^2 IV. The BSA is 2.0 m^2. The label on the vial reads 200 mg/mL. Add the prescribed amount of drug to 250 mL D$_5$W and infuse at a rate of 11 milliliters per hour. At what time will the infusion finish if it begins at 10 A.M.? _____

15. Cefuroxime 33.5 mg/kg q12h added to 200 mL NS IVPB. Weight is 95 pounds. Read the label in Figure 11.12.

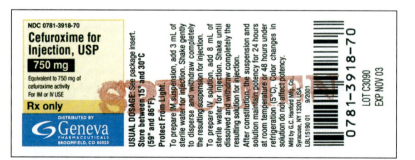

Figure 11.12 Drug label for cefuroxime.
(Courtesy of Geneva Pharmaceuticals.)

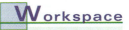

a. How many milliliters will you add to the vial? _____

b. Calculate the flow rate in milliliters per minute required to infuse in 30 minutes. _____

16. The order is Narcan (a narcotic antidote) 2 mg IV push. The vial reads 0.4 mg/mL. How many milliliters will you give the patient? _____

17. Prescriber order:

Sufentanil 6 mcg/kg IVPB in 100 mL D₅W, infuse over 30 minutes. Weight 172 lb.

Read the label in Figure 11.13.

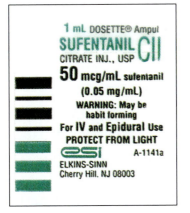

Figure 11.13 Drug label for Sufentanil.
(Courtesy of ESI Lederle, a Business Unit of Wyeth Pharmaceuticals, Philadelphia, PA.)

a. How many milliliters contain the prescribed dose? _____

b. How many ampules of this drug will you need? _____

c. How many microdrops are infused per minute? _____

18. The prescriber ordered morphine sulfate 50 mg to be added to 250 mL of 0.9% NS IVPB. Infuse in 5 hours. Read the label in Figure 11.14.

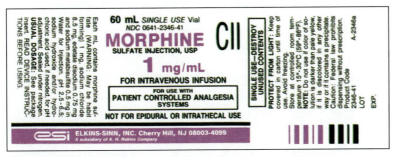

Figure 11.14 Drug label for morphine sulfate.
(Courtesy of ESI Lederle, a Business Unit of Wyeth Pharmaceuticals, Philadelphia, PA.)

a. How many milliliters contain the prescribed dose? _____

b. Calculate the flow rate in milliliters per hour. _____

c. After 90 minutes the patient had breakthrough pain and the physician increased the morphine to 15 mg/h. Recalculate the flow rate. _____

19. The prescriber ordered 500 units of regular insulin added to 250 mL 0.45% NS q12h. Read the information on the label in Figure 11.15.

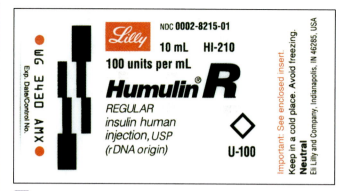

Figure 11.15 Drug label for regular insulin.
(Courtesy of Eli Lilly and Company.)

Calculate the dose and flow rate in milliliters per hour. _____

20. You have an infusion of heparin 50,000 units in 500 mL D₅W. The patient is receiving 1500 units per hour. What is the setting on the pump? _____

Additional Exercises

Now, on your own, test yourself! The answers to the *Additional Exercises* can be found on the companion Website or ask your instructor.

1. Read the information in the third medication order in Figure 11.16. Calculate the rate of flow in drops per minute when the drop factor is 10 drops per milliliter. _____

⊕ GENERAL HOSPITAL ⊕

PRESS HARD WITH BALLPOINT PEN. WRITE DATE & TIME AND SIGN EACH ORDER

DATE	TIME	A.M. P.M.
9/30/03	10	A.M.

IMPRINT
506713   9/30/03
Jason Vuu   6/22/40
26 Marin Dr.   RC
Thousand Oaks, Ore.   Aetna
80413

Dr. A. Giangrasso

1. *clindamycin phosphate 600 mg IVPB q6h × 5 days*

2. *solu-Medrol 1 g in 250 mL 5% D/W, IV*

   infuse 20 mg/hr

3. *aminophylline 1 g in 250 mL 5% D/W, IV*

   infuse 0.15 g/hr

ORDERS NOTED
DATE 9/30/03 TIME 10   A.M. P.M.

❑ MEDEX ❑ KARDEX

NURSE'S SIG. *L. Ablon RN*

SIGNATURE
                    A. Giangrasso M.D.

FILLED BY   DATE

PHYSICIAN'S ORDERS

Figure 11.16 Physician's order sheet.

---

2. The prescriber has ordered 3.1 grams of ticarcillin disodium (Timentin), an antibiotic, IVPB in 100 milliliters of 5% D/W. The directions are as follows: Add 13 mL to vial, 15 mL = 3.1 g. (Total amount of fluid IV: 115 milliliters.) This IV is to be infused in 60 minutes; the drop factor is 15 drops per milliliter. Calculate the flow rate. _____

3. A patient is to receive 500 milliliters of 5% D/W with 20 units of synthetic oxytocin (Pitocin) IV at a rate of 0.002 unit per minute. How many milliliters per hour will your patient receive? _____

4. The order reads: Cefizox 18 mg/kg IVPB q8h. The patient weighs 120 pounds. The directions read: Add 100 mL 0.9% NS to vial (1 g). a. How many milligrams will equal the ordered dose? b. How many milliliters will you administer? _____

5. The order reads: 500 mg of lidocaine in 250 mL 5% D/W. Infuse at 25 μgtt/min. Read the label in Figure 11.17, and (a) calculate the amount of lidocaine you will add to the 250 milliliters of 5% D/W; (b) calculate the flow rate in milliliters per hour; and (c) if the IV order is changed to infuse in 5 hours, determine the flow rate in milliliters per hour.

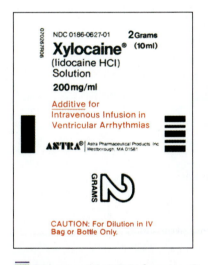

Figure 11.17 Lidocaine 2 g.
(Courtesy of Astra Zeneca Corp.)

6. The physician ordered cisplatin 20 mg/m² IV for a patient with a BSA of 1.7 m². The label of Cisplatin reads 10 mg = 10 mL. (a) How many milligrams should the patient receive? (b) How many milliliters contain the prescribed dose? (c) Add the correct amount of cisplatin to 1000 mL 0.22% N.S., and calculate the rate of flow in milliliters per hour if you infuse in 8 hours. _____

7. Calculate the flow rate in milliliters per hour for a patient receiving an IV of 250 milliliters of 5% D/W with 250 milligrams of aminophylline. The medication order is 0.006 milligram per kilogram per minute and the patient weighs 66 kilograms. _____

8. The prescriber has ordered 250 milliliters of 5% D/W with 2500 units of heparin; the patient is to receive 50 milliliters per hour IV. How many units per hour will your patient receive? _____

9. The order states that 200 milligrams of morphine are to be added to 250 milliliters of 5% D/W, and this solution is to be infused at a rate of 10 milligrams per hour. How many milliliters per hour will your patient receive? _____

10. The medication order is for 180 milligrams of morphine sulfate to be added to 250 milliliters of 5% D/W. If your patient is to receive 0.005 milligram per kilogram per minute IV, how many milligrams per hour should a patient who weighs 100 pounds receive? _____

11. The antifungal drug, Diflucan, has been prescribed for a patient who weighs 70 kg at 4.8 micrograms per kilogram per minute IV. Read the label in Figure 11.18. Calculate the flow rate in milliliters per hour. _____

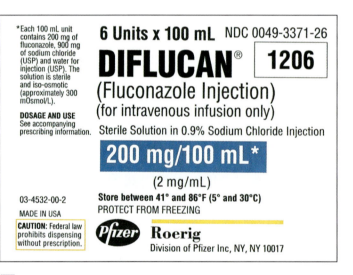

Figure 11.18 Drug label for Diflucan.
(Registered Trademark of Pfizer Inc. Reproduced with permission.)

12. The prescriber ordered dopamine hydrochloride (Intropin) at a rate of 0.003 milligram per kilogram per minute; the patient weighs 122 pounds. The directions are as follows: Add 160 mg (1 mL) to 250 mL of 5% D/W. Calculate the flow rate in milliliters per hour for this infusion.

_____

13. A medication order states that 50 milliliters of asparaginase (Elspar) are to be added to 100 milliliters of 5% D/W (total 150 milliliters). Calculate the flow rate in microdrops so that your patient, who weighs 60 kilograms, receives 1 milliliter per kilogram per hour of this antineoplastic drug. _____

14. The prescriber has ordered 500 milliliters normal saline with 100 units of Humulin R insulin (1 milliliter). Infuse at a rate of 0.7 milliliter per minute. How many hours will it take to complete this infusion?

_____

15. The order reads:

    500 mL of D/5/W with 2 g of lidocaine

    Read the label in Figure 11.19. The flow rate is 15 mL/h. How many milligrams per minute will the patient receive? _____

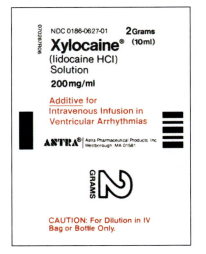

Figure 11.19 Drug label for lidocaine.
(Courtesy Astra Zeneca Corp.)

16. An infusion of 1000 milliliters of 5% D/W is started at 11 A.M. The flow rate is 20 drops per minute, and the drop factor is 20 drops per milliliter. At what time will this infusion finish? _____

17. The prescriber ordered Vibramycin 200 mg in 50 milliliters of Lactated Ringer's solution 0.08 mg/kg/min IV. The patient weighs 74 kilograms and the drop factor is 10 drops per milliliter. Calculate the flow rate in drops per minute. _____

18. Calculate the flow rate in milliliters per hour for a patient receiving an IV of 250 milliliters of 5% D/W with 200 milligrams of methyldopa (Aldomet) 0.005 milligram per kilogram per minute. The patient weighs 200 pounds. _____

19. The medication order states that 12,000 units of heparin are to be added to 250 milliliters of 5% D/W. The patient is to receive 1200 units per hour IV. How many milliliters per hour will your patient receive?

_____

20. The prescriber ordered: amikacin sulfate 120 mg/m^2/hr IV. The package insert directions are as follows: Add 250 mg to 100 mL 5% D/W. Calculate the flow rate in milliliters per hour if the patient's BSA is 0.9 square meter. _____

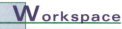

Review your mastery of earlier chapters.

1. The patient weighs 130 pounds. The medication order for a drug is 150 micrograms per kilogram of body weight. The label reads 2 milligrams per milliliter. How many milliliters of solution is equal to the medication order? _____

2. The prescriber ordered 0.02 mg of Methergine IM. How many milliliters of this drug will you prepare if the label reads 20 mcg/mL?

   _____

3. The patient must receive 1,500,000 units of penicillin IM, and the vial contains 20,000,000 units (in powdered form). The directions are as follows: Add 38.7 mL to vial; 1 mL = 500,000 units. How many milliliters will equal 1,500,000 units?

   _____

4. A patient must receive grain $\frac{1}{120}$ of scopolamine sc, a parasympathetic depressant. The label on the ampule reads 0.6 milligram per milliliter.

   How many minims will you administer to this patient? _____

5. The prescriber ordered cefprozil 0.275 g po q12h. The bottle is labeled 125 mg = 5 mL. How many milliliters of this antibiotic will you give your patient?

   _____

6. If you have a vial labeled 120 milligrams per milliliter, how many milliliters would equal 1.2 grams? _____

7. The physician has ordered 0.5 gram of clarithromycin (Biaxin) po. The tablets are 250 milligrams each. How many tablets equal 0.5 gram of this antibiotic? _____

8. The prescriber has requested that you give 40 milliequivalents of potassium chloride (K-Lor) po to a patient from a bottle labeled 10 milliequivalents per 5 milliliters. How many milliliters are needed? _____

9. gr $\frac{1}{500}$ = _____ mg

10. 0.6 mg = gr _____

11. 25 g = gr _____

12. gr $\frac{1}{200}$ = _____ g

13. 1 mL = _____ gtt

14. 1 T = _____ tsp

15. 45 mL = _____ oz

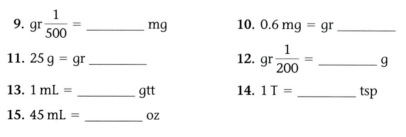

Additional questions, web links, matching exercises, fill-in-the-blanks, and glossary for this chapter can be found on the companion Website at www.prenhall.com/olsen. Click on Chapter 11 to select the activities for this chapter.

CHAPTER TWELVE

Calculating Pediatric Dosages

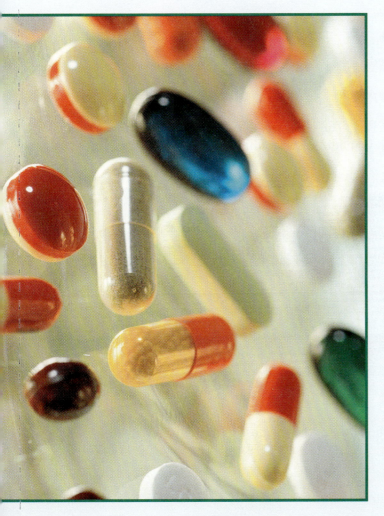

Objectives

After completing this chapter, you will be able to

- Calculate pediatric dosages based on body weight.
- Calculate pediatric dosages based on body surface area.
- Determine body surface area using a pediatric nomogram.
- Calculate pediatric intravenous dosages.

The prescriber must determine the proper kind and amount of medication for a patient. However, the dosage for infants and children is usually less than the adult dosage because their body mass is smaller and their metabolism different from that of adults. In this chapter, you will be introduced to methods of calculating pediatric dosages.

For many years, pediatric dosage calculations used pediatric formulas such as Fried's rule, Young's rule, and Clark's rule. These formulas are based on the weight of the child in pounds, or on the age of the child in months, and the normal adult dose of a specific drug. By using these formulas, one could determine how much should be prescribed for a particular child.

At the present time, the most accurate methods of determining an appropriate pediatric dose are by weight and body surface area (see Appendix G). You **must** know whether the amount of a prescribed pediatric dosage is the safe or appropriate amount for a particular patient. If this information is not on the drug label, it can be found on the package insert, in the hospital formulary, *Physician's Desk Reference* (PDR), *United States Pharmacopeia,* Harriet Lane handbook or in pharmacology texts.

Calculating Drug Dosages by Body Weight

Drug manufacturers sometimes recommend a dosage based on the weight of the patient. You were introduced to this idea in Chapter 6.

Example 12.1

The medication order reads:

> erythromycin 10 mg/kg po q8h

Read the label in Figure 12.1. The child weighs 40 kilograms. How many milliliters of the drug will you administer to this child?

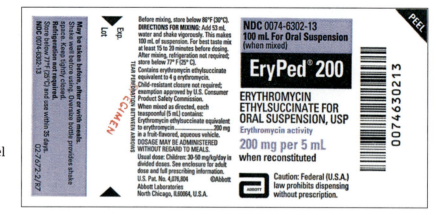

Figure 12.1 Drug label for Erythromycin.
(Reproduced with permission of Abbott Laboratories.)

You want to convert the body weight to the dose in milliliters.

$$40\,\text{kg} \longrightarrow ?\,\text{mL}$$

Do this problem on one line as follows:

$$40\,\text{kg} \times \frac{?\,\text{mg}}{?\,\text{kg}} \times \frac{?\,\text{mL}}{?\,\text{mg}} = ?\,\text{mL}$$

Because $10\,mg = 1\,kg$, the first equivalent fraction is $\dfrac{10\,mg}{1\,kg}$. Because $5\,mL = 200\,mg$, the second equivalent fraction is $\dfrac{5\,mL}{200\,mg}$. You cancel the kilograms and milligrams and obtain the dose in milliliters.

$$40\,\cancel{kg} \times \frac{25\,\cancel{mg}}{1\,\cancel{kg}} \times \frac{5\,mL}{200\,\cancel{mg}} = 10\,mL$$

So, the child should receive 10 milliliters of Erythromycin.

Example 12.2

How many milligrams of the antibiotic, ceftazidime (Fortaz) po, would you administer to a child po with a body weight of 25 kilograms if the order is 50 milligrams per kilogram?

You want to convert body weight to dose in milligrams.

$$25\,kg \longrightarrow ?\,mg$$

$$25\,kg \times \frac{?\,mg}{?\,kg} = ?\,mg$$

Because $50\,mg = 1\,kg$, the equivalent fraction is $\dfrac{50\,mg}{1\,kg}$. You cancel the kilograms and obtain the dose in milligrams.

$$25\,\cancel{kg} \times \frac{50\,mg}{\cancel{kg}} = 1250\,mg$$

So, the child would receive 1250 milligrams of ceftazidime.

Example 12.3

Compute the dose of vancomycin hydrochloride (Vancocin), an antibiotic drug, for a child who weighs 48 kilograms. The is prescribed order 10 milligrams per kilogram po in divided doses per day, bid.

You want to convert body weight to dose in milligrams.

$$48\,kg \longrightarrow ?\,mg$$

$$48\,kg \times \frac{?\,mg}{?\,kg} = ?\,mg$$

Because $10\,mg = 1\,kg$, the equivalent fraction is $\dfrac{10\,mg}{1\,kg}$. You cancel the kilograms and obtain the dose in milligrams.

$$48\,\cancel{kg} \times \frac{10\,mg}{\cancel{kg}} = 480\,mg$$

So, the child should receive 480 milligrams of vancomycin hydrochloride in divided doses per day, bid. So, the child receives 240 mg bid.

Example 12.4

Read the information on the label in Figure 12.2. The prescriber ordered:

cefaclor 15 mg/kg po q8h

The child weighs 18 kilograms. How many milliliters of this antibiotic will you prepare?

Figure 12.2 Drug label for Ceclor.

(Courtesy of Eli Lilly and Company.)

You want to convert the body weight to a dose in milliliters.

$$18\,kg \longrightarrow ?\,mL$$

Do this on one line as follows:

$$18\,kg \times \frac{?\,mg}{?\,kg} \times \frac{?\,mL}{?\,mg} = ?\,mL$$

Because $15\,mg = 1\,kg$, the first equivalent fraction is $\dfrac{15\,mg}{1\,kg}$. Because $125\,mg = 5\,mL$, the second equivalent fraction is $\dfrac{5\,mL}{125\,mg}$.

$$18\,\cancel{kg} \times \frac{15\,\cancel{mg}}{\cancel{kg}} \times \frac{5\,mL}{125\,\cancel{mg}} = 10.8\,mL$$

So, you would prepare 10.8 milliliters of cefaclor.

Example 12.5

You have an order for 5 milligrams per kilogram of ibuprofen (Motrin) q8h. How many grains would you administer to a child who weighs 15 kilograms?

You want to convert the body weight to a dose in grains.

$$15\,kg \longrightarrow gr\,?$$

Do this on one line as follows:

$$15\,kg \times \frac{?\,mg}{?\,kg} \times \frac{gr\,?}{?\,mg} = gr\,?$$

Because $5\,\text{mg} = 1\,\text{kg}$, the first equivalent fraction is $\dfrac{5\,\text{mg}}{1\,\text{kg}}$. Because $60\,\text{mg} = \text{gr}\,1$, the second equivalent fraction is $\dfrac{\text{gr}\,1}{60\,\text{mg}}$.

$$15\,\text{kg} \times \frac{5\,\text{mg}}{\text{kg}} \times \frac{\text{gr}\,1}{60\,\text{mg}} = \text{gr}\,1\frac{1}{4}.$$

So, the dose of this analgesic drug is grains $1\frac{1}{4}$.

Example 12.6

The order reads:

morphine sulfate 0.3 mg IM stat

The recommended dose is 0.01 milligram per kilogram. Is this a safe dose for a child who weighs 31 kilograms?

Again, you want to convert the body weight to a dose in milligrams.

$$31\,\text{kg} \longrightarrow \text{?}\,\text{mg}$$

$$31\,\text{kg} \times \frac{\text{?}\,\text{mg}}{\text{?}\,\text{kg}} = \text{?}\,\text{mg}$$

You cancel the kilograms and obtain the dose in milligrams.

$$31\,\text{kg} \times \frac{0.01\,\text{mg}}{1\,\text{kg}} = 0.31\,\text{mg}$$

So, 0.3 milligram is a safe dose for this child.

Example 12.7

The prescriber ordered 0.37 milligram po of digoxin (Lanoxin). Is this a safe dose for an infant who weighs 15 pounds, and the recommended dose is 0.025 milligram per pound.

You want to convert the body weight to a dose in milligrams.

$$15\,\text{lb} \longrightarrow \text{?}\,\text{mg}$$

$$15\,\text{lb} \times \frac{\text{?}\,\text{mg}}{\text{?}\,\text{lb}} = \text{?}\,\text{mg}$$

You cancel the pounds and obtain the dose in milligrams.

$$15\,\text{lb} \times \frac{0.025\,\text{mg}}{1\,\text{lb}} = 0.375\,\text{mg}$$

Therefore, 0.37 milligram is a safe dose.

Example 12.8

The prescriber ordered:

digoxin 0.012 mg/kg po qd

The child weighs 24 kilograms. Read the label in Figure 12.3. How many milliliters would you prepare.

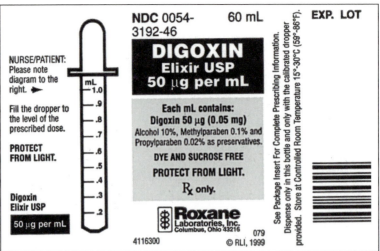

Figure 12.3 Drug label for Digoxin.

(Used with permission of Roxane Laboratories, Inc.)

You want to convert the body weight to a dose in milliliters.

$$24 \, \text{kg} \longrightarrow ? \, \text{mL}$$

$$24 \, \text{kg} \times \frac{? \, \text{mg}}{? \, \text{kg}} \times \frac{? \, \text{mL}}{? \, \text{mg}} = ? \, \text{mL}$$

You cancel the kilograms and milligrams and obtain the dose in milliliters.

$$24 \, \text{kg} \times \frac{0.012 \, \text{mg}}{\text{kg}} \times \frac{1 \, \text{mL}}{0.05 \, \text{mg}} = 5.76 \, \text{mL}$$

So, you would prepare 5.8 milliliters of digoxin.

Example 12.9

The prescriber ordered the antibiotic, cefpodoxime (Vantin) po for a child with a weight of 51 kilograms. The order is 4 milligrams per kilogram. Read the label in Figure 12.4. What would be the dose in milliliters?

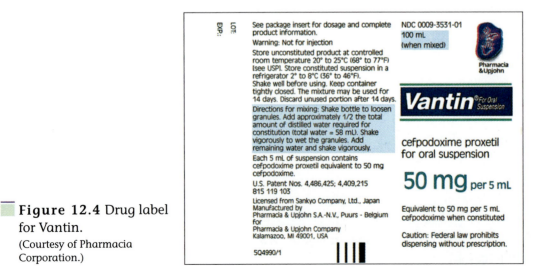

Figure 12.4 Drug label for Vantin.

(Courtesy of Pharmacia Corporation.)

You want to convert the body weight to dose in milliliters.

$$51\,kg \longrightarrow ?\,mL$$

Do this on one line as follows:

$$51\,kg \times \frac{?\,mg}{?\,kg} \times \frac{?\,mL}{?\,mg} = ?\,mL$$

You cancel the kilograms and milligrams and obtain the dose in milliliters.

$$51\,\cancel{kg} \times \frac{4\,\cancel{mg}}{1\,\cancel{kg}} \times \frac{\overset{1}{\cancel{5}}\,mL}{\underset{10}{\cancel{50}}\,\cancel{mg}} = 20.4\,mL$$

So, the prescribed dose is 20.4 milliliters of Vantin.

Example 12.10

The prescriber ordered:

Meclizine HCl 0.83 mg/kg qd po for 5 days

An adolescent weighs 50 kilograms. Read the information on the label in Figure 12.5, and calculate the dose in tablets for this antiemetic drug.

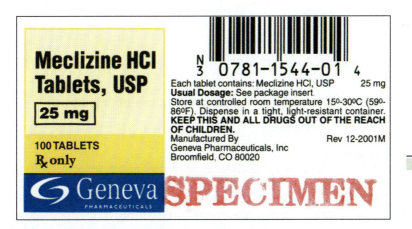

You want to convert the body weight to dose in tablets.

$$55\,kg \longrightarrow ?\,tab$$

Do this on one line as follows:

$$55\,kg \times \frac{?\,mg}{?\,kg} \times \frac{?\,tab}{?\,mg} = ?\,tab$$

The order is 0.83 milligram per kilogram, so the first equivalent fraction is $\frac{0.83\,mg}{1\,kg}$. Because 25 mg = 1 mL, the second equivalent fraction is $\frac{1\,mL}{25\,mg}$.

$$55\,\cancel{kg} \times \frac{0.83\,\cancel{mg}}{1\,\cancel{kg}} \times \frac{1\,tab}{25\,\cancel{mg}} = 1.8\,tabs\ or\ 2\,tabs$$

So, the prescribed dose is 2 tablets of Meclizine.

Calculating Drug Dosages by Body Surface Area

Drug manufacturers often recommend a pediatric dosage based on body surface area (BSA). You have already been introduced to this idea in Chapter 6.

Example 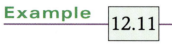 12.11

The prescriber ordered: digoxin $0.72\,mg/m^2$ po stat as a loading dose. The child's BSA is 0.9 square meter. How many milligrams would you administer to this child?

You want to convert the body surface area to a dose in milligrams.

$$0.9\,m^2 \longrightarrow ?\,mg$$

$$0.9\,m^2 \times \frac{?\,mg}{?\,m^2} = ?\,mg$$

Because $0.72\,mg = 1\,m^2$, the equivalent fraction is $\dfrac{0.72\,mg}{1\,m^2}$. You cancel the square meter and obtain the dose in milligrams.

$$0.9\,\cancel{m^2} \times \frac{0.72\,mg}{1\,\cancel{m^2}} = 0.648 \quad or \quad 0.65\,mg$$

So, the child should receive 0.65 milligram of digoxin.

Example 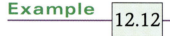 12.12

If a child has a BSA of 0.75 square meter and the medication order is for 2.5 milligrams per square meter of dactinomycin (Cosmegen) IVPB. How many milligrams of this antineoplastic drug should the child receive?

You want to convert the body surface area to a dose in milligrams.

$$0.75\,m^2 \longrightarrow ?\,mg$$

$$0.75\,m^2 \times \frac{?\,mg}{?\,m^2} = ?\,mg$$

Because the order is for $2.5\,mg = 1\,m^2$, the equivalent fraction is $\dfrac{2.5\,mg}{1\,m^2}$. You cancel the square meters and obtain the dose in milligrams.

$$0.75\,\cancel{m^2} \times \frac{2.5\,mg}{1\,\cancel{m^2}} = 1.875\,mg \ or \ 1.9\,mg$$

So, the child should receive 1.9 milligrams of Cosmegen.

BSA Pediatric Nomogram

In Chapter 6, you used the adult nomogram to determine BSA. For children, you can use the pediatric nomogram (Figure 12.6).

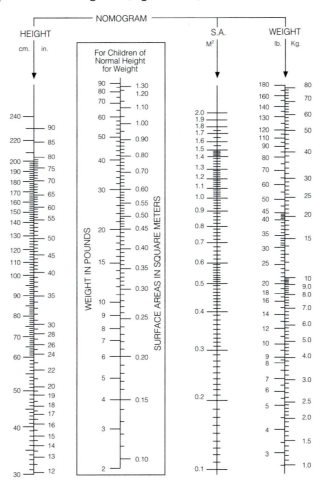

Figure 12.6 Pediatric nomogram for determining BSA.

The body surface area is shown in the column labeled SA in Figure 12.6. A straight line is drawn between the child's height (first column) and the child's weight (last column). The point at which the line crosses the SA column is the estimated *BSA in square meters*. The boxed column listing weight on the left and surface in square meters on the right can be used when a child is of normal height for his or her weight. For additional information concerning a pediatric nomogram, see a pediatric text.

Example 12.13

Estimate the BSA of a child who weighs 40 pounds and is 90 centimeters tall.

Using the nomogram in Figure 12.7, connect the 90 cm mark in the left column and the 40 lb mark in the right column with a straight line. This line crosses the SA column at 0.72 square meter.

So, the child's estimated BSA is 0.72 square meter.

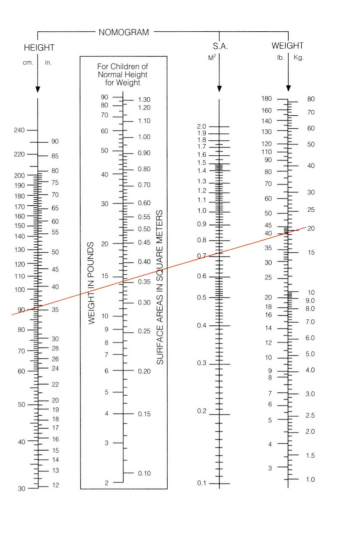

NOMOGRAM

HEIGHT   S.A.   WEIGHT

cm.   in.   M²   lb. │ Kg.

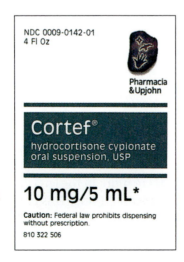

Figure 12.7 Pediatric nomogram for determining BSA for Example 12.13.

Example 12.14

The prescriber has ordered 15 milligrams per square meter of Cortef po. The child weighs 40 kilograms and is 45 inches tall. Read the label in Figure 12.8 and determine how many milliliters this child should receive.

NDC 0009-0142-01
4 Fl Oz

Pharmacia
&Upjohn

Cortef®
hydrocortisone cypionate
oral suspension, USP

10 mg/5 mL*

Caution: Federal law prohibits dispensing without prescription.

810 322 506

Figure 12.8 Drug label for Cortef.
(Courtesy of Pharmacia Corporation.)

You want to find the body surface area and convert it to dose in milliliters.

$$\text{BSA} \longrightarrow ?\,\text{mL}$$

$$\text{m}^2 \times \frac{?\,\text{mg}}{?\,\text{m}^2} \times \frac{?\,\text{mL}}{?\,\text{mg}} = ?\,\text{mL}$$

Using the nomogram, the child has a BSA of approximately 1.16 square meter. The equivalent fraction is $\dfrac{15\,\text{mg}}{1\,\text{m}^2}$. You cancel the square meter and milligrams to obtain the dose in milliliters.

$$1.16\ \cancel{\text{m}^2} \times \frac{15\ \cancel{\text{mg}}}{1\ \cancel{\text{m}^2}} \times \frac{\overset{1}{\cancel{5}}\,\text{mL}}{\underset{2}{\cancel{10}}\ \cancel{\text{mg}}} = 8.7\,\text{mL}$$

So, the child should receive 8.7 milliliters.

Example 12.15

Methylphenidate (Ritalin HCL), a CNS stimulant, has been ordered for a child. How many tablets will you administer to a child who is 50 inches tall and weighs 75 pounds. The order is 10 milligrams per square meter po. Read the label in Figure 12.9, and use the formula to calculate the BSA.

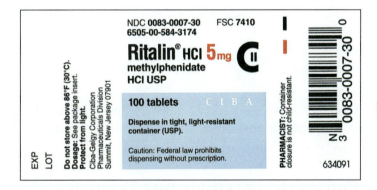

Figure 12.9 Drug label for Ritalin.

(Copyright Novartis Pharmaceuticals Corporation. Reprinted with permission.)

The formulas for calculating pediatric BSA are the same as for adults (see Chapter 6). So, in this problem you use the household formula:

$$\text{BSA} = \sqrt{\frac{\text{Weight} \times \text{Height}}{3131}}$$

$$\text{BSA} = \sqrt{\frac{75 \times 50}{3131}}$$

$$\text{BSA} = \sqrt{1.1977}$$

$$\text{BSA} = 1.09\,\text{m}^2$$

You want to convert body surface area to dose in tablets. According to the formula, the child's BSA is 1.09 square meters.

$$1.09\,\text{m}^2 = ?\,\text{tab}$$

Do this on one line as follows:

$$1.09\,m^2 \times \frac{?\,mg}{?\,m^2} \times \frac{?\,tab}{?\,mg} = ?\,tab$$

$$1.09\,m^2 \times \frac{10\,mg}{m^2} \times \frac{1\,tab}{5\,mg} = 2.18\,tab$$

So, you will administer 2 tablets of Ritalin to the child.

Example 12.16

The prescriber has ordered 250 milligrams po qid of the antiviral drug zidovudine (AZT, Retrovir). Is this a safe dose for a child whose BSA is 1.11 square meter and the recommended dose for the drug is 100 to 180 milligrams per square meter?

You want to convert the body surface area to a dose in milligrams.

$$11.2\,m^2 \longrightarrow ?\,mg$$

First, use the *minimum* recommended dose of 100 milligrams per square meter.

$$1.11\,m^2 \times \frac{100\,mg}{1\,m^2} = 111\,mg$$

Second, use the *maximum* recommended dose of 180 milligrams per square meter.

$$1.11\,m^2 \times \frac{180\,mg}{1\,m^2} = 199.8 \quad or \quad 200\,mg$$

Therefore, any prescribed amount in the range of 111 to 200 milligrams would be acceptable. So, 250 milligrams is *not* a safe dose.

Pediatric Intravenous Dosages

Example 12.17

The prescriber ordered 300 mg/m^2 of Trovan IVPB to infuse in 90 minutes. Read the label in Figure 12.10. Add the Trovan to 100 mL of 5% D/W. How many milliliters per hour would be given to a child who weighs 15 kilograms and is 77 centimeters tall?

Figure 12.10 Drug label for Trovan.

(Registered Trademark of Pfizer Inc. Reproduced with permission.)

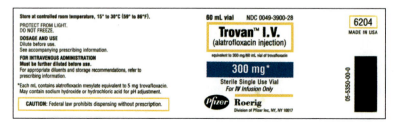

The BSA can be estimated using either the pediatric nomogram or the formula. Using the metric BSA formula yields

$$\text{BSA} = \sqrt{\frac{\text{Weight} \times \text{Height}}{3600}}$$

$$= \sqrt{\frac{15 \times 77}{3600}}$$

$$= \sqrt{0.3208}$$

$$= 0.57 \, \text{m}^2$$

Since the 60 mL vial contains 300 mg of Trovan, when the entire contents of the vial is added to the 100 mL of 5% D/W, the solution formed will be 160 mL with 300 mg of Trovan.

You want to change the BSA of 0.57 m² to milliliters.

$$0.57 \, \cancel{\text{m}^2} \times \frac{\cancel{300 \, \text{mg}}}{\cancel{\text{m}^2}} \times \frac{160 \, \text{mL}}{\cancel{300 \, \text{mg}}} = 91.2 \, \text{mL}$$

The 91.2 mL must infuse in 90 minutes. Now, convert $\dfrac{91.2 \, \text{mL}}{90 \, \text{minutes}}$ to mL/h.

$$\frac{91.2 \, \text{mL}}{90 \, \cancel{\text{min}}} \times \frac{60 \, \cancel{\text{min}}}{1 \, \text{h}} = 60.8 \, \frac{\text{mL}}{\text{h}}$$

So, you would administer 60.8 milliliters per hour of Trovan to the child.

Example 12.18

The prescriber ordered the antibiotic chloramphenicol (Chloromycetin) 250 mg in 100 mL of D/5W IV for a child who weighs 34.6 kilograms. The dose is 0.2 mg/kg/min. The drop factor is 15 drops per milliliter. Calculate the flow rate.

You want to change the weight (34.6 kg) to the flow rate (gtt/min).

$$34.6 \, \cancel{\text{kg}} \times \frac{0.2 \, \cancel{\text{mg}}}{\cancel{\text{kg}} \times \text{min}} \times \frac{\overset{2}{\cancel{100}} \, \cancel{\text{mL}}}{\underset{5}{\cancel{250}} \, \cancel{\text{mg}}} \times \frac{15 \, \text{gtt}}{\cancel{\text{mL}}} = 41.5 \, \frac{\text{gtt}}{\text{min}}$$

So, the flow rate is 42 drops per minute.

Case Study 12.1

A 10-year-old boy is admitted to the hospital with a diagnosis of sickle cell crisis, asthma, and pneumonia. He is complaining of severe pain in his abdomen, back, knees, and elbows; fatigue, and shortness of breath. He has inspiratory and expiratory wheezes and diminished breath sounds. He is 48 inches tall, weighs 58 pounds, and is allergic to peanuts, fish, dogs, and cats. Vital signs are: T 102°; BP 104/74; P 100; R 34. His orders include:

- Bedrest
- Diet as tolerated, encourage po fluids after respirations decrease to 24 respirations per minute
- Fluids 1800 mL/m²/day
- Morphine sulfate 0.2 mg/kg IV q3h
- Aminophylline loading dose: 1 mg/kg/h IV drip for 12 h. Take a blood theophylline level 30 minutes after beginning loading dose. Reduce dose to 0.8 mg/kg/h after 12 h
- Cleocin (clindamycin phosphate) 250 mg IVPB q8h in 30 cc of D/5/W, infuse over 45 minutes
- Tylenol 240 mg po q4h prn temp over 101°
- Proventil (albuterol sulfate) 2 mg po tid
- Folic acid 1000 mcg po od

1. The label on the morphine sulfate reads 10 mg/mL. How many milliliters will you administer?

2. How many milligrams of Aminophylline will the child receive per hour in the loading dose?

3. Aminophylline is available in D/5/0.45% NS labeled 500 mg/500 mL. What rate in milliliters per hour will you set the infusion pump for the second 12 hours?

4. The safe dose range for Cleocin is 20–30 mg/kg/24 h divided q8h. Is the dose ordered within the safe and therapeutic range?

5. The Cleocin is available in a vial labeled 150 mg/mL. How many milliliters will you prepare?

6. Calculate the milliliters per hour that you will need to set the infusion pump to administer the Cleocin.

7. Calculate the child's 24-hour fluid requirement.

8. Folic acid is available in 1 mg tablets. How many tablets will you administer?

9. Proventil is available in 50 cc bottles labeled 2 mg/mL. How many milliliters will you prepare?

10. The physician orders one unit (270 mL) of packed red blood cells to be infused in 4 h. The blood is to infuse at 50 mL/h for the first 30 minutes.

   a. Calculate the flow rate in drops per minute for the first 30 minutes. The drop factor is 10 gtt/mL.

   b. The blood has been infusing without any adverse effects for 30 minutes. Calculate the new rate in milliliters per hour necessary to complete the transfusion within the time frame ordered.

11. The child had a temperature of 102° F. The label on the Tylenol reads 160 mg/5 mL. How many milliliters will you prepare?

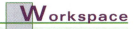
The answers to *Try These for Practice, Exercises,* and *Cumulative Review Exercises* appear in Appendix A at the back of the book. The answers to the *Additional Exercises* can be found on the companion Website or ask your instructor.

Try These for Practice

Test your comprehension after reading this chapter.

1. The following order has been given for a child who weighs 45 kilograms:

   Humulin R insulin 0.14 unit/kg sc bid ac breakfast and dinner

   How many units will this child receive of this insulin in 24 h? _____

2. Read the information on the label in Figure 12.11. What would the prescribed dose in milliliters of zidovudine (Retrovir) be for a patient who weighs 40 pounds. The order is 2.5 milligrams per kilogram? _____

Each 5 mL (1 teaspoonful) contains zidovudine 50 mg and sodium benzoate 0.2% added as a preservative.

See package insert for Dosage and Administration.

Store at 15° to 25°C (59° to 77°F).

GlaxoSmithKline
Research Triangle Park, NC 27709
Made in Canada

4143469   Rev. 11/01

240 mL   NDC 0173-0113-18

gsk **GlaxoSmithKline**

RETROVIR®
(zidovudine)
Syrup

℞ only

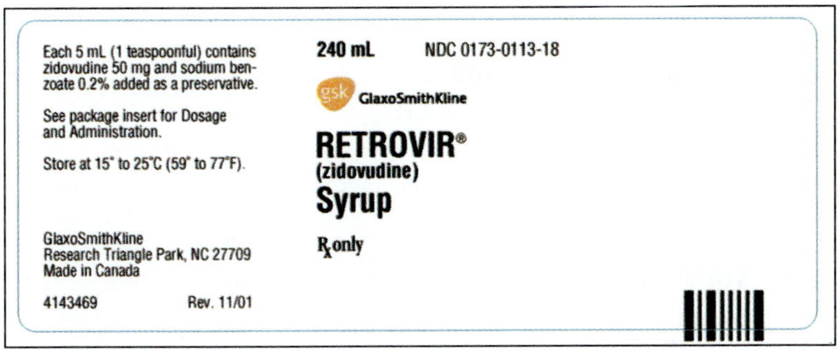

Figure 12.11 Drug label for Retrovir.
(Reproduced with permission of GlaxoSmithKline.)

3. A child must receive meperidine hydrochloride (Demerol). The child's BSA is 0.8 square meter. How many milliliters will you administer to the child if the order is 30 milligrams per square meter IM q3–4h and the label reads 50 milligrams per milliliter? _____

4. Read the information on the label in Figure 12.12. How many milliliters of codeine would you administer to a child who weighs 40 kilograms when the order is 0.3 milligrams per kilogram po q4h.

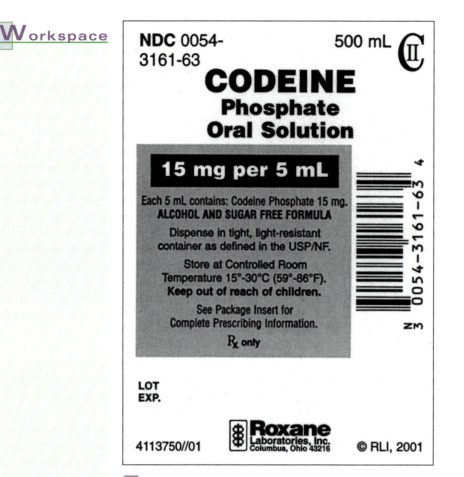

Figure 12.12 Drug label for codeine.
(Used with permission of Roxane Laboratories, Inc.)

5. The order reads: zidovudine $180 \, mg/m^2$ po q6h. The label reads
   $50 \, mg = 5 \, mL$. How many milliliters would you administer to a child
   whose BSA is 0.9 square meter? _____

Exercises

Reinforce your understanding in class or at home.

1. The antiretroviral medication didanosine (Videx) has been prescribed
   for a child with a BSA $0.9 \, m^2$. The order is 100 mg po per m^2 and the
   label reads 240 milliliters contains 2 grams. How many milliliters will
   you administer to the child? _____

2. Physician's order:

   Lamivudine (Epivir) 4 mg/kg po bid

   The label reads 10 mg/mL. How many milliliters will you prepare for
   an infant who weighs 16 pounds? _____

3. Physician's order:

   *Digoxin (Lanoxin) 0.035 mg/kg IV push as a loading dose, divided into
   3 doses in 24 h*

The label reads 0.05 milligrams per milliliter, and the infant weighs 7 pounds. How many milliliters will you prepare for this infant? _____

4. Order:

   Calcitriol (Rocaltrol) 0.04 mg/kg po daily

   The label reads 1 mcg/mL. How many milliliters will you prepare for a child who weighs 35 kg? _____

5. Physician's order:

   Acetazolomide (Diamox) 8 mg/kg IV push q6h

   The label reads 500 mg in 5 mL. How many milliliters will you prepare for a child with acute angle-closure glaucoma who weighs 56 pounds? _____

6. Physician's order:

   Cholera vaccine 0.5 mL IM for 2 doses

   The vial label reads 1.5 mL. How many milliliters will you prepare for each dose? _____

7. The order for hepatitis A vaccine, inactivated (Havrix), is 720 Elisa units (EL. units) sc. The label reads 1440 EL. units/mL. How many milliliters will you prepare? _____

8. The physician ordered 120 mg of guaifenesin po q4h prn. The label reads 100 mg in 5 mL.

   a. How many milliliters will you prepare? _____
   b. If the order is changed to 200 mg how many drams will you prepare? _____

9. The order for Regular insulin is 0.1 units per kilogram IV bolus stat. The child weighs 18 kilograms and the label reads 100 units per milliliter.

   a. How many units will you administer? _____
   b. How many milliliters will you prepare? _____

10. Physician's order:

    Add 100 units of Regular insulin to 100 milliliters of normal saline. Infuse at a rate of 0.1 units per kilogram per hour IV.

    The child weighs 50 pounds; how many milliliters per hour will the child receive? _____

11. Loracarbef (Lorabid) has been prescribed for a 2-year-old child with acute otitis media. The order is 30 milligrams per kilogram po and the child weighs 21 pounds. The oral suspension is labeled 100 milligrams in 5 milliliters. How many milliliters will you give this child in divided doses (q12h)? _____

12. Clarithromycin (Biaxin) 300 milligrams per square meter po has been ordered for a child with a BSA of 0.68 m². The label reads 125 milligrams in 5 milliliters. How many milliliters will you prepare? _____

13. Physician's order:

    Apply 0.025% tretinon (vitamin A acid) solution to affected skin once daily at hour of sleep.

    How many milligrams of vitamin A are in 4 milliliters of solution? _____

14. The BSA of a child is 0.5 m² and the order is 400 mg/m² of Augmentin po. The label reads 250 mg in 5 mL. How many milliliters will you prepare for this child? _____

15. The normal dose range for erythromycin, an antibiotic, is 30–50 mg/kg po in divided doses q6h. The physician ordered 250 mg po q6h for a child who weighs 30 kg. Is this a safe dose for this child? _____

16. Prescriber's order:

    Cefoxitin (Mefoxin) 35 mg/kg IVPB 60 minutes before surgery. The postoperative order is 35 mg/kg q6h for 24 h

    The child weighs 35 kg. What is the total amount in grams that the child will receive preoperatively and postoperatively? _____

17. Order:

    150 mg cefpodoxime (Vantin) po q12h

    The label reads 50 mg/5 mL. How many milliliters will you prepare? _____

18. The prescriber ordered 1.0 gram of ceftriaxone (Rocephin) IVPB stat. The label on the vial reads 1 g in 10 mL of D/5/W. Add to 90 mL D/5/W. Infuse total amount in 30 minutes. Calculate the amount in microdrops per minute. _____

19. Physician's order:

    Vancomycin (Vancocin hcL) 200 mg po q6h

    Read the information on the label in Figure 12.13. How many milliliters will you give the child? _____

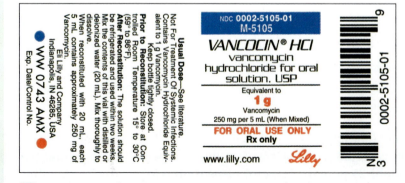

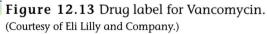

Figure 12.13 Drug label for Vancomycin.
(Courtesy of Eli Lilly and Company.)

20. Ampicillin 25 mg/kg po qid has been prescribed for a child who weighs 42 pounds. The label reads 250 mg = 5 mL. Calculate the dose for this child. _____

Additional Exercises

Now, on your own, test yourself! The answers to the *Additional Exercises* can be found on the companion Website or ask your instructor.

1. Read the first order in the medication administration record shown in Figure 12.14. The label reads 25 milligrams per 5 milliliters. How many teaspoons will you administer? _____

2. Read the second order in the MAR shown in Figure 12.14. The label on the bottle of Tylenol reads 125 mg in 5 mL. How many milliliters will you administer to this patient? _____

✚ GENERAL HOSPITAL ✚

Year 2003	Month 11		Day	24	25	26			
Medication Dosage and Interval				Initials* and Hours	Initials and Hours	Initials and Hours	Initials and Hours	Initials and Hours	Initials and Hours
Date started: 11/24/03 Vistaril 0.025 g qid PO		I		JO	JO	JO			
		AM		10	10	10			
		I		LD LD LD	LD LD LD	LD LD LD			
Discontinued: 11/30/03		PM		2 6 10	2 6 10	2 6 10			
Date started: 11/24/03 Tylenol 125 mg po q4h prn		I		JO	AG JO	AG JO			
		AM		10	1 9	7 11			
		I		JO LD	JO LD LD	LD LD			
Discontinued: 11/30/03		PM		2 8	2 6 10	3 12			
Date started: 11/24/03 Keflex 6.25 mg/kg po qid		I		JO	JO	JO			
		AM		10	10	10			
		I		LD LD LD	LD LD LD	LD LD LD			
Discontinued: 11/30/03		PM		2 6 10	2 6 10	2 6 10			

Allergies: (Specify)

PATIENT IDENTIFICATION

Init*	Signature
JO	June Olsen RN
LD	Larissa Dingman RN
AG	Anthony Giangrasso RN

0312578
Mary Johnson
2183 Avantlar Ave
Phoenix, AZ
85031

Leon Ablon, M.D.

11/24/03

6/21/89
Prot
Aetna

MEDICATION ADMINISTRATION RECORD

Figure 12.14 Medication administration record.

3. Read the third order in Figure 12.14. The child weighs 40 kilograms. How many milliliters of Keflex will you give the child if the label reads 125 milligrams per 5 milliliters? _____

4. The prescriber has ordered 3.3 micrograms per kilogram IM of fentanyl citrate (Sublimaze) as a preoperative medication. The label on the vial reads 50 micrograms per milliliter. How many milliliters will you administer to this child whose weight is 30 kilograms?

_____

5. The normal dose of a drug for a child is 0.3 milligram per square meter. If the child's BSA is 0.6 square meter, how many milligrams should this child receive? _____

6. A child's BSA is 0.93 square meters, and 100 milligrams per square meter of the antineoplastic drug procarbazine HCl (Matulane) has been ordered po. How many milligrams should this child receive?

_____

7. A child's BSA is 1.1 square meters. How many milligrams of the antibiotic gentamicin sulfate (Garamycin) should this child receive if the prescribed amount is 45 milligrams per square meter po? _____

8. A long-acting anti-inflammatory medication, dexamethasone (Decadron), has been ordered for a child with a BSA of 1.04 square meters po. How many milligrams should this child receive if the prescribed amount is 50 milligrams per square meter? _____

9. The anticholinergic medication, scopolamine (Triptone), has been ordered IM for a child with a BSA of 0.8 square meter. How many milliliters will you prepare if the order is for 0.2 milligram per square meter and the ampule reads 0.2 milligram per milliliter?

_____

10. Atropine sulfate has been ordered for a child who weighs 35 kilograms. The prescribed dose is 0.01 milligram per kilogram IM. Read the medication label in Figure 12.15. How many milliliters equal the prescribed dose? _____

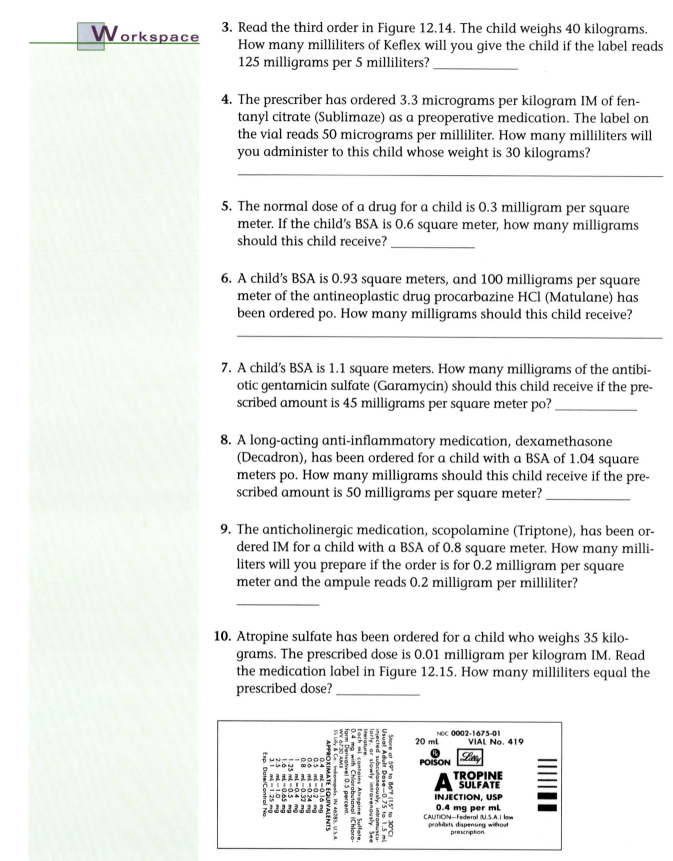

Figure 12.15 Drug label for atropine sulfate.
(Courtesy of Eli Lilly and Company.)

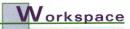

11. The anticonvulsant medication, phenytoin sodium (Dilantin), is ordered po for a child with a BSA of 1.25 square meters. The prescribed dose is 250 milligrams per square meter. How many milliliters should this child receive if the oral suspension is 125 milligrams per milliliter? _____

12. The order states that a child is to receive 1% lidocaine 0.5 mg/kg IV bolus. How many milliliters will you prepare for this child whose weight is 45 kilograms? _____

13. The prescriber orders 0.54 unit per kilogram of NPH insulin (Humulin N) sc. The child weighs 44 kilograms, how many milliliters will you prepare of the insulin in Figure 12.16. _____

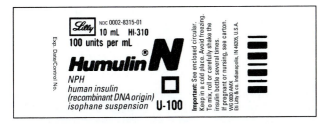

Figure 12.16 Drug label for Humulin N insulin.
(Courtesy of Eli Lilly and Company.)

14. The prescriber ordered Lasix 2 mg/kg po stat. If the child weighs 42 kilograms and the label reads 10 milligrams per milliliter, how many milliliters will you give to the child? _____

15. A 10-year-old child has a fever of 101° F, and 0.4 gram po of the antipyretic acetaminophen (Tylenol) has been ordered. If the elixir is labeled 160 milligrams per 5 milliliters, how many teaspoons will you give to the child? _____

16. A child has to receive an IV bolus of 2% lidocaine, 1 milligram per kilogram. How many milliliters will you prepare for a child with a weight of 50 kilograms? _____

17. Read the information on the label in Figure 12.17. The prescriber has ordered Terramycin IM for a child. The child weighs 42 kilograms and the prescribed dose is 1.2 milligrams per kilogram. How many milliliters will you administer to this child? _____

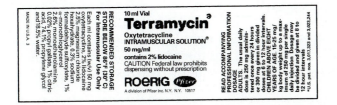

Figure 12.17 Drug label for Terramycin.
(Registered Trademark of Pfizer Inc. Reproduced with permission.)

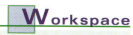

18. The prescriber has ordered a stat dose of the gastrointestinal stimulant, metoclopramide HCl (Reglan), IV 0.1 milligram per kilogram direct IV push. If the vial is labeled 5 milligrams per milliliter and the child weighs 38 kilograms, how many milliliters will you prepare?

_____

19. Meperidine HCl (Demerol) has been prescribed for a child whose weight is 75 pounds. The label on the vial reads 100 milligrams per milliliter. How many milliliters would you prepare of this narcotic analgesic if the prescribed amount is 1.04 milligrams per kilogram?

_____

20. A child must receive the antineoplastic drug melphalan (Alkeran) po × 1. The scored tablets are 2 milligrams each. What would be the correct dose if the order is 3 milligrams per square meter and the child's BSA is 1.02 square meters? _____

CUMULATIVE REVIEW EXERCISES

Review your mastery of earlier chapters.

1. How many milligrams po of ethambutol HCl (Myambutal), an antitubercular drug, would you administer if the prescribed dose is 15 milligrams per kilogram and the child weighs 35 kilograms?

_____

2. How many units of Regular insulin sc would you prepare for a child who weighs 30 kilograms if the order is 1 unit per kilogram? _____

3. The order reads:

Cefixime 8 mg/kg q8h po

a. How many milligrams of this antibiotic would you administer to a child whose weight is 25 kilograms?

b. Each tablet contains 0.2 g _____

c. How many tablets will you administer? _____

4. The order reads:

50 units of Lente insulin sc ac breakfast

The vial is labeled 100 units per milliliter. How many milliliters would you administer to the patient? _____

5. The prescriber has ordered 10 million units of penicillin G IVPB q12h. The 20-million-unit vial of powder has these instructions: add 40 mL of sterile water. How many milliliters equal 10,000,000 units?

_____

6. The order is for 0.3 gram of Ranitidine po. Read the label in Figure 12.18. How many capsules equal the prescribed dose? _____

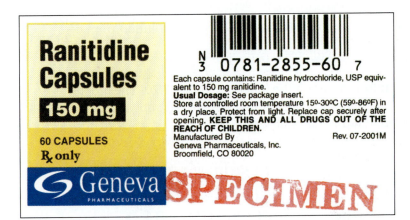

Figure 12.18 Drug label for Ranitidine.
(Courtesy of Geneva Pharmaceuticals.)

7. The order reads:

   Amrinone lactate 0.75 mg/kg IV bolus

   How many milligrams will you prepare of this inotropic drug if the patient weighs 180 pounds? _____

8. The prescriber ordered 900 mL of 5% D/W IV in 5 h. Calculate the flow rate in drops per minute when the drop factor is 20 drops per milliliter. _____

9. The order reads:

   Cimetidine 300 mg IV in 50 mL of 5% D/W. Infuse in 20 minutes.

   Calculate the flow rate in milliliters per minute for this histamine 2 receptor antagonist drug. _____

10. The prescriber ordered 1000 mL 5% D/W at 17 gtt/min IV. The infusion began at 9:00 P.M. At what time will this solution be completed? The drop factor is 15 drops per milliliter. _____

11. 0.002 g = gr _____

12. Read the information on the label in Figure 12.19. How many tablets of Naproxen would you administer po to an adult with a BSA of 1.9 square meters if the order is 200 milligrams per square meter? _____

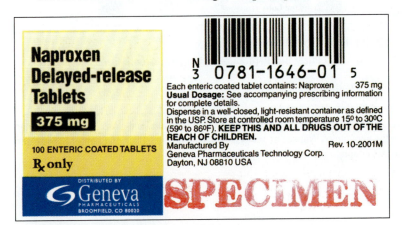

Figure 12.19 Drug label for Naproxen.
(Courtesy of Geneva Pharmaceuticals.)

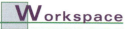

13. Describe how to prepare 100 milliliters of a $\frac{1}{3}$ solution from a $\frac{1}{2}$ solution. _____

14. Read the information on the label in Figure 12.20. The order is 0.04 gram of verapamil po. How many tablets will you administer of this calcium channel blocker drug? _____

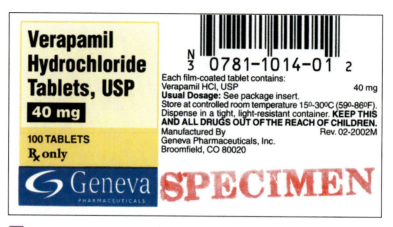

Figure 12.20 Drug label for Verapamil.
(Courtesy of Geneva Pharmaceuticals.)

15. The order for a child with a BSA of 1.2 square meters reads: Zithromax 175 mg/m² po. Read the label in Figure 12.21 and determine how many milliliters the child will receive. _____

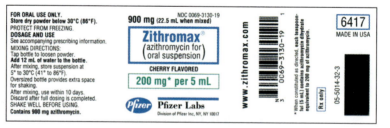

Figure 12.21 Drug label for Zithromax.
(Registered Trademark of Pfizer Inc. Reproduced with permission.)

Additional questions, web links, matching exercises, fill-in-the-blanks, and glossary for this chapter can be found on the companion Website at www.prenhall.com/olsen. Click on Chapter 12 to select the activities for this chapter.

Comprehensive
Self-Tests

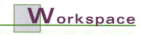

Answers to *Comprehensive Self-Tests* 1–7 can be found in Appendix A at the back of the book.

Comprehensive Self-Test 1

1. Order: Fluoxetine HCl (Prozac), an antipsychotic drug, 40 mg daily (qd) po. Read the information on the label in Figure S.1. How many grams would be contained in 500 pulvules?

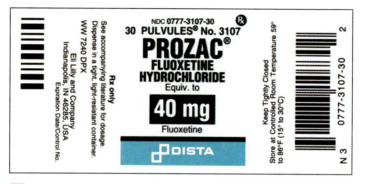

Figure S.1 Drug label for Prozac.
(Courtesy of Eli Lilly and Company.)

2. Using the information in Figure S.2, calculate the number of grams of Naproxen in 1 tablet.

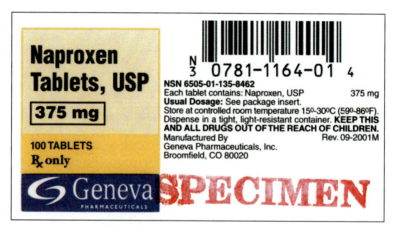

Figure S.2 Drug label for Naproxen.
(Courtesy of Geneva Pharmaceuticals.)

3. Look at the label in Figure S.3. How many micrograms of Fentanyl are contained in 1 milliliter?

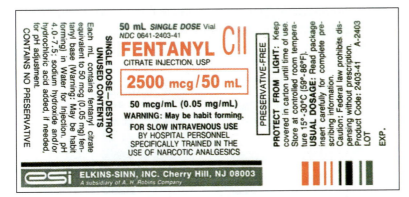

Workspace

Figure S.3 Drug label for Fentanyl.

(Courtesy of ESI Lederle, a Business Unit of Wyeth Pharmaceuticals, Philadelphia, PA.)

4. Order: cimetidine (Tagamet) 0.8 g bid po. Read the label in Figure S.4. How many milligrams of this drug will the patient receive in one day?

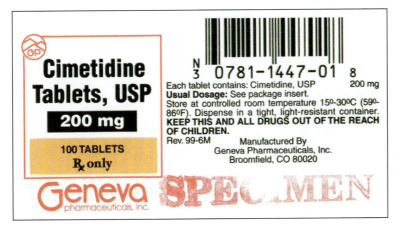

Figure S.4 Drug label for cimetidine.

(Courtesy of Geneva Pharmaceuticals.)

5. The prescriber ordered desipramine HCl (Norpramin) 0.15 g bid po. Read the label in Figure S.5 and determine the number of tablets you will prepare for your patient.

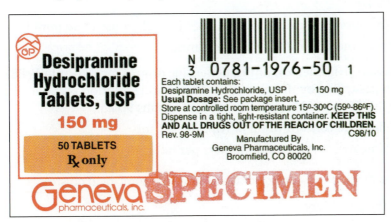

Figure S.5 Drug label for desipramine.

(Courtesy of Geneva Pharmaceuticals.)

6. The order for trovafloxacin (Trovan), an antibiotic, is 600 mg bid po. Read the label in Figure S.6 and calculate the number of tablets you will give your patient.

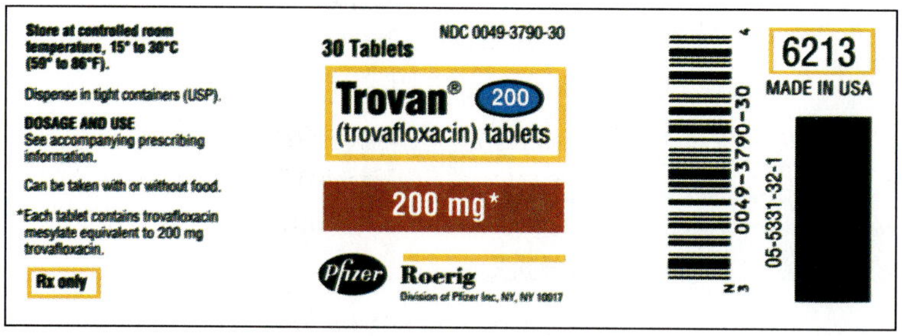

Store at controlled room temperature, 15° to 30°C (59° to 86°F).

Dispense in tight containers (USP).

DOSAGE AND USE
See accompanying prescribing information.

Can be taken with or without food.

*Each tablet contains trovafloxacin mesylate equivalent to 200 mg trovafloxacin.

Rx only

NDC 0049-3790-30

30 Tablets

Trovan® 200
(trovafloxacin) tablets

200 mg*

Pfizer **Roerig**
Division of Pfizer Inc, NY, NY 10017

6213
MADE IN USA

0049-3790-30
05-5331-32-1

Figure S.6 Drug label for Trovan.
(Reg. Trademark of Pfizer Inc. Reproduced with permission.)

7. Order: Dexamethasone 1.5 mg po for 5 days. Read the label in Figure S.7. How many milliliters will you administer each day?

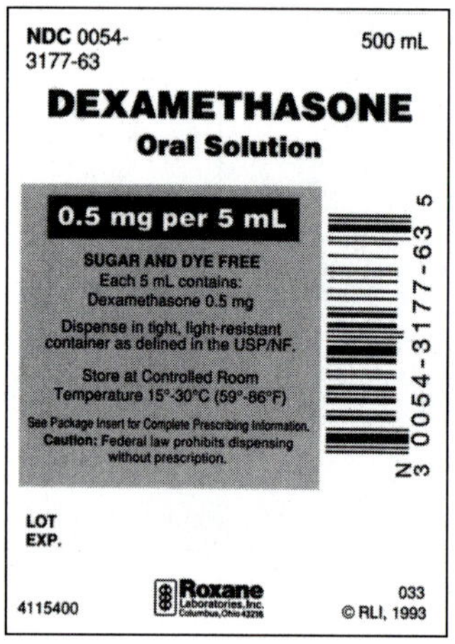

NDC 0054-3177-63

500 mL

DEXAMETHASONE
Oral Solution

0.5 mg per 5 mL

SUGAR AND DYE FREE
Each 5 mL contains:
Dexamethasone 0.5 mg

Dispense in tight, light-resistant container as defined in the USP/NF.

Store at Controlled Room Temperature 15°-30°C (59°-86°F)

See Package Insert for Complete Prescribing Information.
Caution: Federal law prohibits dispensing without prescription.

0054-3177-63

LOT
EXP.

4115400

Roxane
Laboratories, Inc.
Columbus, Ohio 43228

033
© RLI, 1993

Figure S.7 Drug label for dexamethasone.
(Used with permission of Roxane Laboratories, Inc.)

8. Order: Desmopressin acetate (Stimate), a posterior pituitary hormone, 0.3 mcg/kg IVPB. The label reads 4 mcg/mL and the patient weighs 90 kg:

   a. Add the appropriate dose to 50 mL 0.9% NaCl; infuse in 30 minutes.

   b. Calculate the flow rate in milliliter/minute.

9. Nitroprusside (Nipride), an antihypertensive drug, 4 mcg/kg/min IVPB has been prescribed by the physician. The Nipride solution is 250 mL D/5/W with 50 mg of Nipride. The patient weighs 90 kg:

   a. Calculate the concentration of Nipride in 1 mL.

   b. Calculate the flow rate in milliliters per hour.

10. Prepare 400 mL of $\frac{1}{2}$% boric acid solution from boric acid crystals.

   Explain the procedure.

11. A client has an order for glipizide 0.01 g po qd ac breakfast. Each tablet contains 5 mg. How many tablets will you administer?

12. The prescriber ordered ibutilide fumarate (Corvert) 0.01 mg/kg IVPB in 50 mL of 0.9% NaCl; infuse in 10 min. The label reads 1 mg/10 mL.

The patient weighs 130 pounds:

a. How many milliliters of Corvert will you need?

b. Calculate the flow rate in milliliters per minute.

Read the information on the physician's order sheet in Figure S.8 to answer questions 13 through 22.

Utopia General Hospital
Vermont

PRESS HARD WITH BALLPOINT PEN. WRITE DATE AND TIME AND SIGN EACH ORDER.

Date Time AM/PM 5/5/03 10:00 AM	IMPRINT Jones, Allan 5/5/03	
BRP, Ambulate prn	22 Cigar Lane Episcopalian	
Low-sodium diet	Underhill, VT BCBS	
CBC & Electrolytes (fasting)	05489 7/28/46	
Cardura 6 mg daily po		
	A. Giangrasso, MD	
Bumex 2 mg daily po	**ORDERS NOTED**	
K-Tab 20 mEq daily po	DATE 5/5/03 TIME 10:30 AM/PM	
Norvasc 10 mg daily po	☒ MEDEX ☐ KARDEX NURSE'S SIG. *D. Shrimpton RN*	
Signature *A. Giangrasso* MD	FILLED BY DATE Jason Orr 5/5/03	
DATE TIME AM/PM 5/5/03 10.00 AM	IMPRINT	
Tylenol 1g q4h po for fever >39.2°C		
Digoxin 0.125 mg daily po		
Trovan 400 mg BID po		
Elavil 50 mg qhs po		
Glucotrol XL 5 mg po ac breakfast qday		
Feldene 40 mg po daily in AM	**ORDERS NOTED**	
	DATE 5/5/03 TIME 10:30 AM/PM	
	☒ MEDEX ☐ KARDEX NURSE'S SIG. *D. Shrimpton RN*	
Signature *A. Giangrasso* MD	FILLED BY DATE Jason Orr 5/5/03	
DATE TIME AM/PM 5/9/03 10.00 AM	IMPRINT	
Discontinue Trovan, give 600 mg Zithromax po stat and BID for 4 days		
	ORDERS NOTED	
	DATE 5/9/03 TIME 10:30 AM/PM	
	☒ MEDEX ☐ KARDEX NURSE'S SIG. *D. Shrimpton RN*	
Signature *A. Giangrasso* MD	FILLED BY DATE Jason Orr 5/9/03	

Figure S.8 Physician's order sheet.

13. a. Mr. Jones is to receive seven medications daily qd in the morning. Identify each medication and its dose.

b. Name the medication that will be given BID.

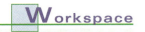

14. a. Which medication is to be administered after a stat dose for 4 days?

   b. The label for the Zithromax reads 5 mL = 200 mg. How many milliliters will you give your patient?

15. Read the label in Figure S.9. How many milligrams of potassium chloride will you administer?

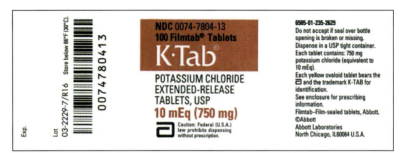

Figure S.9 Drug label for potassium chloride.
(Reproduced with permission of Abbott Laboratories.)

16. How many micrograms of Glucotrol X L will you administer?

17. The label reads 200 mg per tablet of Trovan. Calculate the number of tablets you will give your patient.

18. The label for piroxicam (Feldene) reads 40 mg per capsule. How many capsules will you give your patient?

19. Change the order for Digoxin to micrograms.

20. Which medication is to be given at the hour of sleep?

21. The patient received Bumex daily for 7 days. How many grams did the patient receive in 7 days?

22. Cardura is available in the following strengths: 2 mg, 4 mg, 8 mg. Which tablets would be the most appropriate to use?

23. The physician ordered cisplatin (Platinol) 0.15 mg/kg IV. The cisplatin label reads 1 mg/mL and the patient weighs 95 pounds.

   a. How many grams of Platinol will you prepare for the patient?

   b. Add the correct amount of Platinol to 500 mL of 0.225% NS and calculate the flow rate in milliliters per hour. Infuse in 6 hours.

24. The prescriber ordered 0.3 mg/kg of amphotericin B in 250 mL D/5/W IVPB, to infuse over a 6-hour period. The label on the drug reads 50 mg in 10 mL, and the patient weighs 74 kg.

   a. How many milliliters of amphotericin B will you add to the 250 mL of D5W?

   b. Set the flow rate on the infusion pump in milliliters per hour.

25. Physician's order:

   midazolam HCl (Versed) 0.08 mg/kg IM 60 min before surgery

   The label on the vial reads: 5 mg/mL. How many milliliters will you prepare for a patient who weighs 220 pounds?

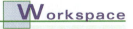

1. Loratadine (Claritin) 0.01 g po q8h has been prescribed for a client. Each milliliter contains 1 mg. How many milliliters contain 0.01 gram?

2. The prescriber ordered 0.04 gram of the antiulcer drug, esomeprazole magnesium (Nexium) po. Each capsule contains 20 milligrams. How many capsules contain the prescribed dose?

3. Order:

   Digoxin 250 mcg po stat

   Each tablet is labeled 0.125 mg. How many tablets will you prepare?

4. Zidovudine (Retrovir), an antiviral drug, 0.3 gram q6h po has been prescribed for a patient with HIV. Each capsule contains 100 mg.

   a. How many capsules will you administer?

   b. How many capsules of Retrovir will you need for 30 days.

5. The prescriber has changed a daily dose of fluoxetine (Prozac), 20 mg po to a weekly dose of 0.09 gram. How many milligrams will the patient now receive each week?

6. Raloxifene (Evista), a drug used to treat postmenopausal osteoporosis, has been prescribed for your client. Each tablet contains 60 milligrams. The order is for 60,000 micrograms po qd. How many tablets will you prepare?

7. Prescriber's order:

   Cimetidine (Tagamet) 0.8 gram ac meals po.

   Read the information on the label in Figure S.10 and calculate the number of tablets you should prepare.

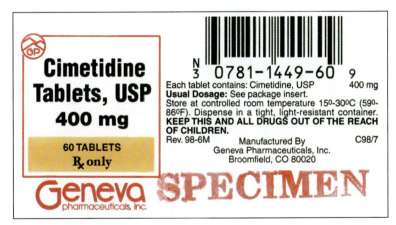

Figure S.10 Drug label for cimetidine.
(Courtesy of Geneva Pharmaceuticals.)

8. Cefoxitin sodium (Mefoxin) 2 gram IVPB has been prescribed. The label reads: Add 20 milliliters of D/5/W to vial and further dilute to a total of 100 mL. Infuse in 2 hours. Set the rate on the infusion pump in milliliters per hour.

9. Aredia, an antihypercalcemic drug, 90 mg IVPB has been ordered for your patient. Instructions are: dilute 90 mg of the drug with 10 mL of

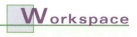

sterile water and add total volume to 1000 mL of 0.45% normal saline. Infuse in 24 hours. Calculate the flow rate in milliliters per hour.

10. How many milligrams of Phospholine Iodide are contained in 3 milliliters of a 0.03% opthalmic solution?

11. The physician writes an order for 50 mcg of zinc sulfate added to a TPN solution. The vial reads 20 mcg/mL. How many milliliters will you prepare?

12. Ritodrine HCL (Yutopar), a medication used to inhibit uterine contractions 0.05 mg/min IVPB is prescribed. The label reads 150 mg/500 mL D/5/W. How many milliliters per minute will this patient receive?

13. Prescriber's order:

    Erythrocin 500 mg IVPB q6h for 3 days

    Directions: Add 2 mL of sterile normal saline to 500-mg vial, further dilute with 200 mL of normal saline (NaCl). Infuse in one hour. The drop factor is 20 gtt/mL. What is the flow rate in drops per minute?

14. The physician changed the order in Exercise 13 to 20 mg/kg of Erythrocin. The patient weighs 110 pounds. How many milligrams of Erythrocin will you prepare for this patient?

15. An order for Streptomycin 12 mg/kg IM has been written for a patient, who weighs 94 pounds. Read the information on the label in Figure S.11. How many milliliters will you administer to your patient?

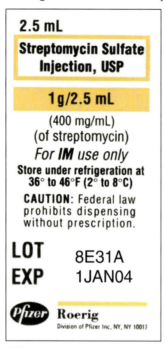

Figure S.11 Drug label for Streptomycin.
(Registered Trademark of Pfizer Inc. Reproduced with permission.)

16. Prescriber's order:

    Cefonicid (Monocid) 1 g IVPB 30 minutes prior to dental surgery

    The vial is labeled 1 g in 100 mL. Infuse in 15 minutes. How many milliliters per minute will the patient receive?

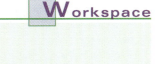

17. Prescriber's order:

> *Ciprofloxacin (Cipro) 800 mg IVPB in 200 mL D5W, infuse in 60 min.*

Calculate the flow rate in milliliters per minute.

18. Order:

> *Acyclovir (Zovirax) 500 mg IVPB q8h*

Directions: Add 9.7 mL to vial; 1 mL = 50 mg. How many milliliters will you prepare for this patient?

Questions 19 through 25 refer to the medication administration record (MAR) in Figure S.12 and to the drug labels in Figure S.13.

UTOPIA GENERAL HOSPITAL

**DAILY MEDICATION
ADMINISTRATION RECORD**

IMPRINT	
Mason Smith	9/1/03
35 Hillcrest Lane	4/23/33
Jericho, VT	Baptist
75098	Oxford
Dr. John Lindsey	

PATIENT NAME **Mason Smith**
ROOM #   42A
ALLERGIC TO (RECORD IN RED):   *NKDA*

DATES GIVEN

Order Date	Initials	Exp Date	MEDICATION, DOSAGE FREQUENCY, & ROUTE	HOURS	9/ 1	9/ 2	9/ 3	9/ 4	9/ 5	9/ 6	9/ 7	9/ 8	9/ 9	9/ 10
9/1		9/5	*Trovan 300 mg in 60 mL D/5/W q8h IVPB*	6am	JO	JO	JO	JO	JO	/	/	/	/	/
				2am	CP	CP	CP	CP	CP	/	/	/	/	/
				10am	JO	JO	JO	JO	JO	/	/	/	/	/
9/1		9/5	*Cardura 6 mg/day po*	10am	CP	CP	CP	CP	CP	/	/	/	/	/
9/1		9/7	*Inderal LA 120 mg po qd*	9pm	BS	BS	BS	BS	BS	BS	BS			
9/1		9/7	*Ferous gluconate 2 tab po qd*	10am	CP	CP	CP	CP	CP	CD	CD			
9/1		9/7	*Glucotrol 10 mg po qd*	10am	CP	CP	CP	CP	CP	CD	CD			
9/1		9/2	*Heparin 25,000 units in 250 mL D/5/W IV @ 1,250 units per hour*	6am	JO	JO	/	/	/	/	/	/	/	/
9/1		9/7	*Meclizine 25 mg po q6h prn vertigo*											
9/6		9/13	*Trovan 200 mg po qd*	10am							JO	JO	JO	JO

Initial	Signature
JO	*Joan Ott RN*
BS	*Bradley Sticks RN*
LO	*Larissa Oppie LPN*
CD	*Carly Dingman RN*
CP	*Christina Petagona RN*

Figure S.12 MAR for questions 19 through 25.

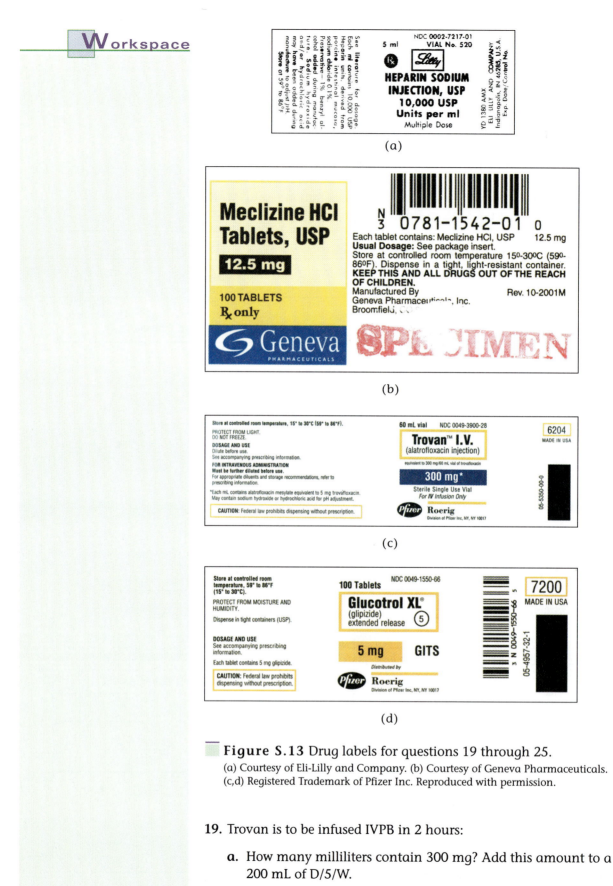

(a)

(b)

(c)

(d)

Figure S.13 Drug labels for questions 19 through 25.

(a) Courtesy of Eli-Lilly and Company. (b) Courtesy of Geneva Pharmaceuticals. (c,d) Registered Trademark of Pfizer Inc. Reproduced with permission.

19. Trovan is to be infused IVPB in 2 hours:

   a. How many milliliters contain 300 mg? Add this amount to a 200 mL of D/5/W.

   b. Calculate the flow rate in milliliters per hour.

20. Read the label for Glucotrol. How many tablets will you administer po?

21. **a.** How many milliliters of heparin will you add to the 250 mL of D/5/W?

  b. Calculate the flow rate in milliliters per hour.

22. How many tablets contain the prescribed dose of Meclizine?

23. How many tablets of ferrous gluconate po will you give the patient in 7 days.

24. How many tablets of Cardura will you give the patient in one day po? Each tablet of Cardura contains 0.002 g.

25. Identify the time for administration of Inderal LA 120 mg.

Comprehensive Self-Test 3

1. The order for Atarax (hydroxyzine HCL) is 15 mg po BID. Read the information on the label in Figure S.14. How many milliliters of Atarax will you give your patient?

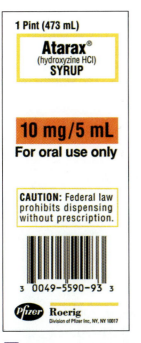

1 Pint (473 mL)

Atarax®
(hydroxyzine HCl)
SYRUP

10 mg/5 mL
For oral use only

CAUTION: Federal law prohibits dispensing without prescription.

3 0049-5590-93 3

Pfizer **Roerig**
Division of Pfizer Inc, NY, NY 10017

Figure S.14 Drug label for Atarax.
(Registered Trademark of Pfizer Inc. Reproduced with permission.)

2. Prepare 60 milligrams of Zantac. Read the information on the label in Figure S.15. How many milliliters contain 60 milligrams?

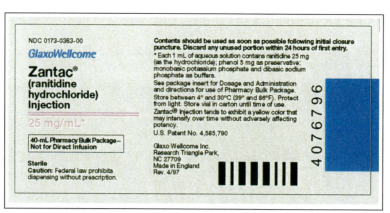

Figure S.15 Drug label for Zantac.
(Reproduced with permission of GlaxoSmithKline.)

3. Prescriber's order:

   Oxacillin 2000 mg in 250 mL of NS IVPB q12h for 5 days. Infuse at 0.28 mg/kg/min. wgt 70 kg

   The vial of oxacillin is labeled 2 g. Calculate the flow rate in micro-drops per minute.

4. The prescriber ordered 500 mg of theophylline (Aminophylline) in 250 mL D/5/W IVPB. The patient is to receive 50 mg/h. Calculate the flow rate in milliliters per hour.

5. An order for penicillin IVPB has been changed to 2,000,000 units per hour. The label reads 20,000,000 units of penicillin in 750 milliliters of D/5/W. Calculate the flow rate in milliliters per hour.

6. Physician's order:

   500 milliliters of NS IV in 2 hours as a fluid challenge

   Calculate the flow rate in microdrops per minute.

7. Prescriber's order:

   Piperacillin 3 g in 100 mL D5W IVPB q8h

   Calculate the flow rate in milliliters per minute. Infuse in 30 minutes.

8. Prepare 200 mL of a 10% boric acid solution from a 50% solution.

9. How many grams of sodium chloride are contained in 2000 mL 0.45% normal saline?

10. Physician's order:

    Floxin 400 mg in 100 mL D5W IVPB q12h. Infuse in 90 minutes.

    The label on the vial reads Floxin 400 mg/10 mL.

    a. How many milliliters of Floxin will you add to the 100 mL D/5/W?

    b. Calculate the flow rate in microdrops per minute.

11. Physician's order:

> *Amoxcillin 300 mg po q8h for 10 days*

The label reads 125 mg/5 mL. How many milliliters will you prepare of this antibiotic for one dose?

12. The anticonvulsant drug valproate sodium (Depakene) 15 mg/kg po qd has been prescribed for your patient, who weighs 60 kg. The drug label reads 200 mg/5 mL. How many milliliters will you prepare?

13. Physician's order:

> *furosemide 0.04 g po BID*

Read the label in Figure S.16. How many milliliters will the patient receive in one day?

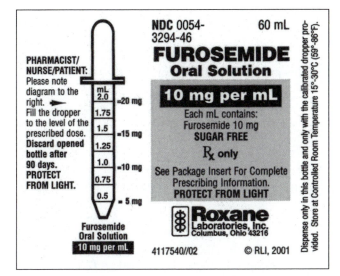

Figure S.16 Drug label for Furosemide.
(Used with permission of Roxane Laboratories Inc.)

14. Physician's order:

> *Talwin 0.02g IV push q3h prn*

The label on the vial reads 30 mg/mL. How many milliliters will you prepare?

15. The antidepressant phenelzine sulfate (Nardil) 60 mg po daily in divided doses has been ordered for your patient. Each tablet contains 15 mg. How many tablets will the patient receive in one day?

16. A child, who weighs 44 pounds, is to receive Motrin 5 mg/kg po. The label reads 100 mg/5 mL. How many milliliters will you give this child?

17. An IV infusion of D/5/W is infusing at a rate of 17 gtt/min. The drop factor is 10 gtt/mL.

a. How many milliliters per hour is the patient receiving?

b. The infusion is completed in $9\frac{1}{2}$ hours. How many milliliters of D/5/W did the patient receive?

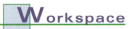

18. The prescriber ordered 0.5 mcg/kg IM of fentanyl citrate (Sublimaze) for a patient who weighs 121 lb. The label reads 50 mcg/mL. How many milliliters will you prepare?

19. Inderal LA 120 mg po qd has been prescribed for your patient. Each capsule is 0.12 g. How many capsules will you give your patient?

20. A patient has an IV of 500 mL D/5/W with 2 g of 1% lidocaine infusing at a flow rate of 20 mL per hour.

    a. What is the concentration of lidocaine in 1 mL?
    b. How many milligrams of lidocaine is the patient receiving per hour?
    c. A volumetric infusion pump is used to administer this solution. How many milligrams of lidocaine is the patient receiving per minute?

21. How would you prepare 2000 mL of a 1% Neosporin solution from 5 g tablets?

22. Tamoxifen 20 mg po qd is ordered for a patient. Each tablet contains gr $\frac{1}{6}$. How many tablets will you give to the patient?

23. Physician's order:

    Kefurox 1.5 g in 50 mL D5W IVPB, infuse in 20 minutes

    Calculate the flow rate; the drop factor is 20 gtts/mL.

24. Change gr $\frac{1}{600}$ to milligrams.

25. The label on the vial of atropine sulfate reads 1.25 mL = 0.5 mg. The client must receive 0.32 mg sc. How many milliliters will you prepare?

Comprehensive Self-Test 4

1. Read the information on the label in Figure S.17. The prescriber ordered Naproxen 275 mg/m^2 po bid. The patient has a BSA of 1.9 m^2. How many tablets will you give the patient?

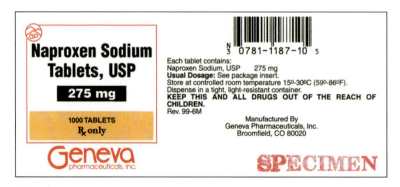

Figure S.17 Drug label for Naproxen.
(Courtesy of Geneva Pharmaceuticals.)

2. Order: Tikosyn 1 mg po q8h. Read the information on the label in Figure S.18. How many capsules will you prepare for the patient?

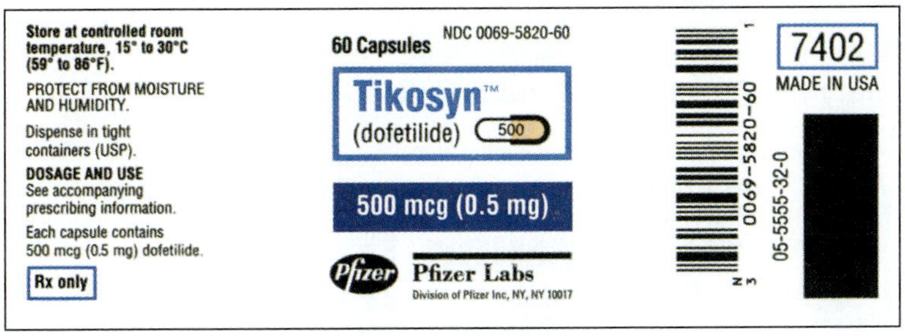

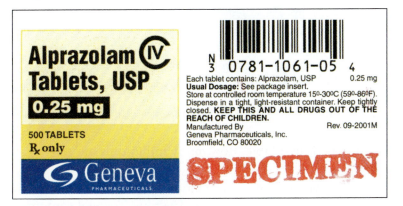

Figure S.18 Drug label for Tikocyn.
(Registered Trademark of Pfizer Inc. Reproduced with permission.)

3. The physician ordered Alprazolam 0.5 mg po q8h prn. Read the information in Figure S.19. How many tablets will you administer to the patient in 24 hours?

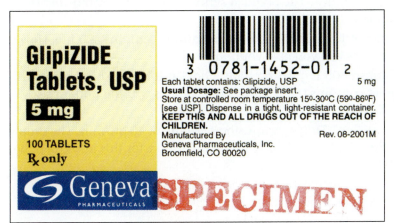

Figure S.19 Drug label for Alprazolam.
(Courtesy of Geneva Pharmaceuticals.)

4. Order: GlipiZIDE 0.01 g po 30 minutes ac breakfast. Read the information on the label in Figure S.20. How many tablets of this drug will you administer?

Figure S.20 Drug label for GlipiZIDE.
(Courtesy of Geneva Pharmaceuticals.)

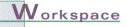
5. The prescriber ordered amiodarone 0.8 g BID po. Each tablet contains 200 mg. How many tablets will you give the patient?

6. Read the label in Figure S.21.
   a. How many milligrams of furosemide in 1 milliliter?
   b. How many milliliters of furosemide in the bottle?

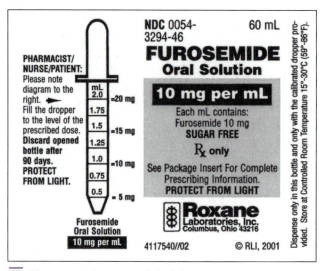

Figure S.21 Drug label for Furosemide.

7. How would you prepare 400 mL of 10% Chlorox solution from a 100% solution?

8. Epinephrine 1:1000 is available. How many milligrams are contained in 2 mL?

9. The prescriber ordered one drop of scopolamine opthalmic solution in the right eye BID. Each milliliter contains 15 drops. The vial contains 2 milliliters and the drug is labeled 0.25% scopolamine.
   a. How many drops are in the vial?
   b. How many days will the vial last?
   c. How many grams of scopolamine are in the vial?

10. Anakinra (Kineret) 0.1 g IM qd has been prescribed for a client with rheumatoid arthritis. The prefilled syringe is labeled 100 mg/mL. How many milliliters will you administer?

11. Order: Tylenol 1.5 g po q8h prn. Each capsule contains 500 mg. How many capsules will you give your patient?

12. Order: Motrin 800 mg q12h po for 5 days prior to onset of menses. Each tablet contains 0.8 g. How many tablets will the patient receive in 5 days?

13. An IV of 1000 mL D/5/W is infusing at a rate of 40 gtt/min. The drop factor is 20 gtt/mL. How many hours will it take for this infusion to be completed?

14. The physician ordered 1800 mg/m² of Cefobid IVPB qd, to infuse in 3 h. The BSA of the patient is 2.2 m². The label on the vial reads 40 mL = 4 g; add to 200 mL D/5/W.
    a. How many milligrams will the patient receive?
    b. Calculate the flow rate in milliliters per hour.

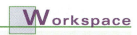

15. Vibramycin 4.4 mg/kg IVPB once a day has been ordered for a child who weighs 80 pounds. The premixed bag of Vibramycin is labeled Vibramycin 200 mg/250 mL D/5/W. Infuse in 4 h.

    a. How many milligrams will the patient receive?

    b. How many milliliters of Vibramycin will the patient receive?

    c. Calculate the flow rate in milliliters per minute.

16. Order: Levofloxacin (Levaquin) 500 mg in 100 mL D/5/W IVPB daily for 14 days. The label reads 0.5 g in 100 mL; infuse in 1 h. Calculate the flow rate in drops per minute; the drop factor is 15 gtt = 1 mL.

17. The physician ordered abciximab (ReoPro) 0.5 mg/kg IVPB to be infused in 12 hours for a patient, who weighs 75 kg. The label reads 2 mg/mL.

    a. How many milligrams will the patient receive?

    b. How many milliliters of ReoPro will you add to 250 mL of normal saline?

    c. Calculate the flow rate in milliliters per hour.

18. 8 tsp = ? oz

19. Your patient must receive grain $\frac{1}{5}$ of morphine sulfate sc stat. Read the label in Figure S.22 and calculate the amount required in milliliters.

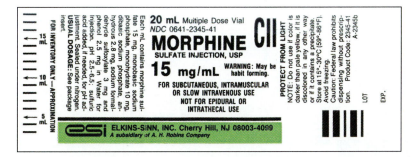

Figure S.22 Drug label for morphine sulfate.

(Courtesy of ESI Lederle, a Business Unit of Wyeth Pharmaceuticals, Philadelphia, PA.)

20. Atenolol is the generic version of Tenormin. The prescriber ordered 100 mg po daily. Read the label in Figure S.23 and calculate the number of tablets you will prepare.

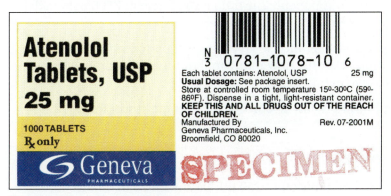

Figure S.23 Drug label for atenolol.

(Courtesy of Geneva Pharmaceuticals.)

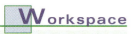
21. The antidepressive drug, amitriptyline (Elavil), 0.025 g po has been ordered by the prescriber. Read the label in Figure S.24 and calculate the number of tablets you will give your patient.

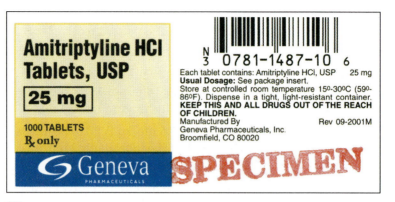

Figure S.24 Drug label for meclizine.
(Courtesy of Geneva Pharmaceuticals.)

22. A patient has an order for 0.6 g of ranitidine po BID for 3 weeks. Read the label in Figure S.25 and calculate the total number of milligrams the patient will receive in 21 days.

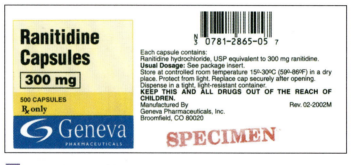

Figure S.25 Drug label for ranitidine.
(Courtesy of Geneva Pharmaceuticals.)

23. The anticoagulant, warfarin (Coumadin) 0.0075 g po qd has been prescribed for your patient. The drug is available in 7500 mcg tablets. How many tablets will you administer?

24. Interferon beta–1a 44 mcg sc TIW has been prescribed for a patient with multiple sclerosis. How many milligrams of this drug will your patient receive in one week?

25. How would you prepare 200 mL of 1/3 strength Isocal from 1/2 strength Isocal?

Comprehensive Self-Test 5

1. A patient has an infusion of 250 mL D5W with 25,000 units of heparin infusing at a flow rate of 20 mL per hour. How many units of heparin per hour is the patient receiving?

2. A patient has an IV of 500 mL D5W with 50,000 units of heparin. The order is 1400 units of heparin per hour. Calculate the flow rate in milliliters per hour.

3. Prescriber's order:

   Melphalan (Alkeran) 16 mg/m² IVPB in 100 mL 0.9% NS q2 weeks for 4 doses. Infuse in 20 minutes.

   The patient's BSA is 1.2 m². Read the information on the labels in Figure S.26.

   a. How many milliliters of diluent will you add to the 50-mg vial?

   b. How many milliliters of Alkeran will you add to 100 mL of 0.9% NS?

   c. Set the flow rate in milliliters per minute of this antineoplastic drug.

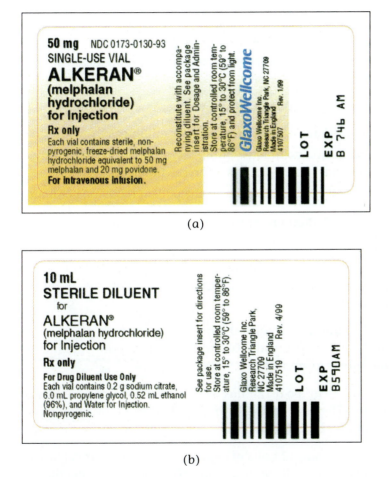

(a)

(b)

■ **Figure S.26a** (a) Drug label for Alkeran, (b) label for sterile diluent. (Reproduced with permission of GlaxoSmithKline.)

4. Order: Protamine sulfate 22 mg IV push in 10 minutes. The label for this heparin antagonist reads 10 mg/mL.

   a. How many milliliters will you prepare?

   b. Add the dose to 25 mL 0.9% NS. At what rate would you set the infusion pump in milliliters per minute?

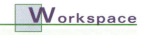

5. A patient is to receive ranitidine (Zantac) 0.05 grams in 100 mL D/5/W IVPB; infuse at a rate of 6.25 mg/h. The label reads 50 mg/ 100 mL. Set the rate on the infusion pump in milliliters per hour.

6. Physician's order:

Ciprofloxacin (Cipro) 0.75 gram po q12h

Each tablet is labeled 250 mg; how many tablets will you administer to the patient per day?

7. Order: Lomefloxacin hydrochloride (Maxaquin) 0.4 g stat. Each tablet contains 400 mg. How many tablets will you administer to your patient?

8. Order: Ofloxacin (Floxin) 600 mg IVPB × 1 dose. The vial is labeled 0.6 g in 100 mL D/5/W; infuse in 90 minutes.

   a. How many grams of Floxin are in 600 mg?

   b. Calculate the flow rate in drops per minute; the drop factor is 10 gtt/mL.

9. A patient has an IV of 500 mL D/5/W with 2 grams of lidocaine.

   a. What is the concentration of lidocaine per milliliter?

   b. The infusion is on a volumetric pump set at 24 mL/h. How many milligrams of lidocaine is the patient receiving per minute?

   c. How many milligrams of lidocaine is the patient receiving per hour?

10. An IV of D/5/NS (1000 mL) is infusing at a rate of 50 mL/h. The infusion started at 1:00 P.M.; at what time will it finish?

11. Order: 500 mL of D/5/W with 50,000 units of heparin IVPB. The patient is to receive 1500 units per hour. Calculate the flow rate in microdrops per minute.

12. Lorabid, an anti-infective drug, 400 mg po q12h has been prescribed for your patient. The label reads 100 mg/5 mL. How many milliliters will you administer to your patient?

13. Lorabid 240 mg per m^2 po q 12h has been ordered for a child who has a BSA of 1.2 m^2. The label reads 200 mg/5 mL. How many milliliters will you administer to the child?

14. Your patient is receiving 12 units of regular insulin per hour IVPB. The solution is labeled 288 units of insulin in 250 mL NS. Calculate the flow rate in milliliters per hour.

15. The physician ordered doxacurium 0.05 mg/kg IVPB 30 minutes before surgery for a patient who weighs 90 kg. The vial reads 1 mg/mL. How many milliliters will you prepare?

16. A child who weighs 40 pounds must have a bronchial lavage procedure. The physician has ordered atracurium besylate (Tracrium) 0.5 mg/kg IV bolus. The vial reads 10 mg/mL. How many milliliters will you prepare?

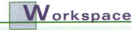

17. Order: Cefazolin (Kefzol) 1 g in 50 mL D/5/W IVPB q6h; infuse in 20 minutes. Read the information on the label in Figure S.27.

    a. How many milliliters of diluent will you add to the vial so that 1 g of Kefzol will be contained in 5 mL of solution?

    b. Calculate the flow rate in milliliters per minute.

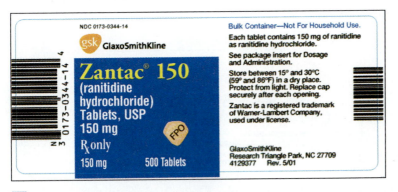

Figure S.27 Drug label for Kefzol.
(Courtesy of Eli Lilly and Company.)

18. A patient is to receive ranitidine HCl (Zantac) 150 mg po BID. Read the information on the label in Figure S.28. How many tablets will the patient receive in 24 hours?

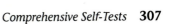

Figure S.28 Drug label for Zantac.
(Reproduced with permission of GlaxoSmithKline.)

19. The order for Zantac has been changed to 0.45 g po qd. Read the information on the label in Figure S.28. How many tablets will you give the patient?

20. Order: The antiparkinsonian drug, trihexyphenidyl hydrochloride (Artane), 3 mg po tid. The label reads 2 mg/5 mL. How many milliliters will you give your patient?

21. The nurse has prepared 7 mg of dexamethasone for IV administration. Read the label in Figure S.29. How many milliliters did she prepare?

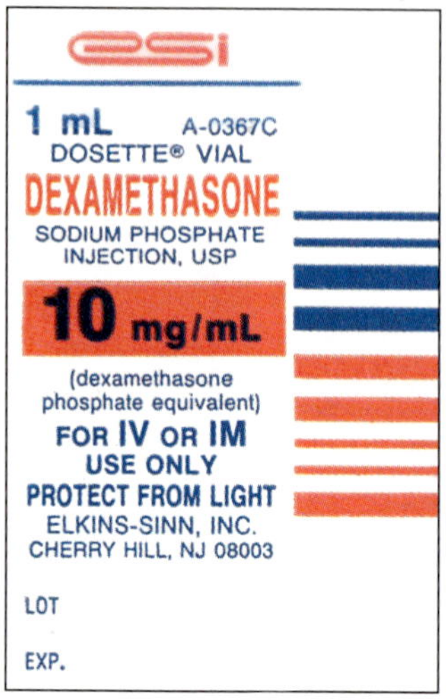

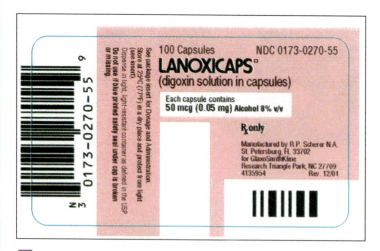

Figure S.29 Drug label for dexamethasone.
(Courtesy of ESI Lederle, a Business Unit of Wyeth Pharmaceuticals, Philadelphia, PA.)

22. The order is for Idamycin 12 mg/m² IVPB; infuse in 15 minutes. The BSA of the patient is 1.2 m². The label reads 1 mg/mL.

a. How many milliliters will you prepare?

b. Calculate the flow rate in milliliters per minute.

23. You need to prepare 0.1 mg of Lanoxin po bid for your patient. Read the information on the label in Figure S.30. How many capsules contain 0.1 mg?

Figure S.30 Drug label for Lanoxin.
(Reproduced with permission of GlaxoSmithKline.)

24. Read the label in Figure S.31. How many grams of Wellbutrin are contained in 3 tablets?

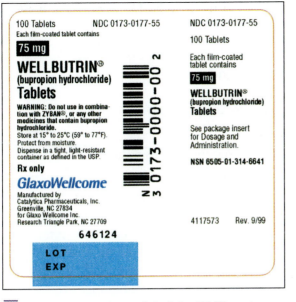

Figure S.31 Drug label for Wellbutrin.
(Reproduced with permission of GlaxoSmithKline.)

25. Read the label in Figure S.32. How many tablets of Avandia contain 8 mg?

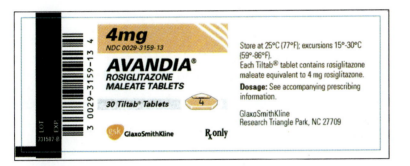

Figure S.32 Drug label for Avandia.
(Reproduced with permission of GlaxoSmithKline.)

Comprehensive Self-Test 6

1. The label reads azithromycin (Zithromax) 200 mg/5 mL. Determine how many milliliters of azithromycin you will give a patient with a BSA of 1.8 m^2. The order is 300 mg per square meter po.

2. The client is to receive 1000 micrograms per m^2 of glucagon IV push for a blood glucose level of 60 (hypoglycemia). The label on the vial reads 1 mg/mL. The BSA of the patient is 1.7 m^2. How many milliliters will you prepare for this patient?

3. The prescriber ordered digoxin 0.2 mg per m^2 po qd for a child who has a BSA of 0.3 m^2. The label on the vial reads 50 μg/mL. How many milliliters will you administer?

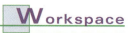

4. The physician ordered 160 mg per m² po q6h of Keflex for a patient who has a BSA of 1.6 m². The bottle reads 125 mg/mL.

   a. How many milligrams of this drug will you prepare?

   b. How many milliliters will you administer?

5. Prepare Rocephin 10 mg/kg IVPB for a patient who weighs 125 pounds. The label reads 2 g/50 mL premixed.

   a. How many milligrams of Rocephin will this patient receive?

   b. How many milliliters will you prepare?

6. The prescriber has ordered 38 milligrams of the antagonist digoxin immune Fab (Digibind) IVPB in 40 mL of sterile water to be infused in 30 minutes. Calculate the flow rate in milliliters per minute.

7. Aminocaproic acid (Amicar) 5 grams in 250 mL of Ringer's Lactate IV has been prescribed for a patient. Infuse in 5 hours. Calculate the flow rate in microdrops per minute.

8. The protease inhibitor Amprenavir (Agenerase) 1200 mg po BID has been prescribed for a client with HIV. Each capsule is labeled 150 mg. How many capsules will you administer?

9. The prescriber ordered acetylcystine (Mucomyst) 150 mg/kg in 200 mL D/5/W IVPB. Infuse in 15 minutes. The patient weighs 200 pounds and the label reads 200 mg/mL.

   a. Calculate the amount of acetylcystine to be added to the D/5/W.

   b. Determine the flow rate in milliliters per minute.

10. Physician's order:

    Vancomycin 1 g in 250 mL D5W IVPB stat, infuse in 90 minutes

    Calculate the flow rate in microdrops per minute.

11. The order for Vancomycin is 500 mg in 250 mL 0.9% NS q6h IVPB. Infuse in 60 minutes. Calculate the flow rate in milliliters per minute.

12. Physician's order:

    Milrinone lactate (Primacor) 50 mcg/kg IV in 10 min IV push. The label reads 200 mcg/mL and the patient weighs 60 kg.

    a. How many milliliters will you administer?

    b. Calculate the flow rate in milliliters per minute.

13. How many grams are equal to the number of milligrams contained in 1 tablet of verapamil hydrochloride shown in Figure S.33.

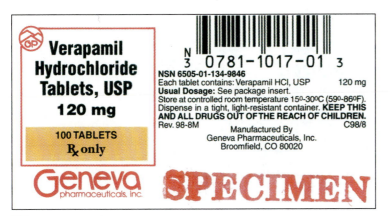

Figure S.33 Drug label for Verapmil.
(Courtesy of Geneva Pharmaceuticals.)

14. Amoxcillin (Amoxil) 8.2 mg/kg po q8h has been prescribed for a patient who weighs 136 pounds. Read the information on the label in Figure S.34. How many tablets will you prepare?

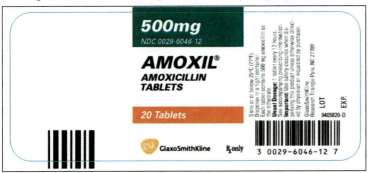

Figure S.34 Drug label for Amoxcillin.
(Reproduced with permission of GlaxoSmithKline.)

15. Order: Enalapril Maleate 20 mg po hs. Read the information on the label in Figure S.35. How many tablets will you give the patient?

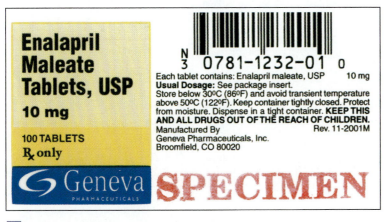

Figure S.35 Drug label for Enalapril.
(Courtesy of Geneva Pharmaceuticals.)

16. Read the information on the label in Figure S.36. Calculate the number of grains in 2 tablets of Prozac.

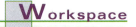
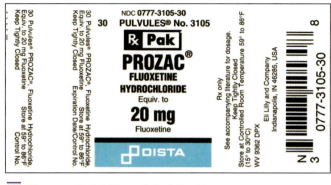

Figure S.36 Drug label for Prozac.
(Courtesy of Eli Lilly and Company.)

Refer to the information in Figure S.37 Medication Administration Record to answer questions 17 through 19.

UTOPIA GENERAL HOSPITAL

IMPRINT
Taylor Keefe   12/4/03
313 Pack St   2/21/46
New Milford, NJ   Baptist
07646   Oxford
D. O'Donavan, MD

**DAILY MEDICATION
ADMINISTRATION RECORD**

PATIENT NAME **Taylor Keefe**
ROOM #   <u>312</u>
ALLERGIC TO (RECORD IN RED): <u>*Cheese*</u>

DATES GIVEN

Order Date	Initials	Exp Date	MEDICATION, DOSAGE FREQUENCY, AND ROUTE	HOURS	12/4	12/5	12/6	12/7	12/8	12/9	12/10
12/4	JJ	12/10	*Zantac 50 mg IVPB in 50 mL D5W q8h, infuse in 20 minutes IVPB*	10am	JJ	JJ	JJ	JJ	MK	MK	MK
				6pm	OT	OT	OT	OT	LR	LR	LR
				2am	LD	LD	LD	LD	CR	CR	CR
12/4	JJ	12/4	*Imitrex 6 mg sc at 10am & 6pm 12/4/03 only*	10am	JJ						
				6pm	OT						
12/4	JJ	12/10	*Regular insulin 24 units sc ac breakfast and 7:30 pm*	7am 7:30 pm	JJ OT	JJ OT	JJ OT	JJ OT	MK LR	MK LR	MK LR
12/4	JJ	12/10	*Sinemet 10/100 BID po*	10am	JJ	JJ	JJ	JJ	MK	MK	MK
				6pm	OT	OT	OT	OT	LR	LR	LR
12/4	JJ	12/10	*Entacapone 200 mg BID po*	10am	JJ	JJ	JJ	JJ	MK	MK	MK
				6pm	OT	OT	OT	OT	LR	LR	LR

Initial	Signature	Title
JJ	*Joan Jok*	RN
MK	*Mike Keefe*	RN
LR	*Lou Rase*	RN
OT	*Olaf Tyson*	LPN
LD	*Lorie Davis*	RN

Figure S.37 MAR for questions 17 through 19.

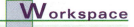

17. **a.** What is the name of the physician?

    b. Which medications are to be administered subcutaneously?

    c. Name the drug(s) that must be administered by mouth.

18. **a.** At what time and what date was the Imitrex given to the patient?

    b. Who administered the Regular insulin at 7:30 P.M. on December 8, 2003?

    c. Identify the drugs given at 10:00 A.M. on December 10, 2003?

    d. How many doses of Entacapone did the patient receive in 4 days?

19. The injectable form of Zantac is labeled 25 mg/mL.

    a. How many milliliters of Zantac will you need?

    b. Calculate the flow rate in milliliters per minute.

20. You are told to infuse 20 milliliters of a solution in 20 minutes. The drop factor is 60 microdrops per milliliter. Determine the flow rate.

21. An infusion of D/5/W has 800 milliliters left in the bag (LIB). The flow rate is 31 drops per minute, and the drop factor is 15 drops per milliliter. How many hours will it take for the remainder of this IV to infuse?

22. Calculate the number of milliliters per hour for an IV of 250 milliliters of D/5/W with 0.5 grams of 1% lidocaine. The order is to administer 2 milligrams per minute.

23. The patient has an order for 25 milligrams IV push of labetalol (Normodyne) in 3 minutes. The vial is labeled 5 milligrams per milliliter. How many milliliters of this antihypertensive drug will the patient receive?

24. The prescriber has ordered 100 milligrams of bretylium tosylate (Bretylate), an adrenergic blocking agent, in 500 milliliters of normal saline solution IVPB. Infuse at a rate of 0.05 milligrams per minute. The total amount of IV solution is 510 milliliters. Calculate the flow rate in milliliters per hour.

25. The patient was admitted to the ER with unstable ventricular tachycardia. The order reads:

    Add 500 mg bretylium tosylate (20 mL) to 50 mL D5W IVPB, infuse at a rate of 0.1 mg/kg/min.

    The patient weighs 220 pounds and the drop factor is 15 gtt/mL.

    a. Calculate the flow rate in drops per minute.

    b. Change the flow rate to milliliters per hour.

Comprehensive Self-Test 7

1. An infant is diagnosed with infectious diarrhea. The prescriber orders neomycin sulfate 25 mg/kg po q6h. The drug is labeled 125 mg/5 mL. How many milliliters will you give this infant who weighs 8 pounds?

2. A child has a urinary tract infection and is to receive Amoxicillin 10 mg/kg po q8h. The label on the vial reads 125 mg/5 mL. How many milliliters will you prepare for this child who weighs 44 pounds?

3. Prescriber's order:

   5% D/W 100 mL per q1h IV

   Calculate the flow rate in drops per minute; the drop factor is 15 gtt/mL.

4. Prepare 3000 mL of a 1% neosporin solution from a 5% neosporin solution.

5. You have a 2-milliliter ampule of Epinephrine 1:1000. Calculate the amount of milligrams of Epinephrine in 0.5 mL.

6. Prescriber's order:

   Dynapen (dicloxacillin) 250 mg q6h po

   The label reads 62.5 mg/5 mL. How many milliliters will you administer to your patient?

7. Physician's order:

   Gentamycin 2.5 mg/kg IVPB in 200 mL of D5W, infuse in 90 minutes

   The label reads 225 mg/10 mL and the client weighs 90 kg.

   a. How many milligrams will you prepare for your patient?

   b. Calculate the flow rate in milliliters per hour.

8. Tenofovir (Viread) 0.3 g po qd has been ordered for a patient with an HIV infection. The bottle is labeled 300 mg per tablet. How many tablets of this antiviral drug will you prepare?

9. Physician's order:

   Saquinavir (Fortovase) 1200 mg TID pc meals po

   Each soft-gel capsule contains 0.2 gram. How many capsules will you give your client?

10. Prescriber's order:

    Relfinavir (Virocept) 750 mg po TID with food

    Each tablet contains 0.25 gram. How many tablets will you administer?

11. Prescriber's order:

    Tamiflu 0.075 g q12h po for 5 days

    Each capsule contains 75 mg. How many capsules of this antiflu drug will the patient receive in 5 days?

12. The antidiabetic drug, peoglitazone HCl (Actos), 30 mg po qid has been ordered for your patient. Each tablet contains 0.015 g. How many tablets will you administer to your patient?

13. Aceon (perindopril erbumine) 0.008 g po BID has been ordered for your patient. Each tablet contains 8 mg. How many tablets of this ACE inhibitor drug will you prepare for your patient?

14. Amiodarone HCl (Cordarone) 10 mg/kg IV over 24 hours has been prescribed for a patient who weighs 174 pounds. The label on the vial reads 50 mg/mL and the directions are to add the required amount of Cordarone to 250 mL of D/5/W.

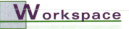

a. How many milliliters of Cordarone will you add to the IV solution?

b. Set the rate on the infusion pump in milliliters per hour.

15. A patient has to receive lidocaine 1% 0.05 mg/kg IV push. How many cubic centimeters of the lidocaine will you prepare for the patient who weighs 90 kg?

16. A patient has to receive phenytoin 0.1 gram IM prior to surgery. Read the information on the label in Figure S.38. How many milliliters will you give the patient?

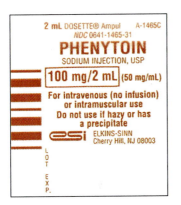

Figure S.38 Drug label for phenytoin.
(Courtesy of ESI Lederle, a Business Unit of Wyeth Pharmaceuticals, Philadelphia, PA.)

17. The physician ordered 0.5 mg IM of Glucagon for a patient. The label reads 1 mg = 1 mL. How many milliliters will you give the patient?

18. A patient needs to receive 6 mg of adenosine IV push bolus in 2 seconds. The label on the vial reads 3 mg/mL. How many milliliters will you give the patient?

19. The label on the bottle reads 50 mL of 25% albumin. The physician ordered 25 grams; how many bottles will you need?

20. Cephapirin (Cefadyl) 2 g IVPB in 100 mL NS has been prescribed for perioperative prophylaxis. Infuse at a rate of 100 mL in 2 hours.

a. How many milligrams of this antibiotic are in 100 mL?

b. How many microdrops per minute are necessary to infuse as ordered?

21. The antiarrythmic drug, sotalol HCl (Betapace), 320 mg po daily has been prescribed for a patient. Each tablet is labeled 160 mg. How many tablets will you administer to the patient?

22. Physician's order:

Somatropin (Nutropin), human growth hormone, 0.06 mg/kg sc weekly

The label on the vial reads 5 mg/5 mL and the child weighs 34 kg.

a. How many milligrams contain the prescribed medication?

b. How many milliliters will you administer?

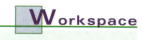

23. The physician ordered ciprofloxacin (Cipro) 400 mg IVPB q12h, infuse in 60 minutes. The label reads 400 mg of ciprofloxacin in 200 mL D/5/W.

    a. How many milliliters contain the prescribed dose?

    b. Calculate the flow rate in milliliters per hour.

24. Physician's order:

    Calcium carbonate 1875 mg po daily

Read the label in Figure S.39. How many milliliters contain the prescribed dose?

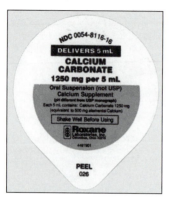

Figure S.39 Drug label for Calcium Carbonate.
(Used with permission of Roxane Laboratories, Inc.)

25. gr $\dfrac{1}{1000}$ = ? mg

APPENDICES

APPENDIX A

Answer Section

Included in this section are the answers to the *Diagnostic Test of Arithmetic, Try These for Practice, Exercises, Cumulative Review Exercises, Case Studies,* and *Comprehensive Self-Tests.* The answers to the *Additional Exercises* can be found on the companion Website or ask your instructor.

Diagnostic Test of Arithmetic

1. $\dfrac{5}{8}$ 2. 2.75   3. 4.8

4. 0.67   5. 40   6. 326.7

7. 4.251   8. 1300   9. 2

10. $\dfrac{2}{9}$ 11. $\dfrac{4}{3}$ or $1\dfrac{1}{3}$ 12. $\dfrac{1}{16}$

13. $\dfrac{7}{20}$ 14. 0.025   15. $\dfrac{23}{5}$

Chapter 1

Try These for Practice

1. 0.6   2. 0.2   3. 22.11

4. 1   5. 0.045

Exercises

1. $0.62 = \dfrac{62}{100} = \dfrac{31}{50}$ 2. $5\dfrac{75}{100} = 5\dfrac{3}{4}$

3.
$$
\begin{array}{r}
.375 \Rightarrow 0.375 \\
8\overline{)3.000} \\
\underline{2\,4} \\
60 \\
\underline{56} \\
40 \\
\underline{40}
\end{array}
$$

4.
$$
\begin{array}{r}
.28 \Rightarrow 0.28 \\
25\overline{)7.00} \\
\underline{5\,0} \\
2\,00 \\
\underline{2\,00}
\end{array}
$$

5.
$$
\begin{array}{r}
.2 \Rightarrow 0.2 \\
5\overline{)1.0} \\
\underline{1\,0}
\end{array}
$$

6.
$$
\begin{array}{r}
.0033 \Rightarrow 0.00333\ldots \\
300\overline{)1.0000} \\
\underline{900} \\
1000 \\
\underline{900} \\
100
\end{array}
$$

7.
$$\begin{array}{r} .0066 \Rightarrow 0.00666\ldots \text{ or } 0.007 \\ 150\overline{)1.0000} \\ \underline{900} \\ 1000 \\ \underline{900} \\ 100 \end{array}$$

8. $\dfrac{92\cancel{0}\cancel{0}\cancel{0}}{1\cancel{0}\cancel{0}} = 92$

9. Move decimal 3 places to the left: 0.00375.

10.
$$\begin{array}{r} 27.62 \Rightarrow 27.6 \\ 7\overline{)193.40} \\ \underline{14} \\ 53 \\ \underline{49} \\ 4\,4 \\ \underline{4\,2} \\ 20 \\ \underline{14} \\ 6 \end{array}$$

11.
$$\begin{array}{r} .9 \Rightarrow 0.9 \\ 0.\underbrace{4}\overline{)0.3\,6} \\ \underline{3\,6} \\ 0 \end{array}$$

12.
$$\begin{array}{r} .9 \Rightarrow 0.9 \\ 0.0\,\underbrace{4}\overline{)0.0\,3\,6} \\ \underline{3\,6} \\ 0 \end{array}$$

13. $278.\underbrace{2} \Rightarrow 27{,}820$

14.
$$\begin{array}{r} 10.175 \\ \times \quad 10.3 \\ \hline 3\,0525 \\ 0\,000 \\ \underline{101\,75} \\ 104.8025 \end{array}$$

15. $64.7\underbrace{3} \Rightarrow 64{,}730$

16.
$$\begin{array}{r} 19\,0\,0. \Rightarrow 1900 \\ 0.0\,5\overline{)95.0\,0} \\ \underline{5} \\ 45 \\ \underline{45} \\ 0\,0 \\ \underline{0} \\ 0\,0 \\ \underline{0} \\ 0 \end{array}$$

17.
$$\begin{array}{r} 1\,9\,0. \Rightarrow 190 \\ 0.0\,5\overline{)9.5\,0} \\ \underline{5} \\ 4\,5 \\ \underline{4\,5} \\ 0\,0 \\ \underline{0} \\ 0 \end{array}$$

18. $\dfrac{7}{\cancel{15}_{3}} \times \dfrac{\cancel{20}^{\overset{2}{\cancel{4}}}}{1} \times \dfrac{1}{\cancel{2}_{1}} = \dfrac{14}{3}$ or $4\dfrac{2}{3}$

19. $\dfrac{7}{2} \div \dfrac{6}{1} = \dfrac{7}{2} \times \dfrac{1}{6} = \dfrac{7}{12}$

20. $\dfrac{13}{1} \div \dfrac{7}{3} = \dfrac{13}{1} \times \dfrac{3}{7} = \dfrac{39}{7}$ or $5\dfrac{4}{7}$

21. $6.35 = 6\dfrac{35}{100}$ or $6\dfrac{7}{20}$

$6\dfrac{7}{20} \times \dfrac{1}{5} = \dfrac{127}{20} \times \dfrac{1}{5} = \dfrac{127}{100} = 1\dfrac{27}{100}$

22. $\dfrac{1}{500} \times \dfrac{175}{1} \times \dfrac{1}{0.5} = \dfrac{175}{250} = \dfrac{7}{10}$

23. $7.75 \times \dfrac{1}{0.5} = \dfrac{7.75}{0.5} \times \dfrac{100}{100} = \dfrac{\overset{31}{\cancel{775}}}{\underset{2}{\cancel{50}}} = 15\dfrac{1}{2}$ or 15.5

24. $7 \div \dfrac{3}{8} = \dfrac{7}{1} \times \dfrac{8}{3} = \dfrac{56}{3}$ or $18\dfrac{2}{3}$

But $\dfrac{2}{3} = 0.6666$ and $18.666\ldots$ is 18.7 to the nearest tenth.

25. $\dfrac{\frac{1}{5}}{4} \times \dfrac{9}{1} = \dfrac{\frac{9}{5}}{4}$

$\dfrac{9}{5} \div \dfrac{4}{1} = \dfrac{9}{5} \times \dfrac{1}{4} = \dfrac{9}{20}$ or 0.45

26. $\dfrac{\frac{2}{3} \times 170}{\frac{3}{8}} = \dfrac{\frac{340}{3}}{\frac{3}{8}} = \dfrac{340}{3} \div \dfrac{3}{8}$

$\dfrac{340}{3} \times \dfrac{8}{3} = \dfrac{2720}{9}$ or $302\dfrac{2}{9}$ or 302.2

27. $5\overline{)3.0}$ So $24\dfrac{3}{5}\% = 24.6\%$.

$\underline{3\,0}$

0

Move the decimal two places left: 0.246.

28. $63\% = \underset{\smile}{6\,3} = 0.63$

29. $2.75\% = \dfrac{2.75}{100}$

$\dfrac{2.75}{100} \times \dfrac{100}{100} = \dfrac{275}{10,000} = \dfrac{11}{400}$

30. $7.5\% = \dfrac{7.5}{100}$

$\dfrac{7.5}{100} \times \dfrac{10}{10} = \dfrac{75}{1000}$ or $\dfrac{3}{40}$

Chapter 2

Try These for Practice

1. po
2. 60
3. 80 mg
4. Atarax
5. 20 mg

Exercises

1. olanzapine
2. Geodon
3. quinidine gluconate
4. by mouth
5. Atarax

Name of Drug	Dose	Route of Administration	Time of Administration	Date Started	Expiration Date
Celebrex	100 mg	po	8 AM 8 PM q12h	12/7/03	12/18/03
Flomax	0.4 mg	po	30 min ac dinner 5 PM	12/7/03	12/13/03
Ditropan	0.005 g	po	8 AM qd	12/7/03	12/13/03
Zoloft	0.1 g	po	8 AM q AM	12/8/03	12/14/03
Seraquel	100 mg	po	Hs 9 PM	12/7/03	12/13/03
Valium	10 mg	po	Hs 9 PM prn	12/9/03	12/16/03
Fluconazole	400 mg	IV	q12h 8 AM 8 PM	12/8/03	12/15/03

6. a. Celebrex   b. 4   c. fluconazole
   d. one, Flomax   e. 8 A.M.   f. Robert Graham
   g. Seraquel   h. Dr. A. Giangrasso

7. a. transdermal, through the skin   b. Vioxx
   c. Nitroglycerine, Diabenase, Vioxx, Monopril
   d. Vioxx, furosemide   e. Cefaclor
   f. Diabenase

8. a. cefazolin   b. 330 mg/mL   c. intravenous
   d. 500 mg q12h

Chapter 3

Try These for Practice

1. 195 min
2. 104 oz
3. 6 ft
4. 20 yd
5. $6\frac{1}{2}$ yr

Exercises

1. $\overset{9}{\cancel{540}} \text{ sec} \times \dfrac{1 \text{ min}}{\underset{1}{\cancel{60} \text{ sec}}} = 9 \text{ min}$

2. $1.25 \text{ yr} \times \dfrac{12 \text{ mon}}{1 \text{ yr}} = 15 \text{ mon}$

3. $4 \text{ d} \times \dfrac{24 \text{ hr}}{1 \text{ d}} = 96 \text{ h}$

4. $4 \text{ lb} \times \dfrac{16 \text{ oz}}{1 \text{ lb}} = 64 \text{ oz}$

5. $\dfrac{3 \text{ min}}{4} \times \dfrac{\overset{15}{\cancel{60}} \text{ sec}}{1 \text{ min}} = 45 \text{ sec}$

6. $\dfrac{5 \text{ yr}}{\underset{1}{\cancel{3}}} \times \dfrac{\overset{4}{\cancel{12}} \text{ mon}}{1 \text{ yr}} = 20 \text{ mon}$

7. $\dfrac{3 \text{ yd}}{2} \times \dfrac{3 \text{ ft}}{1 \text{ yd}} = \dfrac{9 \text{ ft}}{2} = 4\dfrac{1}{2} \text{ ft}$

8. $\overset{3}{\cancel{12}} \text{ oz} \times \dfrac{1 \text{ lb}}{\underset{4}{\cancel{16}} \text{ oz}} = \dfrac{3}{4} \text{ lb}$

9. $\overset{40}{\cancel{480}} \text{ in} \times \dfrac{1 \text{ ft}}{\underset{1}{\cancel{12} \text{ in}}} = 40 \text{ ft}$

10. $\overset{2}{\cancel{6}} \text{ ft} \times \dfrac{1 \text{ yd}}{\underset{1}{\cancel{3} \text{ ft}}} = 2 \text{ yd}$

11. $8 \text{ lb} \times \dfrac{16 \text{ oz}}{1 \text{ lb}} = 128 \text{ oz}$

12. $\overset{3}{\cancel{18}} \text{ hr} \times \dfrac{1 \text{ d}}{\underset{4}{\cancel{24} \text{ hr}}} = \dfrac{3}{4} \text{ d}$

13. $\overset{4}{\cancel{48}} \text{ in} \times \dfrac{1 \text{ ft}}{\underset{1}{\cancel{12} \text{ in}}} = 4 \text{ ft}$

14. $50 \text{ min} \times \dfrac{1 \text{ h}}{60 \text{ min}} = \dfrac{5}{6} \text{ h}$

15. $\overset{5}{\cancel{30}} \text{ mo} \times \dfrac{1 \text{ yr}}{\underset{2}{\cancel{12} \text{ mo}}} = \dfrac{5}{2} \text{ or } 2\dfrac{1}{2} \text{ yr}$

16. $2.25 \text{ h} \times \dfrac{60 \text{ min}}{1 \text{ h}} = 135 \text{ min}$

17. $55 \text{ min} \times \dfrac{60 \text{ sec}}{1 \text{ min}} = 3300 \text{ sec}$

18. $5 \text{ ft} \times \dfrac{12 \text{ in}}{1 \text{ ft}} = 60 \text{ in}$

19. $\dfrac{5 \text{ lb}}{\underset{1}{\cancel{2}}} \times \dfrac{\overset{8}{\cancel{16}} \text{ oz}}{1 \text{ lb}} = 40 \text{ oz}$

20. $9 \text{ d} \times \dfrac{24 \text{ h}}{1 \text{ d}} = 216 \text{ h}$

Chapter 4

Try These for Practice

1. a. 2 pt
   b. ℥ 16
   c. ℥ 8
   d. m 60
   e. ℥ 8
   f. ℥ 8
   g. ℥ 6
   h. 2 T
   i. 3 t
   j. 60 gtt
   k. 16 oz
   l. 1000 cc
   m. 1 cc = 1 cm³
   n. 1000 mL
   o. 1000 g
   p. 1000 mg
   q. 1000 μg
   r. 1000 mcg
   s. 1 mcg

2. 0.075 g
3. 50 mcg
4. 66.7 oz

5. dram 16

Exercises

1. $\cancel{℥ 32}^{4} \times \dfrac{℥ 1}{\cancel{℥ 8}_{1}} = ℥ 4$

2. $0.05 \,\cancel{g} \times \dfrac{1000 \,\text{mg}}{1 \,\cancel{g}} = 50 \,\text{mg}$

3. $0.04 \,\cancel{g} \times \dfrac{1000 \,\text{mg}}{1 \,\cancel{g}} = 40 \,\text{mg}$

4. $4.75 \,\cancel{L} \times \dfrac{1000 \,\text{cc}}{1 \,\cancel{L}} = 4750 \,\text{cc}$

5. $\cancel{\text{dram } 3} \times \dfrac{\text{minim } 60}{\cancel{\text{dram } 1}} = \text{minim } 180$

6. $℥ 64 \times \dfrac{ʒ 8}{℥ 1} = ʒ 512$

7. 120 cc

8. $100{,}000 \,\cancel{\text{mcg}} \times \dfrac{1 \,\text{mg}}{\cancel{1000 \,\text{mcg}}} = 100 \,\text{mg}$

9. $\dfrac{7}{2}\,\cancel{t} \times \dfrac{\text{m } 60}{1 \,\cancel{t}} = \text{m } 210$

10. $6 \,\cancel{T} \times \dfrac{3 \,t}{1 \,\cancel{T}} = 18 \,t$

11. $8 \,\cancel{\text{pt}} \times \dfrac{1 \,\text{qt}}{2 \,\cancel{\text{pt}}} = 4 \,\text{qt}$

12. $0.26 \,\cancel{\text{kg}} \times \dfrac{1000 \,\text{g}}{1 \,\cancel{\text{kg}}} = 260 \,\text{g}$

13. $100 \,\cancel{\text{mg}} \times \dfrac{1 \,\text{g}}{1000 \,\cancel{\text{mg}}} = 0.1 \,\text{g}$

14. $30 \,\cancel{\text{mg}} \times \dfrac{1 \,\text{g}}{1000 \,\cancel{\text{mg}}} = 0.03 \,\text{g}$

15. $0.3 \,\cancel{g} \times \dfrac{1000 \,\text{mg}}{1 \,\cancel{g}} = 300 \,\text{mg}$

16. $\dfrac{1}{2}\,\cancel{\text{pt}} \times \dfrac{16 \,\text{oz}}{\cancel{\text{pt}}} = 8 \text{ ounces every 2 hours}$

17. $0.5 \,\cancel{\text{mg}} \times \dfrac{1 \,\text{g}}{1000 \,\cancel{\text{mg}}} = \dfrac{0.5}{1000} = 0.0005 \,\text{g}$

18. $150 \,\cancel{\text{mg}} \times \dfrac{1 \,\text{g}}{1000 \,\cancel{\text{mg}}} = 0.15 \,\text{g}$

19. $2.8 \,\cancel{\text{kg}} \times \dfrac{1000 \,\text{g}}{1 \,\cancel{\text{kg}}} = 2800 \,\text{g}$

20. $1.5 \,\cancel{g} \times \dfrac{1000 \,\text{mg}}{1 \,\cancel{g}} = 1500 \,\text{mg}$

Answers to Cumulative Exercises

1. 7800 mg

2. 250 μg

3. ʒ 4

4. ℥ 224

5. 1 t

6. 7600 g

7. 0.75 L

8. 12 t

9. 1000 mg

10. 0.25 g

11. 650 mcg

12. 6 t

13. $\dfrac{1}{4}\,t$

14. 0.25 L

15. 32 mg

Chapter 5

Try These for Practice

1. a. $1\,cm^3$ b. 1000 mL   c. 1000 g

   d. 1 g   e. 1 mg   f. 1 mcg

   g. ℥ 8   h. ʒ 6   i. 2 T

   j. 3 t   k. 60 gtt   l. 16 oz

   m. 12 in   n. 2 pt   o. ℥ 16

   p. ʒ 8   q. ♏ 60

   r. ʒ 1 = 1 t = ♏ 60 = 60 gtt = 4 or 5 mL

   s. ℥ 1 = 2 T = ʒ 8 = 30 or 32 mL

   t. 1 measuring cup = 1 glass = ℥ 8 = $\dfrac{1}{2}$ pt

   u. 60 mg   v. gr 15   w. 15 gtt

   x. 2.2 lb   y. 0.45 kg   z. 2.5 cm

2. grains 11   3. 77.4 kg or 78.2 kg

4. gr $\dfrac{1}{8}$ 5. 0.24 mg

Exercises

1. $3200\ \cancel{mcg} \times \dfrac{1\ mg}{1000\ \cancel{mcg}} = 3.2\ mg$ 2. $250\ \cancel{g} \times \dfrac{1000\ mg}{1\ \cancel{g}} = 250{,}000\ mg$

3. $0.005\ \cancel{g} \times \dfrac{1000\ mg}{1\ \cancel{g}} = 5\ mg$ 4. $0.004\ \cancel{mg} \times \dfrac{1000\ mcg}{1\ \cancel{mg}} = 4\ mcg$

5. $\dfrac{\cancel{gr\ 15}}{2} \times \dfrac{1\ g}{\cancel{gr\ 15}} = 0.5\ g$ 6. $0.006\ \cancel{mg} \times \dfrac{gr\ 1}{60\ \cancel{mg}} = gr\ \dfrac{1}{10{,}000}$

7. $0.7\ \cancel{mg} \times \dfrac{1\ g}{1000\ \cancel{mg}} = 0.0007\ g$ 8. $8.25\ \cancel{L} \times \dfrac{1000\ mL}{1\ \cancel{L}} = 8250\ mL$

9. $10{,}075\ \cancel{mL} \times \dfrac{1\ L}{1000\ \cancel{mL}} = 10.075\ L$

10. $\dfrac{\cancel{gr\ 15}}{4} \times \dfrac{60\ mg}{\cancel{gr\ 1}} = 225\ mg$ or $gr\ 3\dfrac{3}{4} = 250\ mg$ is an equivalence.

11. $1\ \cancel{mL} \times \dfrac{12\ mg}{5\ \cancel{mL}} = 2.4\ mg$ of codeine phosphate

12. $0.5\ \cancel{g} \times \dfrac{1000\ mg}{1\ \cancel{g}} = 500\ mg$

13. $150\ \cancel{mg} \times \dfrac{1\ mL}{30\ \cancel{mg}} = 5\ mL$ of Chlorpromazine

14. $30 \text{ mg} \times \dfrac{5 \text{ mL}}{20 \text{ mg}} = 7.5 \text{ mL of Prozac}$

15. $500 \text{ mg} \times \dfrac{1 \text{ tab}}{250 \text{ mg}} = 2 \text{ tablets of Ery-Tab}$

16. $10 \text{ mL} \times \dfrac{1 \text{ t}}{5 \text{ mL}} = 2 \text{ t of Benadryl}$

17. $150 \text{ \textmu g} \times \dfrac{1 \text{ mL}}{50 \text{ \textmu g}} = 3 \text{ mL of Digoxin}$

18. $\dfrac{0.3 \text{ mg}}{\text{dose}} \times \dfrac{1 \text{ tab}}{0.1 \text{ mg}} \times \dfrac{2 \text{ dose}}{\text{day}} = \dfrac{0.6}{0.1} = 6 \text{ tablets per day of Clonidine 0.1 mg}$

19. $200 \text{ mg} \times \dfrac{1 \text{ tab}}{100 \text{ mg}} = 2 \text{ tablets of Diabinese}$

20. $\text{gr } 45 \times \dfrac{1 \text{ g}}{\text{gr } 15} = 3 \text{ grams}$

Cumulative Review

1. 125 mcg
2. 9 mg
3. 5650 g

4. 100 mcg
5. 60 mg
6. 225 or 250 mg

7. 7750 mL
8. 600 mcg
9. 1.25 L

10. $\text{gr } \dfrac{1}{2}$
11. $\text{gr } 2\dfrac{1}{4} \text{ or } 2\dfrac{1}{2}$
12. 0.15 g

13. 0.01 g
14. 0.01 g
15. 0.09 g

Chapter 6

Practice Reading Labels

1. $0.01 \text{ g} \times \dfrac{1000 \text{ mg}}{1 \text{ g}} \times \dfrac{1 \text{ cap}}{10 \text{ mg}} = 1 \text{ capsule of Feldene}$

2. $0.12 \text{ g} \times \dfrac{1000 \text{ mg}}{1 \text{ g}} \times \dfrac{1 \text{ tab}}{60 \text{ mg}} = 2 \text{ tablets of Evista}$

3. $0.5 \text{ g} \times \dfrac{\overset{2}{\cancel{1000}} \text{ mg}}{1 \text{ g}} \times \dfrac{1 \text{ tab}}{\underset{1}{\cancel{500}} \text{ mg}} = 1 \text{ tablet of Relafen}$

4. $245 \text{ mg} \times \dfrac{5 \text{ mL}}{375 \text{ mg}} = 3.27 \text{ or } 3.3 \text{ milliliters of Ceclor}$

5. $0.01 \text{ g} \times \dfrac{1000 \text{ mg}}{1 \text{ g}} \times \dfrac{1 \text{ tab}}{10 \text{ mg}} = 1 \text{ tablet of Hytrin}$

6. $\overset{2}{\cancel{200}}\text{ mg} \times \dfrac{1\text{ tab}}{\underset{1}{\cancel{100}\text{ mg}}} = 2$ tablets of Thorazine

7. $75\text{ mg} \times \dfrac{5\text{ mL}}{187\text{ mg}} = 2$ milliliters of Ceclor

8. $\text{gr } 3 \times \dfrac{60\text{ mg}}{\text{gr }1} \times \dfrac{5\text{ mL}}{200\text{ mg}} = 4.5$ milliliters of Zovirax

9. $\text{gr }\dfrac{1}{\underset{1}{\cancel{6}}} \times \dfrac{\overset{10}{\cancel{60}}\text{ mg}}{\text{gr }1} \times \dfrac{1\text{ mL}}{1\text{ mg}} = 10$ milliliters of alprazolam

10. $75\cancel{00}\text{ }\mu\text{g} \times \dfrac{1\text{ mg}}{10\cancel{00}\text{ }\mu\text{g}} \times \dfrac{1\text{ tab}}{7.5\text{ mg}} = 1$ tablet of Zyprexa

11. $0.5\text{ g} \times \dfrac{\overset{4}{\cancel{1000}}\text{ mg}}{1\text{ g}} \times \dfrac{1\text{ tab}}{\underset{1}{\cancel{250}\text{ mg}}} = 2$ tablets of Biaxin

12. $0.999\text{ g} \times \dfrac{1000\text{ mg}}{1\text{ g}} \times \dfrac{1\text{ tab}}{333\text{ mg}} = 3$ tablets of Erythromycin

13. $\overset{3}{\cancel{6}}\text{ mg} \times \dfrac{1\text{ cap}}{\underset{1}{\cancel{2}\text{ mg}}} = 3$ capsules of Detrol LA

14. $1.2\text{ g} \times \dfrac{1000\text{ mg}}{1\text{ g}} \times \dfrac{1\text{ tab}}{600\text{ mg}} = 2$ tablets of Zyflo

15. $\overset{4}{\cancel{200}}\text{ mg} \times \dfrac{5\text{ mL}}{\underset{1}{\cancel{50}\text{ mg}}} = 20$ milliliters of Vantin

16. $0.02\text{ g} \times \dfrac{1000\text{ mg}}{1\text{ g}} \times \dfrac{1\text{ tab}}{10\text{ mg}} = 2$ tablets of methadone HCl

17. $0.2\text{ mg} \times \dfrac{\overset{10}{\cancel{1000}}\text{ mcg}}{1\text{ mg}} \times \dfrac{1\text{ tab}}{\underset{1}{\cancel{100}\text{ mcg}}} = 2$ tablets of Cytotec

18. 5 milliliters of codeine phosphate.

19. $\overset{2}{\cancel{800}}\text{ mg} \times \dfrac{1\text{ tab}}{\underset{1}{\cancel{400}\text{ mg}}} = 2$ tablets of Erythromycin

20. $10\text{ mg} \times \dfrac{\overset{1}{\cancel{5}}\text{ mL}}{\underset{1}{\cancel{5}\text{ mg}}} = 10$ milliliters of Diazepam

21. $0.45\text{ g} \times \dfrac{1000\text{ mg}}{1\text{ g}} \times \dfrac{1\text{ cap}}{150\text{ mg}} = 3$ capsules of Mycobutin

22. $0.01\text{ g} \times \dfrac{1000\text{ mg}}{1\text{ g}} \times \dfrac{1\text{ tab}}{10\text{ mg}} = 1$ tablet of Glucotrol XL

23. $\dfrac{\cancel{\text{gr } 1}}{\underset{1}{\cancel{6}}} \times \dfrac{\overset{10}{\cancel{60}} \text{ mg}}{\cancel{\text{gr } 1}} \times \dfrac{1 \text{ tab}}{10 \text{ mg}} = 1$ tablet of Provera

24. $0.0375 \text{ g} \times \dfrac{1000 \text{ mg}}{1 \text{ g}} \times \dfrac{1 \text{ tab}}{37.5 \text{ mg}} = 1$ tablet of Cylert

25. $\overset{3}{\cancel{150}} \text{ mg} \times \dfrac{5 \text{ mL}}{\underset{4}{\cancel{200}} \text{ mg}} = 3.75$ milliliters of Zithromax

26. $0.02 \text{ g} \times \dfrac{1000 \text{ mg}}{1 \text{ g}} \times \dfrac{1 \text{ tab}}{20 \text{ mg}} = 1$ tablet of Lipitor

27. $1 \text{ g} \times \dfrac{\overset{2}{\cancel{1000}} \text{ mg}}{1 \text{ g}} \times \dfrac{1 \text{ tab}}{\underset{1}{\cancel{500}} \text{ mg}} = 2$ tablets of Biaxin

28. $0.005 \text{ g} \times \dfrac{\overset{200}{\cancel{1000}} \text{ mg}}{1 \text{ g}} \times \dfrac{1 \text{ tab}}{\underset{1}{\cancel{5}} \text{ mg}} = 1$ tablet of Hytrin

29. $\overset{4}{\cancel{400}} \text{ mg} \times \dfrac{2.5 \text{ mL}}{\underset{1}{\cancel{100}} \text{ mg}} = 10$ milliliters of EryPed

30. $0.05 \text{ g} \times \dfrac{1000 \text{ mg}}{1 \text{ g}} \times \dfrac{1 \text{ tab}}{25 \text{ mg}} = 2$ tablets of Cyclophosphamide

31. $\overset{6}{\cancel{60}} \text{ mg} \times \dfrac{1 \text{ mL}}{\underset{1}{\cancel{10}} \text{ mg}} = 6$ milliliters of Diflucan

32. $0.01 \text{ g} \times \dfrac{1000 \text{ mg}}{1 \text{ g}} \times \dfrac{1 \text{ tab}}{10 \text{ mg}} = 1$ tablet of Glucotrol XL

33. $\overset{3}{\cancel{375}} \text{ mg} \times \dfrac{5 \text{ mL}}{\underset{1}{\cancel{125}} \text{ mg}} = 15$ milliliters of Ceclor

34. $0.004 \text{ g} \times \dfrac{\overset{500}{\cancel{1000}} \text{ mg}}{1 \text{ g}} \times \dfrac{1 \text{ tab}}{\underset{1}{\cancel{2}} \text{ mg}} = 2$ tablets of Cardura

35. 2.5 ml of contains acetaminophen 60 mg and codeine 6 mg

36. $\overset{2}{\cancel{400}} \text{ mg} \times \dfrac{1 \text{ cap}}{\underset{1}{\cancel{200}} \text{ mg}} = 2$ capsules of Placidyl

37. $0.2 \text{ g} \times \dfrac{1000 \text{ mg}}{1 \text{ g}} \times \dfrac{1 \text{ cap}}{100 \text{ mg}} = 2$ capsules of Nembutal

38. $1.25 \text{ g} \times \dfrac{1000 \text{ mg}}{1 \text{ g}} \times \dfrac{5 \text{ ml}}{1250 \text{ mg}} = 5$ milliliters of calcium carbonate

39. $\overset{2}{\cancel{50}} \text{ mg} \times \dfrac{1 \text{ tab}}{\underset{1}{\cancel{25}} \text{ mg}} = 2$ tablets of amitriptyline

40. $\text{gr } \dfrac{1}{\cancelto{1}{60}} \times \dfrac{\cancelto{1}{60} \text{ mg}}{\text{gr } 1} \times \dfrac{1 \text{ tab}}{1 \text{ mg}} = 1$ tablet of Hytrin

41. $\text{gr } \dfrac{1}{\cancelto{1}{6}} \times \dfrac{\cancelto{10}{60} \text{ mg}}{\text{gr } 1} \times \dfrac{1 \text{ tab}}{5 \text{ mg}} = 2$ tablets of Ambien

42. $0.0375 \text{ g} \times \dfrac{1 \text{ tab}}{37.5 \text{ mg}} \times \dfrac{1000 \text{ mg}}{1 \text{ g}} = 1$ tablet of Cyclert

43. $\cancelto{2}{40} \text{ mg} \times \dfrac{1 \text{ tab}}{\cancelto{1}{20} \text{ mg}} = 2$ tablets of furosemide

44. $2 \text{ g} \times \dfrac{\cancelto{2}{1000} \text{ mg}}{1 \text{ g}} \times \dfrac{1 \text{ tab}}{\cancelto{1}{500} \text{ mg}} = 4$ tablets of Azulfidine

45. $60 \text{ mg} \times \dfrac{1 \text{ mL}}{40 \text{ mg}} = 1.5$ milliliters of Diflucan

46. $\cancelto{5}{50} \text{ mg} \times \dfrac{5 \text{ mL}}{\cancelto{1}{10} \text{ mg}} = 25$ milliliters of Cortef

47. $2500 \text{ mcg} \times \dfrac{1 \text{ mg}}{1000 \text{ mcg}} \times \dfrac{1 \text{ tab}}{2.5 \text{ mg}} = 1$ tablet of Micronase

48. $\dfrac{20 \text{ mg}/25 \text{ mg}}{1} \times \dfrac{1 \text{ tab}}{10 \text{ mg}/12.5 \text{ mg}} = \dfrac{20/25 \text{ tab}}{10/12.5} = 2$ tablets of Lotensin 10 mg/12.5 mg

49. $\cancelto{2}{180} \text{ mg} \times \dfrac{1 \text{ tab}}{\cancelto{1}{90} \text{ mg}} = 2$ tablets of Procardia XL

50. $0.1 \text{ g} \times \dfrac{\cancelto{20}{1000} \text{ mg}}{1 \text{ g}} \times \dfrac{1 \text{ tab}}{\cancelto{1}{50} \text{ mg}} = 2$ tablets of atenolol

51. $\cancelto{2}{500} \text{ mg} \times \dfrac{1 \text{ tab}}{\cancelto{1}{250} \text{ mg}} = 2$ tablets of erythromycin

52. $0.25 \text{ mg} \times \dfrac{1 \text{ tab}}{0.125 \text{ mg}} = \dfrac{0.25}{0.125} = 2$ tablets of Halcion

53. $1.8 \text{ g} \times \dfrac{1000 \text{ mg}}{1 \text{ g}} \times \dfrac{1 \text{ tab}}{600 \text{ mg}} = 3$ tablets of Zyvox

54. $\text{gr } \dfrac{2}{3} \times \dfrac{\cancelto{3}{60} \text{ mg}}{\text{gr } 1} \times \dfrac{1 \text{ cap}}{\cancelto{2}{40} \text{ mg}} = \dfrac{6 \text{ cap}}{6}$ or 1 capsule of Geodon

55. $\cancelto{5}{5000} \text{ µg} \times \dfrac{1 \text{ mg}}{1000 \text{ µg}} \times \dfrac{1 \text{ tab}}{\cancelto{1}{5} \text{ mg}} = 1$ tablet of Haloperidol

56. $0.005 \; \cancel{g} \times \dfrac{1000 \; \cancel{mg}}{1 \; \cancel{g}} \times \dfrac{1 \; tab}{5 \; \cancel{mg}} = 1$ tablet of fluophenazine Hcl

57. $0.3 \; \cancel{mg} \times \dfrac{1000 \; \cancel{mcg}}{1 \; \cancel{mg}} \times \dfrac{1 \; tab}{100 \; \cancel{mcg}} = 3$ tablets of Cytotec

58. $0.1 \; \cancel{g} \times \dfrac{1000 \; \cancel{mg}}{1 \; \cancel{g}} \times \dfrac{1 \; tab}{100 \; \cancel{mg}} = 1$ tablet of Rescriptor

59. $\overset{4}{\cancel{100}} \; \cancel{mg} \times \dfrac{1 \; tab}{\underset{1}{\cancel{25} \; \cancel{mg}}} = 4$ tablets of Viagra

60. $4 \; \cancel{mg} \times \dfrac{5 \; mL}{0.5 \; \cancel{mg}} = \dfrac{20 \; mL}{0.5} = 40$ milliliters of Dexamethasone

Case Study 6

1. $1200 \; mL + 200 \; mL + 150 \; mL = 1550 \; mL$

2. $\dfrac{\overset{2}{\cancel{500}} \; \cancel{mg}}{6 \; \cancel{h}} \times \dfrac{1 \; cap}{\underset{1}{\cancel{250} \; \cancel{mg}}} \times 24 \; \cancel{h} = 8$ capsules of Zithromax in 24 hours

3. 1 capsule of Tikocyn a day

4. $200 \; \cancel{mg} \times \dfrac{15 \; mL}{150 \; \cancel{mg}} = 20 \; mL$ of Colace

5. 1 tablet of atenolol

6. $10 \; \cancel{mg} \times \dfrac{5 \; cc}{5 \; \cancel{mg}} = 10 \; cc$ of diazepam

7. $\dfrac{25 \; \cancel{mg}}{\cancel{dose}} \times \dfrac{1 \; tab}{25 \; \cancel{mg}} \times \dfrac{2 \; \cancel{doses}}{day} = 2$ tablets per day of Zoloft

   $\dfrac{2 \; tab}{\cancel{day}} \times \dfrac{21 \; \cancel{days}}{3 \; wk} = 42$ tablets in 3 weeks

8. $0.5 \; \cancel{g} \times \dfrac{1000 \; \cancel{mg}}{\cancel{g}} \times \dfrac{1 \; tab}{500 \; \cancel{mg}} = 1$ tablet of clarithromicin

9. 30 tablet of famotidine

10. $5 \; \cancel{mg} \times \dfrac{1 \; tab}{2.5 \; \cancel{mg}} = 2$ tablets of glipizide

11. $\dfrac{0.015 \; \cancel{g}}{\cancel{dose}} \times \dfrac{1 \; tab}{15 \; \cancel{mg}} \times \dfrac{1000 \; \cancel{mg}}{\cancel{g}} \times \dfrac{2 \; \cancel{doses}}{day} = 2$ tablets per day of Tranxene

Try These for Practice

1. 2 tab   2. 40 mL   3. 12 mL

4. 4 tab   5. 4 mg and 2 mg tab

Answers to Exercises

1. $40\ \text{mg} \times \dfrac{1\ \text{g}}{1000\ \text{mg}} \times \dfrac{1\ \text{tab}}{0.02\ \text{g}} = 2$ tablets of Paxil

2. $\overset{13}{65}\ \text{kg} \times \dfrac{0.55\ \text{mg}}{1\ \text{kg}} \times \dfrac{1\ \text{mL}}{\underset{6}{30}\ \text{mg}} = 1.19$ or 1.2 milliliters of Chlorpromazine

3. $0.85\ \text{g} \times \dfrac{1000\ \text{mg}}{1\ \text{g}} \times \dfrac{1\ \text{tab}}{850\ \text{mg}} = 1$ tablet of Glucophage

4. $5\ \text{mg} \times \dfrac{1\ \text{tab}}{2.5\ \text{mg}} = 2$ tablets of Glyburide

5. $66\ \text{kg} \times \dfrac{0.015\ \text{mg}}{1\ \text{kg}} \times \dfrac{1\ \text{tab}}{1\ \text{mg}} = 0.99$ or 1 tablet of (Robinol) glycopyrrolate

6. $0.005\ \text{g} \times \dfrac{1000\ \text{mg}}{1\ \text{g}} \times \dfrac{1\ \text{tab}}{2.5\ \text{mg}} = 2$ tablets of Norvasc

7. Select a 2.5 mg and a 5 mg tablet for this dose of Vasotec.

8. $0.5\ \text{mg} \times \dfrac{1\ \text{mL}}{1\ \text{mg}} = 0.5$ milliliters of Alprazolam

9. $0.01\ \text{g} \times \dfrac{1\ \text{tab}}{0.005\ \text{g}} = 2$ tablets of Ambien

10. $2.5\ \text{mg} \times 3\ \text{days} = 7.5\ \text{mg}$
    $1\ \text{mg} \times 4\ \text{days} = \underline{4.0\ \text{mg}}$
    $\qquad\qquad\qquad$ 11.5 mg of Coumadin per week

11. $0.5\ \text{g} \times \dfrac{1\ \text{tab}}{0.25\ \text{g}} = 2$ tablets of Ticlid

12. $\dfrac{3\ \text{mg}}{12\ \text{h}} \times \dfrac{1\ \text{tab}}{1.5\ \text{mg}} \times 24\ \text{h} = 4$ tab of Decadron in 24 h

13. $0.08\ \text{g} \times \dfrac{1000\ \text{mg}}{1\ \text{g}} \times \dfrac{1\ \text{tab}}{20\ \text{mg}} = 4$ tablets of Furosemide

14. $\overset{1}{200}\ \text{mg} \times \dfrac{1\ \text{g}}{\underset{5}{1000}\ \text{mg}} \times \dfrac{1\ \text{tab}}{0.2\ \text{g}} = 1$ tablet of Papaverine

15. $\dfrac{0.8\ \text{g}}{\text{dose}} \times \dfrac{\overset{5}{1000}\ \text{mg}}{1\ \text{g}} \times \dfrac{1\ \text{caplet}}{\underset{2}{400}\ \text{mg}} \times \dfrac{3\ \text{dose}}{\text{days}} \times \dfrac{5\ \text{days}}{1} = 30$ caplet of Motrin

16. $\dfrac{\text{gr}\ \dfrac{1}{100}}{\text{dose}} \times \dfrac{60\ \text{mg}}{\text{gr}\ 1} \times 8\ \text{dose} = 4.8$ milligrams in 8 hours of colchicine

17. $\overset{2}{100}\ \text{mg} \times \dfrac{5\ \text{mL}}{\underset{1}{50}\ \text{mg}} = 10$ milliliters of Zidovudine

18. $\sqrt{\dfrac{90\,\text{kg} \times 160\,\text{cm}}{3600}}$

$= \sqrt{4}$

$= 2\,\text{m}^2$

$2\,\text{m}^2 \times \dfrac{500\,\text{mg}}{\text{m}^2} \times \dfrac{3}{\text{day}} = 3000\,\text{mg/day}$

19. $148\,\text{lb} \times \dfrac{0.45\,\text{kg}}{1\,\text{lb}} \times \dfrac{3\,\text{mg}}{1\,\text{kg}} \times \dfrac{1\,\text{tab}}{50\,\text{mg}} = 3.996$ or 4 tablets of Cytoxan

20. $1.65\,\text{m}^2 \times \dfrac{30\,\text{mg}}{\text{m}^2} \times \dfrac{1\,\text{tab}}{50\,\text{mg}} = 0.99$ or 1 tablet of prednisone

Cumulative Answers

1. 1 tab	2. 10 mL	3. gr 3
4. 400 mg	5. 0.12 mg	6. 450 or 500 mg
7. ℥ 5	8. 10.6 mL	9. 1 cap
10. 4 tab	11. 3 tab	12. 3 tab
13. 0.2 g	14. 2 tab	15. 5 mL

Case Study 7

1. a. Draw line at the 1 mL mark of each syringe.

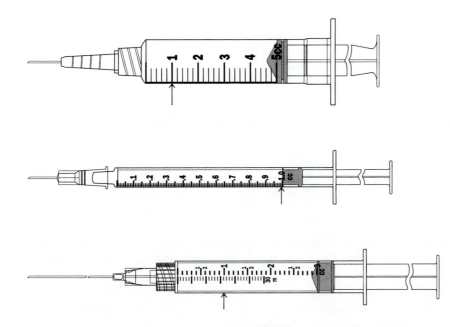

   b. The tuberculin syringe is the best syringe to most accurately measure small quantities of medication for injection.

2. a. $0.4 \text{ mg} \times \dfrac{\text{gr } 1}{60 \text{ mg}} \times \dfrac{1 \text{ mL}}{\text{gr } \dfrac{1}{150}} = 1 \text{ mL of Atropine}$

   b. The 3 cc syringe

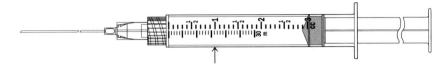

3. a. $\overset{70}{154 \text{ lb}} \times \dfrac{1 \text{ kg}}{\underset{1}{2.2 \text{ lb}}} \times \dfrac{0.07 \text{ mg}}{\text{kg}} = 4.9 \text{ mg or 5 mg of Versed}$

   b. Use the 5 mg/mL vial of Versed and the 50 mg/mL prefilled syringe of Demerol. Draw the 1 mL of Versed into the prepackaged 50 mg/mL syringe.

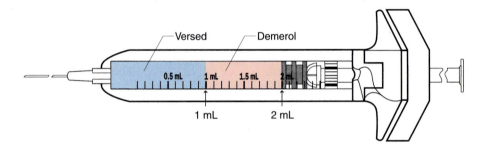

4. $0.005 \text{ g} \times \dfrac{1000 \text{ mg}}{1 \text{ g}} \times \dfrac{1 \text{ mL}}{5 \text{ mg}} \times \dfrac{\text{m } 15}{1 \text{ mL}} = \text{m } 15 \text{ of Compazine}$

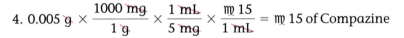

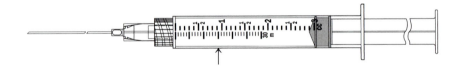

5. Draw a line at the 10 cc mark on the 20 cc syringe.

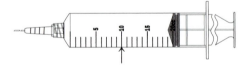

6. a. Use the 50 unit Lo-Dose insulin syringe for doses less than 50 units of insulin. Draw a line at the 6 unit mark and the 12 unit mark.

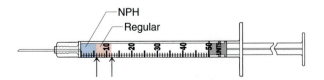

b. The patient is receiving 8 units of regular insulin in the morning plus 6 units of regular insulin before dinner for a total of 14 units of regular insulin per day.

7. $\overset{70}{\cancel{154}}$ $\cancel{lb} \times \dfrac{1\,\cancel{kg}}{2.2\,\cancel{lb}} \times \dfrac{1\,mg}{\cancel{kg}} = 70\,mg$ of Lovenox

Use the 80 mg/0.8mL vial.

$70\,\cancel{mg} \times \dfrac{0.8\,mL}{80\,\cancel{mg}} = 0.7$ mL of Lovenox; therefore draw a line at the 0.7 mL mark on the tuberculin syringe

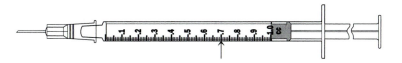

Try These for Practice

1. _____Tuberculin_____ syringe: 0.7 cc

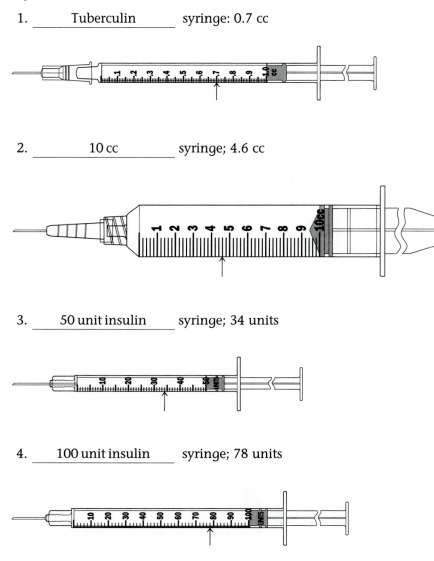

2. _____10 cc_____ syringe; 4.6 cc

3. ___50 unit insulin___ syringe; 34 units

4. ___100 unit insulin___ syringe; 78 units

5. $5 \text{ mg} \times \dfrac{1 \text{ mL}}{2 \text{ mg}} = 2.5 \text{ mL}$

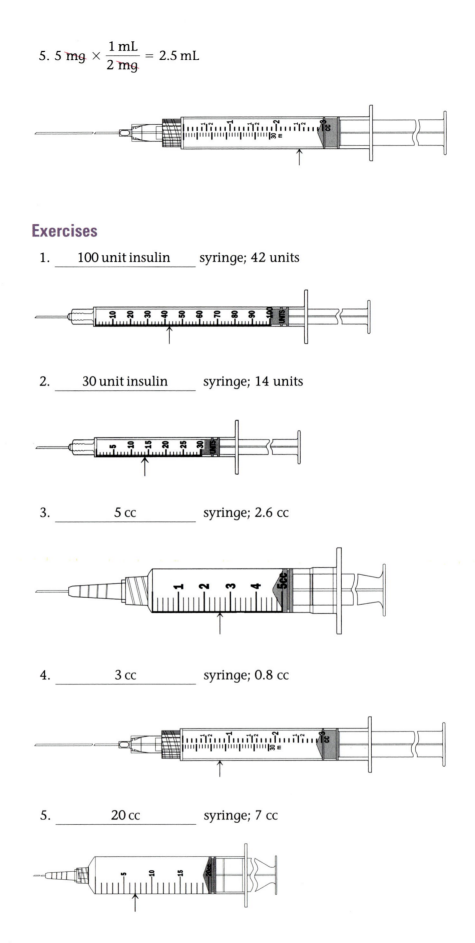

Exercises

1. _____100 unit insulin_____ syringe; 42 units

2. _____30 unit insulin_____ syringe; 14 units

3. _____5 cc_____ syringe; 2.6 cc

4. _____3 cc_____ syringe; 0.8 cc

5. _____20 cc_____ syringe; 7 cc

6. _____20 cc_____ syringe; 16 cc

7. _____50 unit insulin_____ syringe; 12 units

8. _____100 unit insulin_____ syringe; 54 units

9. _____Tuberculin_____ syringe; 0.3 cc

10. _____50 unit insulin_____ syringe; 45 units

11. _____10 cc_____ syringe; 3.8 cc

12. _____50 unit insulin_____ syringe; 16 units

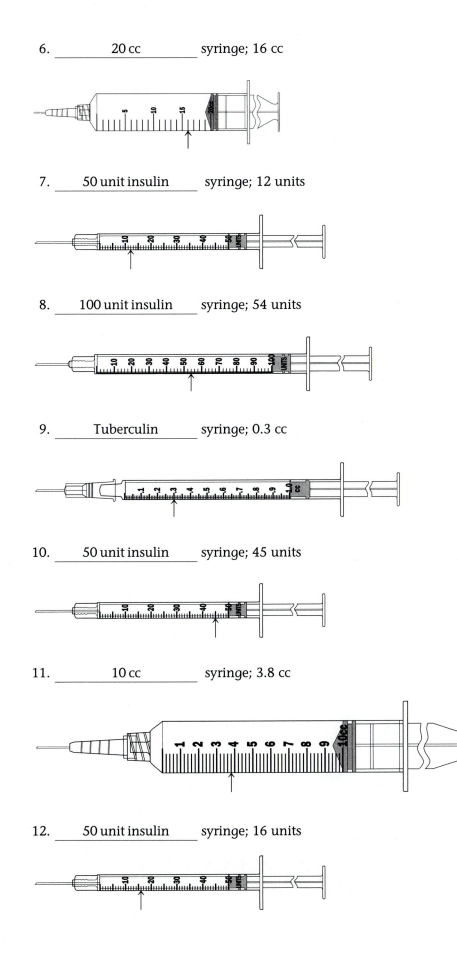

13. _____10 cc_____ syringe; 7.8 cc

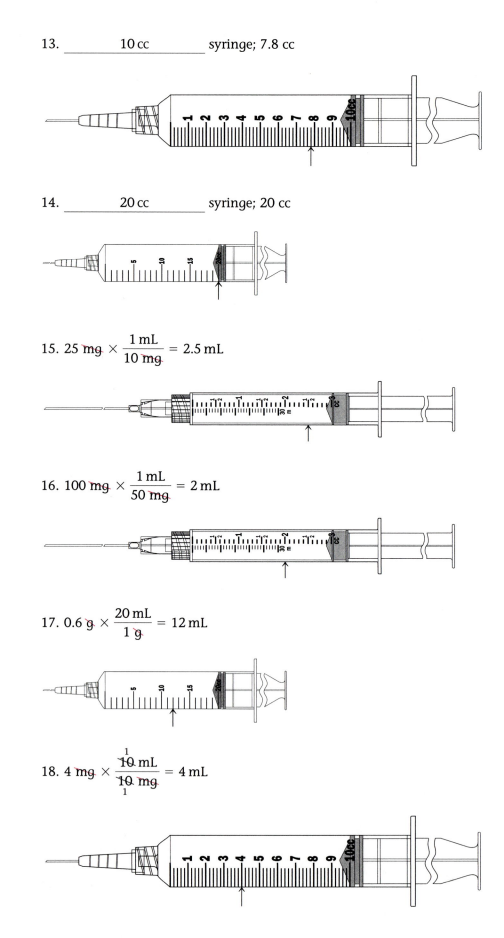

14. _____20 cc_____ syringe; 20 cc

15. 25 m̶g̶ × $\dfrac{1\ mL}{10\ m̶g̶}$ = 2.5 mL

16. 100 m̶g̶ × $\dfrac{1\ mL}{50\ m̶g̶}$ = 2 mL

17. 0.6 g̶ × $\dfrac{20\ mL}{1\ g̶}$ = 12 mL

18. 4 m̶g̶ × $\dfrac{\overset{1}{1̶0̶}\ mL}{\underset{1}{1̶0̶}\ m̶g̶}$ = 4 mL

19. $1.6 \text{ mg} \times \dfrac{1 \text{ mL}}{2 \text{ mg}} = 0.8 \text{ mL}$

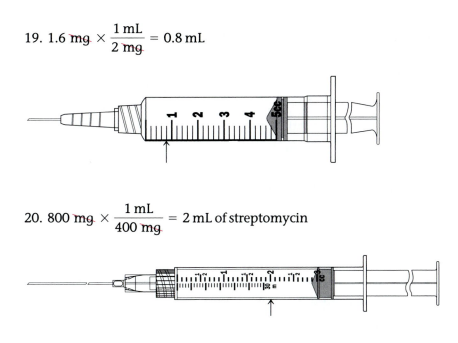

20. $800 \text{ mg} \times \dfrac{1 \text{ mL}}{400 \text{ mg}} = 2 \text{ mL of streptomycin}$

Cumulative Review Exercises

1. 1200 mg

2. 1.6 L

3. 1 capsule of Prilosec

4. 7.5 mg of morphine sulfate

5. 4 mL of Biaxin

6. 0.12 mg

7. 4 ounces every 2 hours for 10 hours

8. ℥ 3

9. gr $\dfrac{1}{150}$

10. gr $\dfrac{3}{50}$ or gr $\dfrac{1}{15}$

11. 2 tablets of Cardura

12. 3 tablets of clonidine

13. 1 tablet of Detrol

14. 175 mg of Trovan

15. 0.8 mL of phenobarbital

Case Study 8

1. $40 \text{ mg} \times \dfrac{1 \text{ g}}{1000 \text{ mg}} \times \dfrac{1 \text{ tab}}{0.04 \text{ g}} = 1 \text{ tab of Inderal three times a day}$

2. a $\dfrac{20 \text{ mg}}{\text{dose}} \times \dfrac{2 \text{ dose}}{\text{day}} = 40 \text{ mg/day which is } 0.04 \text{ g/day}$

   b. $\dfrac{0.04 \text{ g}}{\text{day}} \times \dfrac{7 \text{ day}}{\text{week}} = 0.28 \text{ g per week}$

3. $20 \text{ mEq} \times \dfrac{4 \text{ oz}}{\overset{40 \text{ mEq}}{\underset{2}{}}} \times \dfrac{30 \text{ mL}}{\text{oz}} = \dfrac{120 \text{ mL}}{2} = 60 \text{ mL will contain } 20 \text{ mEq K-Lor}$

4. $600 \text{ mg} \times \dfrac{1 \text{ tab}}{600 \text{ mg}} = 1$ tab of azithromycin

5. $0.1 \text{ g} \times \dfrac{1000 \text{ mg}}{1 \text{ g}} \times \dfrac{1 \text{ tab}}{100 \text{ mg}} = 1$ tab of trovafloxacin

6. $0.01 \text{ g} \times \dfrac{1000 \text{ mg}}{1 \text{ g}} \times \dfrac{1 \text{ tab}}{10 \text{ mg}} = 1$ tab of glipizide

7. $0.05 \text{ g} \times \dfrac{1000 \text{ mg}}{1 \text{ g}} = 50$ mg; give one tablet of hydroxyzine to patient

Try These for Practice

1. Take 9 g of sodium chloride and add water to the level of 1000 mL.

2. 15 g of epsom salt crystals

3. 1000 mL of the 2% solution

4. Take 60 mL of the 1:5 solution and add water to the level of 300 mL.

5. Take 40 (5 g) tab and add water to the level of 4000 mL.

Exercises

1. $\dfrac{2000 \text{ mL} \times \dfrac{1 \text{ mL}}{50 \text{ mL}}}{\dfrac{100 \text{ mL}}{100 \text{ mL}}} = $ 40 mL of the 100% lysol solution and add water to a level of 2000 mL

2. $\dfrac{\overset{5}{500} \text{ mL} \times \dfrac{0.5 \text{ mL}}{100 \text{ mL}}}{\dfrac{10 \text{ mL}}{100 \text{ mL}}} = $ 25 mL of the 10% Dakin's solution and add water to the level of 500 mL

3. $\dfrac{250 \text{ mL} \times \dfrac{3 \text{ mL}}{100 \text{ mL}}}{\dfrac{15 \text{ mL}}{100 \text{ mL}}} = 250 \text{ mL} \times \dfrac{3 \text{ mL}}{100 \text{ mL}} \times \dfrac{100 \text{ mL}}{\underset{5}{15} \text{ mL}} = 50 \text{ mL of } 15\%$

hydrogen peroxide solution; add water to the level of 250 mL

4. $\dfrac{240 \text{ mL} \times \dfrac{1 \text{ mL}}{2 \text{ mL}}}{\dfrac{100 \text{ mL}}{100 \text{ mL}}} = $ 120 mL of Ensure; add water to the level of 240 mL

5. $\overset{5}{500} \text{ mL} \times \dfrac{8.5 \text{ g}}{\underset{1}{100} \text{ mL}} = $ 42.5 g of amino acid in 500 mL of an 8.5% solution

6. $\overset{5}{\cancel{250}} \text{ mL} \times \dfrac{10 \text{ g}}{\underset{2}{\cancel{100} \text{ mL}}} = 25 \text{ g}$ of lipids in 250 mL of a 10% Introlipid solution

7. $50 \text{ g} \times \dfrac{\overset{5}{\cancel{100} \text{ mL}}}{\underset{1}{\cancel{20} \text{ g}}} = 250 \text{ mL}$ will contain 50 g of glucose

8. $2 \text{ g} \times \dfrac{\overset{2}{\cancel{100} \text{ mL}}}{\underset{1}{\cancel{50} \text{ g}}} = 4 \text{ mL}$ of 50% magnesium sulfate

9. $\overset{2}{\cancel{200} \text{ mL}} \times \dfrac{2000 \text{ mg}}{\underset{1}{\cancel{100} \text{ mL}}} = 4000 \text{ mg}$ of lidocaine are contained in 200 mL of a 2% lidocaine solution.

10. $\overset{1}{\cancel{4} \text{ mL}} \times \dfrac{1 \text{ g}}{\underset{25}{\cancel{100} \text{ mL}}} = 0.04 \text{ g}$ of lidocaine

11. $\overset{1}{\cancel{100} \text{ mL}} \times \dfrac{0.9 \text{ g}}{\underset{1}{\cancel{100} \text{ mL}}} = 0.9 \text{ g}$ of sodium chloride crystals; add water to the level of 100 mL

12. $\cancel{4000} \text{ mL} \times \dfrac{25 \text{ g}}{100 \text{ mL}} = 1000 \text{ g}$ of dextrose are contained in 4000 mL of a 25% dextrose solution

13. $\dfrac{240 \text{ mL} \times \dfrac{1 \cancel{\text{ mL}}}{3 \cancel{\text{ mL}}}}{\dfrac{\cancel{100} \cancel{\text{ mL}}}{\cancel{100} \cancel{\text{ mL}}}} = 80 \text{ mL}$ of Ensure; add water to the level of 240 mL

14. $\dfrac{500 \text{ mL} \times \dfrac{0.25 \cancel{\text{ mL}}}{100 \cancel{\text{ mL}}}}{\dfrac{5 \text{ mL}}{100 \cancel{\text{ mL}}}} = \overset{100}{\cancel{500}} \text{ mL} \times \dfrac{0.25}{\underset{1}{\cancel{100}}} \times \dfrac{\overset{1}{\cancel{100}}}{\underset{1}{\cancel{5}}} = 25 \text{ mL}$ of the 5% solu-

tion; add water to the level of 500 mL

15. $2 \text{ mL} \times \dfrac{10 \text{ g}}{100 \text{ mL}} = 0.2 \text{ g}$ of calcium chloride

16. $0.001 \text{ g} \times \dfrac{1000 \text{ mg}}{1 \text{ g}} \times \dfrac{1 \text{ mL}}{0.1 \text{ mg}} = 10 \text{ mL}$ of Epinephrine 1:1000 will contain 0.001 g of Epinephrine

or

$0.001 \text{ g} \times \dfrac{10,000 \text{ mL}}{1 \text{ g}} = 10 \text{ mL}$

17. $\overset{1}{\cancel{25} \text{ mL}} \times \dfrac{25 \text{ g}}{\underset{4}{\cancel{100} \text{ mL}}} = 6.25 \text{ g}$ of Mannitol are contained in 25 mL of the 25% solution

18. $20 \text{ g} \times \dfrac{30 \text{ mL}}{1 \text{ g}} = 600 \text{ mL}$ of 1:30 acetic acid solution will contain 20 g of acetic acid

19. $\overset{8}{\cancel{4000}}\text{ mL} \times \dfrac{\cancel{4}\text{ g}}{\cancel{100}\text{ mL}} \times \dfrac{1\text{ tab}}{\cancel{5}\text{ g}} = $ 32 tab of potassium permanganate; add H_2O to the level of 4000 mL

20. $3500\text{ mL} \times \dfrac{1\text{ g}}{1000\text{ mL}} \times \dfrac{1\text{ tab}}{0.5\text{ g}} = $ 7 tab of aluminum acetate, add H_2O to the level of 3500 mL

Cumulative Review Exercises

1. 12.5 g of dextrose
2. 60 mL of Levophed
3. 150 mL of Isocal and add H_2O to level of 200 mL
4. 0.25 mg
5. $\dfrac{1}{2}$ oz
6. gr $\dfrac{1}{1000}$
7. 0.6 mg
8. gr $1\dfrac{1}{2}$
9. 0.5 g
10. 0.0004 g of atropine sulfate
11. 250 μg of digoxin
12. 0.2 mg epinephrine
13. 3.6 g of Zithromax
14. 1 tab Tranxene
15. 15 mL of Biaxin

Case Study 9

1. $2\text{ g} \times \dfrac{\cancel{1000}\text{ mg}}{1\text{ g}} \times \dfrac{1\text{ vial}}{\cancel{1000}\text{ mg}} = $ 2 vials labeled 1000 mg/vial

2. $240\text{ mg} \times \dfrac{1\text{ g}}{1000\text{ mg}} \times \dfrac{1\text{ mL}}{0.04\text{ g}} = $ 6 mL of Gentamicin for one dose

3. $\dfrac{300\,\mu g}{\text{mL}} = $ 1 mL (microgram is written as mcg or μg) of Neupogen

4. $\overset{3}{\cancel{1500}}\text{ mg} \times \dfrac{1\text{ g}}{\underset{2}{\cancel{1000}}\text{ mg}} \times \dfrac{\text{vial}}{3\text{ g}} = \dfrac{1}{2}$ vial of Unasyn

5. $\text{gr } 2 \times \dfrac{60\text{ mg}}{\text{gr } 1} \times \dfrac{1\text{ mL}}{65\text{ mg}} = $ 1.8 mL of phenobarbital

6. $0.025\text{ g} \times \dfrac{1000\text{ mg}}{1\text{ g}} \times \dfrac{1\text{ tab}}{25\text{ mg}} = $ 1 tab of atenolol

7. $\overset{1}{\cancel{50}}\text{ mcg} \times \dfrac{2\text{ mL}}{\underset{2}{\cancel{100}}\text{ mcg}} = $ 1 mL of Fentanyl

8. 6 units on a 30 unit Lo-Dose insulin syringe

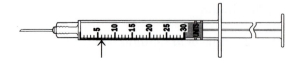

9. $110 \text{ lb} \times \dfrac{0.45 \text{ kg}}{1 \text{ lb}} \times \dfrac{5 \text{ mcg}}{\text{kg}} \times \dfrac{1 \text{ mL}}{300 \text{ mcg}} = 0.8 \text{ mL of Neupogen}$

Try These for Practice

1. 2 mL   2. 0.35 mL   3. 1.5 mL

4. 4 mL   5. minims 8

Exercises

1. $0.75 \text{ g} \times \dfrac{1000 \text{ mg}}{1 \text{ g}} \times \dfrac{7 \text{ mL}}{750 \text{ mg}} = 7 \text{ mL of Kefurox}$

2. $\overset{1}{500} \text{ mg} \times \dfrac{1 \text{ g}}{\underset{2}{1000} \text{ mg}} \times \dfrac{2.5 \text{ mL}}{1 \text{ g}} = \dfrac{2.5 \text{ mL}}{2} = 1.25 \text{ mL of Streptomycin}$

3. $700 \text{ mg} \times \dfrac{\text{minims } 15}{250 \text{ mg}} = \text{minims } 42$

4. $0.2 \text{ mg} \times \dfrac{2 \text{ mL}}{0.5 \text{ mg}} = 0.8 \text{ mL of Digoxin}$

5. $\text{gr} \dfrac{1}{400} \times \dfrac{\text{minims } 15}{\text{gr} \dfrac{1}{150}} = \text{minims } 6 \text{ of atropine sulfate}$

6. $330 \, \mu\text{g} \times \dfrac{1 \text{ mg}}{1000 \, \mu\text{g}} \times \dfrac{1 \text{ mL}}{6.6 \text{ mg}} = 0.05 \text{ mL of Vitrovene}$

7. $0.725 \text{ mg} \times \dfrac{2 \text{ mL}}{2.5 \text{ mg}} = 0.6 \text{ mL of Inapsine}$

8. $\overset{20}{400} \text{ mg} \times \dfrac{1 \text{ mL}}{\underset{1}{20} \text{ mg}} = 20 \text{ mL of Cipro}$

9. $\overset{3}{30} \text{ mg} \times \dfrac{1 \text{ mL}}{\underset{1}{10} \text{ mg}} = 3 \text{ mL of morphine sulfate}$

10. $175{,}000 \text{ units} \times \dfrac{1 \text{ mL}}{50{,}000 \text{ units}} = 3.5 \text{ mL of Urokinase}$

11. $0.45 \text{ g} \times \dfrac{\overset{2}{1000} \text{ mg}}{1 \text{ g}} \times \dfrac{10 \text{ mL}}{\underset{1}{500} \text{ mg}} = 9 \text{ mL of Vancomycin}$

12. $\overset{3}{600} \text{ mg} \times \dfrac{1 \text{ g}}{\underset{5}{1000} \text{ mg}} \times \dfrac{1 \text{ mL}}{0.4 \text{ g}} = \dfrac{3}{2} \text{ or } 1.5 \text{ mL of Cleocin}$

13. $\overset{1}{500} \text{ mg} \times \dfrac{1 \text{ g}}{\underset{2}{1000} \text{ mg}} \times \dfrac{5 \text{ mL}}{1 \text{ g}} = \dfrac{5}{2} \text{ or } 2.5 \text{ mL of Kefzol}$

14. $70 \text{ kg} \times \dfrac{10.7 \text{ mg}}{\text{kg}} \times \dfrac{1 \text{ g}}{1000 \text{ mg}} \times \dfrac{5 \text{ mL}}{1 \text{ g}} = 3.75 \text{ mL of Ancef}$

15. $55 \text{ kg} \times \dfrac{\overset{1}{\cancel{5} \text{ mg}}}{\text{kg}} \times \dfrac{1 \text{ mL}}{\underset{15}{\cancel{75} \text{ mg}}} = 3.7 \text{ mL of cedofovir}$

16. $1.8 \text{ m}^2 \times \dfrac{2000 \text{ mg}}{\text{m}^2} \times \dfrac{1 \text{ mL}}{24 \text{ mg}} = 150 \text{ mL of foscarnet}$

17. $90 \text{ lb} \times \dfrac{0.45 \text{ kg}}{1 \text{ lb}} \times \dfrac{3 \text{ mg}}{\text{kg}} \times \dfrac{3 \text{ mL}}{300 \text{ mg}} = 1.2 \text{ mL of Pentam}$

18. $\overset{6}{\cancel{60}} \text{ kg} \times \dfrac{0.25 \text{ mg}}{\text{kg}} \times \dfrac{10 \text{ mL}}{\underset{5}{\cancel{50} \text{ mg}}} = 3 \text{ mL of Amphotericin B}$

19. $1.5 \text{ g} \times \dfrac{4 \text{ mL}}{2 \text{ g}} = 3 \text{ mL of Mefoxin}$

20. $0.3 \text{ g} \times \dfrac{6 \text{ mL}}{2 \text{ g}} = 0.9 \text{ mL of Ampicillin}$

Cumulative Review Exercises

1. 1 tab of Zithromax   2. 2 tab of Bentyl   3. 2 cap of Inderal SL

4. 1 tab of Viagra   5. Minims 4 of Demerol

6. 3 packets of K-Lor 20mEq   7. 1 tab of Norfloxacin

8. 2 mL of Tagamet   9. 4 cap of Mycobutin 10. 0.5 mL of penicillin G

11. 0.0003 g   12. 3 mg   13. gr $1\dfrac{1}{2}$

14. 150 gtt   15. gr $\dfrac{1}{1000}$

Case Study 10

1. $\dfrac{83 \text{ mL}}{60 \text{ min}} \times \dfrac{10 \text{ gtt}}{1 \text{ mL}} = \dfrac{83}{6} = 13.8 \quad \text{or} \quad 14 \text{ gtt/min}$

2. $\dfrac{83 \text{ mL}}{1 \text{ h}} \times 24 \text{ h} = 1992 \text{ mL of N/S}$

3. a. According to the label, use 16 mL of Sterile Water.

   b. $\cancel{750} \text{ mg} \times \dfrac{16 \text{ mL}}{\cancel{1500} \text{ mg}} = 8 \text{ mL of Cefuroxime}$

   c. $\dfrac{58 \text{ mL}}{\underset{2}{\cancel{30} \text{ min}}} \times \dfrac{\overset{1}{\cancel{15} \text{ gtt}}}{1 \text{ mL}} = \dfrac{58}{2} = 29 \text{ gtt/min}$

4. $\overset{1}{\cancel{5000}} \text{ units} \times \dfrac{1 \text{ mL}}{\underset{4}{\cancel{20,000} \text{ units}}} = \dfrac{1}{4} = 0.25 \text{ mL of Heparin}$

5. Use the TB syringe to measure small amounts of drugs. Place an arrow at the 0.25 mL mark.

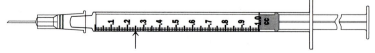

6. $\dfrac{5000 \text{ units}}{\text{dose}} \times \dfrac{2 \text{ doses}}{\text{day}} = 10{,}000$ units each day of heparin

7. $\dfrac{250 \text{ mL}}{60 \text{ min}} \times \dfrac{60 \text{ min}}{1 \text{ h}} = \dfrac{250 \text{ mL}}{\text{h}}$ of Zithromax infusion

8. $\overset{2}{10} \text{ mg} \times \dfrac{1 \text{ tab}}{\underset{1}{5} \text{ mg}} = 2$ tab of Accupril

9. $10 \text{ mg} \times \dfrac{1000 \text{ mcg}}{1 \text{ mg}} = 10{,}000$ mcg of Accupril

10. $0.05 \text{ g} \times \dfrac{\overset{20}{1000} \text{ mg}}{\text{g}} \times \dfrac{1 \text{ tab}}{\underset{1}{50} \text{ mg}} = 1$ tab of Lopressor

Try These for Practice

1. 10 gtt/min   2. 38 gtt/min   3. 106.25 mL/h

4. 148 mL/h   5. 60 μgtt/min

Exercises

1. $\dfrac{3000 \text{ mL}}{24 \text{ h}} \times \dfrac{\overset{1}{10} \text{ gtt}}{\text{mL}} \times \dfrac{1 \text{ h}}{\underset{6}{60} \text{ min}} = 20.8$ or   21 gtt/min

2. $\dfrac{250 \text{ cc}}{8 \text{ h}} \times \dfrac{1 \text{ h}}{\underset{1}{60} \text{ min}} \times \dfrac{\overset{1}{60} \mu\text{gtt}}{\text{cc}} = 31.25$ or   31 μgtt/min

3. $\dfrac{1000 \text{ mL}}{8 \text{ h}} = 125$ mL/h will be the setting on the infusion pump

4. $\dfrac{75 \text{ mL}}{\text{h}} \times \dfrac{1 \text{ h}}{\underset{10}{60} \text{ min}} \times \dfrac{\overset{3}{18} \text{ gtt}}{\text{mL}} = 22.5$ or   23 gtt/min

5. $\dfrac{100 \text{ mL}}{60 \text{ min}} \times \dfrac{60 \mu\text{gtt}}{\text{mL}} = 100 \mu$gtt/min (remember mL/h = microgtts/min)

6. $\dfrac{650 \text{ mL}}{8 \text{ h}} = 81.25$ mL/h; set the infusion pump at 81.25 mL/h

7. $\dfrac{\overset{5}{300} \text{ mL}}{\underset{3}{180} \text{ min}} \times \dfrac{12 \text{ gtt}}{\text{mL}} = 20$ gtt/min

8. 55 mL/h is 55 μgtt/min

9. $\dfrac{2500 \text{ mL}}{24 \text{ h}} =$ set the infusion pump at 104.2 mL/h

10. $\dfrac{850 \text{ mL}}{6 \text{ h}} \times \dfrac{1 \text{ h}}{60 \text{ min}} \times \dfrac{15 \text{ gtt}}{1 \text{ mL}} = 35.4$ or   35 gtt/min

11. 167 μgtt/min is the same as 167 mL/h

12. $\dfrac{17 \text{ gtt}}{\text{min}} \times \dfrac{1 \text{ mL}}{\underset{1}{10} \text{ gtt}} \times \dfrac{\overset{6}{60} \text{ min}}{1 \text{ h}} = 102$ mL/h

13. $\dfrac{250\,cc}{24\,h} = 10.4\,mL/h$

14. a. $50\,\mu gtt/min$ is $50\,mL/h$

    b. $\dfrac{50\,mL}{h} \times 24\,h = 1200\,mL$ in 24 h

15. The patient was receiving 125 mL/h so the infusion pump was stopped after 3 h (375 mL) and stopped for 1 h so there are four hours remaining.

    $\dfrac{625\,mL}{4\,h} = 156.25$ or   156 mL/h

16. $125\,\mu gtt/min$ is 125 mL/h

17. $\dfrac{700\,mL}{10\,h} = 70\,mL/h$

18. a. $\dfrac{1000\,mL}{10\,h} \times \dfrac{1\,h}{60\,min} \times \dfrac{20\,gtt}{mL} = 33.3$ or   33 drops of Ensure per minute

    b. $1000\,mL \times \dfrac{1\,can}{200\,mL} = 5$ cans of Ensure

19. $\dfrac{31\,gtts}{min} \times \dfrac{60\,min}{1\,h} \times \dfrac{1\,mL}{15\,gtt} = 124\,mL/h$

20. $40\,\mu gtt/min$ is 40 mL/h.

    $\dfrac{40\,mL}{h} \times 18\,h = 720\,mL$ in 18 h

Cumulative Review Exercises

1. 80 mL/h   2. 62.5 mL/h   3. 156.25 mL/h

4. 17 drops per minute   5. 0.12 mg   6. 1 cap

7. 4.5 mg   8. 3 mL   9. 1 cap

10. 3.1 mL   11. 12 tsp   12. $gr\dfrac{1}{10}$

13. 150 gtt   14. 0.00067   or   0.0007 g

15. 30 mL

Case Study 11

1. $150\,mg \times \dfrac{5\,mL}{75\,mg} = 10\,mL$ of Cleocin

2. $150\,mg \times \dfrac{1\,mL}{15\,mg} = 10\,mL$ of Zantac

3. $150\,mg \times \dfrac{24\,h}{12\,h} = 300\,mg$ of Zantac each day

4. $\overset{2}{\cancel{100}} \text{ mg} \times \dfrac{1 \text{ mL}}{\underset{1}{\cancel{50} \text{ mg}}} = 2 \text{ mL of Dilantin}$

5. $\dfrac{52 \cancel{\text{mL}}}{\underset{2}{\cancel{30} \text{ min}}} \times \dfrac{\overset{1}{\cancel{15} \text{ gtt}}}{1 \cancel{\text{mL}}} = 26 \text{ gtt/min of N/S}$

6. $\dfrac{\overset{8}{\cancel{480} \cancel{\text{mL}}}}{\underset{1}{\cancel{6} \text{ h}}} \times \dfrac{1 \cancel{\text{h}}}{\underset{1}{\cancel{60} \text{ min}}} \times \dfrac{\overset{3}{\cancel{18} \text{ gtt}}}{1 \cancel{\text{mL}}} = 24 \text{ gtt/min of Ensure}$

7. $\dfrac{\overset{5}{\cancel{100} \cancel{\text{g}}}}{3 \text{ h}} \times \dfrac{100 \text{ mL}}{\underset{1}{\cancel{20} \cancel{\text{g}}}} = \dfrac{500 \text{ mL}}{3 \text{ h}} = 166.7 \text{ mL/h is the rate to set the infusion pump}$

8. $\dfrac{100 \text{ mL}}{\underset{1}{\cancel{30} \cancel{\text{min}}}} \times \dfrac{\overset{2}{\cancel{60} \cancel{\text{min}}}}{1 \text{ h}} = 200 \text{ mL/h is the rate to set the infusion pump}$

9. $178 \cancel{\text{lb}} \times \dfrac{1 \cancel{\text{kg}}}{2.2 \cancel{\text{lb}}} \times \dfrac{7.5 \text{ mg}}{\cancel{\text{kg}}} = 607 \text{ mg of Flagyl every 6 h}$

10. $\dfrac{100 \cancel{\text{mL}}}{\underset{6}{\cancel{60} \text{ min}}} \times \dfrac{\overset{1}{\cancel{15} \text{ gtt}}}{\cancel{\text{mL}}} = \dfrac{100 \text{ gtt}}{6 \text{ min}} = 16.6 \quad \text{or} \quad 17 \text{ gtt/min of Flagyl}$

11. $\dfrac{\text{Ensure } \overset{80}{\cancel{480} } \text{ mL}}{\underset{1}{\cancel{6} \cancel{\text{h}}}} \times \dfrac{24 \cancel{\text{h}}}{\text{day}} = \dfrac{1920 \text{ mL}}{\text{day}}$

$\dfrac{\text{Sterile H}_2\text{O } 50 \text{ mL}}{\underset{1}{\cancel{6} \cancel{\text{h}}}} \times \dfrac{\overset{4}{\cancel{24} \cancel{\text{h}}}}{\text{day}} = \dfrac{200 \text{ mL}}{\text{day}}$

$\dfrac{\text{Ranitidine } 10 \text{ mL}}{\underset{1}{\cancel{12} \cancel{\text{h}}}} \times \dfrac{\overset{2}{\cancel{24} \cancel{\text{h}}}}{\text{day}} = \dfrac{20 \text{ mL}}{\text{day}}$

$\dfrac{\text{Cleocin } 10 \text{ mL}}{\cancel{6} \cancel{\text{h}}} \times \dfrac{\overset{4}{\cancel{24} \cancel{\text{h}}}}{\text{day}} = \dfrac{40 \text{ mL}}{\text{day}}$

Total enteral fluid intake in 24 h = 2180 mL

12. $60 \cancel{\text{mg}} \times \dfrac{1 \cancel{\text{g}}}{1000 \cancel{\text{mg}}} \times \dfrac{30 \text{ mL}}{0.08 \cancel{\text{g}}} = \dfrac{180 \text{ mL}}{8} = 22.5 \text{ mL of furosemide}$

Try These for Practice

1. a. 32 mL of cefuroxime,

   b. 116 microdrops per minute

2. 120 mL/h   3. 28 mL/h   4. 13 h and 9 min

5. a. 1.3 mL

   b. 51 μgtt/min

Exercises

1. a. $145 \text{ lb} \times \dfrac{0.45 \text{ kg}}{\text{lb}} \times \dfrac{6 \text{ mcg}}{\text{kg/min}} \times \dfrac{60 \text{ min}}{1 \text{ h}} \times \dfrac{\overset{1}{500} \text{ mL}}{\underset{1}{500} \text{ mg}} \times \dfrac{1 \text{ mg}}{1000 \text{ mcg}} =$

   23.49   or   23.5 mL/h

   b. $500 \text{ mL} \times \dfrac{1 \text{ h}}{23.5 \text{ mL}} = 21.27 \text{ h}$ or   21 h and 16 min. This infusion will end at 3:16 A.M. on the following day.

2. $160 \text{ mg} \times \dfrac{1 \text{ mL}}{50 \text{ mg}} = 3.2 \text{ mL}$ of amiodarone must be added to 20 mL D_5W; this equals 23.2 mL

   $\dfrac{23.2 \text{ mL}}{\underset{1}{10} \text{ min}} \times \dfrac{\overset{6}{60} \mu\text{gtt}}{\text{mL}} = 139.2$ or   139 μgtt/min

3. $720 \text{ mg} \times \dfrac{1 \text{mL}}{50 \text{mg}} = 14.4 \text{ mL}$ of amiodarone must be added to 500 mL D_5W

   $\dfrac{514.4 \text{ mL}}{24 \text{ h}} = 21.4 \text{ mL/h}$

4. a. $0.09 \text{ g} \times \dfrac{1000 \text{ mg}}{\text{g}} \times \dfrac{10 \text{ mL}}{90 \text{ mg}} = 10 \text{ mL}$ of Aredia

   b. $\dfrac{1010 \text{ mL}}{24 \text{ h}} = 42.08$ or   42.1 mL/h

5. a. $150 \text{ lb} \times \dfrac{0.45 \text{ kg}}{1 \text{ lb}} \times \dfrac{0.75 \text{ mg}}{\text{kg}} \times \dfrac{100 \text{ mL}}{2000 \text{ mg}} = 2.53$ or   2.5 mL of lidocaine

   b. $150 \text{ lb} \times \dfrac{0.45 \text{ kg}}{1 \text{ lb}} \times \dfrac{0.75 \text{ mg}}{\text{kg}} = 50.625 \text{ mg}$; the patient will receive 50.6 mg of 2% lidocaine

   $\dfrac{502.5 \text{ mL}}{50.6 \text{ mg}} \times \dfrac{5 \text{ mg}}{\text{h}} = 49.7 \text{ mL per hour}$

6. a. $210 \text{ lb} \times \dfrac{1 \text{ kg}}{2.2 \text{ lb}} \times \dfrac{0.25 \text{ mg}}{\text{kg}} = \dfrac{52.5}{2.2} = 23.86$ or   23.9 mg of Cardizem

   b. $23.9 \text{ mg} \times \dfrac{1 \text{ mL}}{5 \text{ mg}} = 4.78$ or   4.8 mL

7. a. $\overset{10}{500} \text{ mg} \times \dfrac{1 \text{ mL}}{\underset{1}{50} \text{ mg}} = 10 \text{ mL}$ of Dilantin

   b. $\dfrac{10 \text{ mL}}{10 \text{ min}} \times \dfrac{60 \mu\text{gtt}}{\text{mL}} = 60 \mu\text{gtt/min}$

   The patient has to receive 60 μgtt/min.

8. $0.25 \text{ mg} \times \dfrac{1 \text{ mL}}{0.5 \text{ mg}} = 0.5 \text{ mL}$ of digoxin

9. a. $80 \text{ kg} \times \dfrac{18 \text{ mg}}{\text{kg}} = 1440 \text{ mg of Cefuroxime}$

   b. $1440 \text{ mg} \times \dfrac{8 \text{ mL}}{750 \text{ mg}} = 15.36 \text{ mL of Cefuroxime}$

   c. $\dfrac{215 \text{ mL}}{1.5 \text{ h}} = 143.6 \text{ mL/h}$

10. $\overset{2}{6} \text{ mg} \times \dfrac{1 \text{ mL}}{3 \text{ mg}} = 2 \text{ mL of Adenocor}$

11. a. $\overset{2}{500} \text{ mg} \times \dfrac{8 \text{ mL}}{\underset{3}{750} \text{ mg}} = 5.3 \text{ mL of Cefuroxime}$

   b. $\dfrac{105.3 \text{ mL}}{20 \text{ min}} = 5.27 \text{ mL/min}$

12. $\text{gr} \dfrac{1}{\underset{1}{60}} \times \dfrac{\overset{1}{60} \text{ mg}}{\text{gr}} \times \dfrac{1 \text{ mL}}{0.5 \text{ mg}} = 2 \text{ mL of atropine}$

13. a. $\dfrac{500 \text{ mL}}{\underset{1}{15} \text{ h}} \times \dfrac{\overset{4}{60} \mu\text{gtt}}{1 \text{ mL}} \times \dfrac{1 \text{ h}}{60 \text{ min}} = 33 \,\mu\text{gtt/min}$

   b. $\dfrac{500 \text{ mL}}{15 \text{ h}} = 33.3 \text{ mL/h}$

14. $2 \text{ m}^2 \times \dfrac{1500 \text{ mg}}{\text{m}^2} \times \dfrac{1 \text{ mL}}{200 \text{ mg}} = 15 \text{ mL of calcium EDTA}$

   $265 \text{ mL} \times \dfrac{1 \text{ h}}{11 \text{ mL}} = 24.1 \text{ h}$ or   24 h and 6 min. The IV will be completed at 10:06 A.M. the following morning.

15. a. $95 \text{ lb} \times \dfrac{\text{kg}}{2.2 \text{ lb}} \times \dfrac{33.5 \text{ mg}}{\text{kg}} \times \dfrac{8 \text{ mL}}{750 \text{ mg}} = 15.43$ or   15.4 mL

   b. $\dfrac{215.4 \text{ mL}}{30 \text{ min}} = 7.18$ or   7.2 mL/min

16. $2 \text{ mg} \times \dfrac{1 \text{ mL}}{0.4 \text{ mg}} = 5 \text{ mL of Narcan}$

17. a. $172 \text{ lb} \times \dfrac{\text{kg}}{2.2 \text{ lb}} \times \dfrac{6 \text{ mcg}}{\text{kg}} \times \dfrac{1 \text{ mL}}{50 \text{ mcg}} = 9.38$ or   9.4 mL contain the prescribed dose

   b. $9.4 \text{ mL} \times \dfrac{1 \text{ ampule}}{1 \text{ mL}} = 9.34 \text{ ampules, so you need 10 ampules}$

   c. $\dfrac{109.4 \text{ mL}}{\underset{1}{30} \text{ min}} \times \dfrac{\overset{2}{60} \mu\text{gtt}}{\text{mL}} = 218.8$ or   219 μgtt/min

18. a. $50 \text{ mg} \times \dfrac{1 \text{ mL}}{1 \text{ mg}} = 50 \text{ mL of morphine sulfate}$

   b. $\dfrac{300 \text{ mL}}{5 \text{ h}} = 60 \text{ mL/h}$

   c. $\dfrac{210 \text{ mL}}{\underset{7}{35} \text{ mg}} \times \dfrac{\overset{3}{15} \text{ mg}}{\text{h}} = 90 \text{ mL/h}$

19. $\overset{5}{\cancel{500}\text{ units}} \times \dfrac{1\text{ mL}}{\underset{1}{\cancel{100}\text{ units}}} = 5\text{ mL of Regular insulin is the dose}$

$\dfrac{255\text{ mL}}{12\text{ h}} = 21.3\text{ mL/h is the flow rate}$

20. $\dfrac{\cancel{1500}\text{ units}}{\text{h}} \times \dfrac{\overset{1}{\cancel{500}\text{ mL}}}{\underset{1}{\cancel{50{,}000}\text{ units}}} = 15\text{ mL/h is the setting on the pump}$

Cumulative Review Exercises

1. 4.4 mL of medication

2. 1 mL of Methergine

3. 3 mL of penicillin

4. minims 12.5 or ℳ 13

5. 11 mL

6. 10 mL

7. 2 tab

8. 20 mL

9. 0.12 mg

10. gr $\dfrac{1}{100}$

11. gr 375

12. 0.0003 g

13. 15 gtt

14. 3 tsp

15. $1\dfrac{1}{2}$ oz

Case Study 12

1. $58\ \cancel{\text{lb}} \times \dfrac{1\ \cancel{\text{kg}}}{2.2\ \cancel{\text{lb}}} \times \dfrac{0.2\ \cancel{\text{mg}}}{\cancel{\text{kg}}} \times \dfrac{1\text{ mL}}{10\ \cancel{\text{mg}}} = \dfrac{11.6}{22} = 0.52\quad\text{or}\quad 0.5\text{ mL of morphine sulfate}$

2. $58\ \cancel{\text{lb}} \times \dfrac{1\ \cancel{\text{kg}}}{2.2\ \cancel{\text{lb}}} \times \dfrac{1\text{ mg}}{\cancel{\text{kg}} \times \text{h}} = 26.36\text{ mg/h of Aminophylline}$

3. $58\ \cancel{\text{lb}} \times \dfrac{1\ \cancel{\text{kg}}}{2.2\ \cancel{\text{lb}}} \times \dfrac{0.8\ \cancel{\text{mg}}}{\cancel{\text{kg}} \times \text{h}} \times \dfrac{\cancel{500}\text{ mL}}{\cancel{500}\ \cancel{\text{mg}}} = 21.1\text{ mL/h}$

4. $58\ \cancel{\text{lb}} \times \dfrac{1\ \cancel{\text{kg}}}{2.2\ \cancel{\text{lb}}} \times \dfrac{20\text{ mg}}{\cancel{\text{kg}}} = \dfrac{1160}{2.2} = 527\text{ mg (minimum dose of Cleocin)}$

$58\ \cancel{\text{lb}} \times \dfrac{1\ \cancel{\text{kg}}}{2.2\ \cancel{\text{lb}}} \times \dfrac{30\text{ mg}}{\cancel{\text{kg}}} = \dfrac{1740}{2.2} = 790\text{ mg (maximum dose of Cleocin)}$

$\dfrac{250\text{ mg}}{\cancel{\text{dose}}} \times \dfrac{3\ \cancel{\text{doses}}}{\text{day}} = 750\text{ mg per day}$

Yes, the dose of Cleocin is within the safe and therapeutic range.

5. $\overset{5}{\cancel{250}}\ \cancel{\text{mg}} \times \dfrac{1\text{ mL}}{\underset{3}{\cancel{150}}\ \cancel{\text{mg}}} = 1.7\text{ mL of Cleocin}$

6. $\dfrac{31.7\text{ mL}}{45\ \cancel{\text{min}}} \times \dfrac{60\ \cancel{\text{min}}}{1\text{ h}} = 42.3\text{ mL/h of Cleocin}$

7. $\quad \text{BSA} = \sqrt{\dfrac{58 \times 48}{3131}}$

$\qquad\qquad = \sqrt{\dfrac{2784}{3131}}$

$\qquad\qquad = \sqrt{0.889}$

$\qquad\qquad = 0.94 \, \text{m}^2$

$0.94 \, \cancel{\text{m}^2} \times \dfrac{1800 \, \text{mL}}{\cancel{\text{m}^2} \times \text{day}} = 1692 \, \text{mL/day}$

8. $1000 \, \cancel{\text{mcg}} \times \dfrac{1 \, \cancel{\text{mg}}}{1000 \, \cancel{\text{mcg}}} \times \dfrac{1 \, \text{tab}}{1 \, \cancel{\text{mg}}} = 1$ tab of folic acid

9. $\overset{1}{\cancel{2}} \, \cancel{\text{mg}} \times \dfrac{1 \, \text{mL}}{\underset{1}{\cancel{2}} \, \cancel{\text{mg}}} = 1 \, \text{mL}$ of Proventil

10. a. $\dfrac{50 \, \text{mL}}{\underset{3}{\cancel{30}} \, \text{min}} \times \dfrac{\overset{1}{\cancel{10}} \, \text{gtt}}{1 \, \cancel{\text{mL}}} = \dfrac{50}{3} = 16.6$ or 17 gtt/min

   b. $\dfrac{220 \, \text{mL}}{3.5 \, \text{h}} = 63 \, \text{mL/h}$ to complete the infusion in the time frame ordered

11. $\overset{6}{\cancel{240}} \, \cancel{\text{mg}} \times \dfrac{5 \, \text{mL}}{\underset{4}{\cancel{160}} \, \cancel{\text{mg}}} = \dfrac{30}{4} = 7.5 \, \text{mL}$ of Tylenol

Try These for Practice

1. 6.3 units of insulin bid in 24 h
   mL
2. 4.5 or 4.6

3. 0.5 mL   4. 4 mL   5. 16.2 mL

Exercises

1. $0.9 \, \cancel{\text{m}^2} \times \dfrac{100 \, \cancel{\text{mg}}}{\cancel{\text{m}^2}} \times \dfrac{1 \, \cancel{\text{g}}}{1000 \, \cancel{\text{mg}}} \times \dfrac{240 \, \text{mL}}{2 \, \cancel{\text{g}}} = 10.8 \, \text{mL}$ of Videx

2. $16 \, \cancel{\text{lb}} \times \dfrac{0.45 \, \cancel{\text{kg}}}{1 \, \cancel{\text{lb}}} \times \dfrac{\overset{2}{\cancel{4}} \, \cancel{\text{mg}}}{\cancel{\text{kg}}} \times \dfrac{1 \, \text{mL}}{\underset{5}{\cancel{10}} \, \cancel{\text{mg}}} = 2.88$ or 2.9 mL of Epivir

3. $7 \, \cancel{\text{lb}} \times \dfrac{0.45 \, \cancel{\text{kg}}}{1 \, \cancel{\text{lb}}} \times \dfrac{0.035 \, \cancel{\text{mg}}}{\cancel{\text{kg}}} \times \dfrac{1 \, \text{mL}}{0.05 \, \cancel{\text{mg}}} = 2.2 \, \text{mL}$ of Lanoxin in 3 divided doses over 24 hours, 0.7 mL/dose

4. $35 \, \cancel{\text{kg}} \times \dfrac{0.04 \, \cancel{\text{mcg}}}{\cancel{\text{kg}}} \times \dfrac{1 \, \text{mL}}{1 \, \cancel{\text{mcg}}} = 1.4 \, \text{mL}$ of Calcitriol

5. $56 \, \cancel{\text{lb}} \times \dfrac{0.45 \, \cancel{\text{kg}}}{\cancel{\text{lb}}} \times \dfrac{\overset{2}{\cancel{8}} \, \cancel{\text{mg}}}{\cancel{\text{kg}}} \times \dfrac{5 \, \text{mL}}{\underset{125}{\cancel{500}} \, \cancel{\text{mg}}} = \dfrac{252 \, \text{mL}}{125} = 2.016$ or 2 mL of acetozolamide

6. Each dose will be 0.5 mL of the cholera vaccine.

7. $\overset{1}{\cancel{720}} \, \cancel{\text{EL units}} \times \dfrac{1 \, \text{mL}}{\underset{2}{\cancel{1440}} \, \cancel{\text{EL units}}} = 0.5 \, \text{mL}$ of the hepatitis A vaccine

8. a. $120 \text{ mg} \times \dfrac{5 \text{ mL}}{100 \text{ mg}} = \dfrac{60 \text{ mL}}{10}$ or   6 mL of guaifenesin

b. $\overset{2}{200} \text{ mg} \times \dfrac{\text{dram } 1}{\underset{1}{100 \text{ mg}}} = \text{dram } 2 \text{ of guaifenesin}$

9. a. $18 \text{ kg} \times \dfrac{0.1 \text{ units}}{\text{kg}} = 1.8 \text{ units}$ or   2 units of insulin

b. 0.02 mL in insulin syringe

10. $50 \text{ lb} \times \dfrac{0.45 \text{ kg}}{1 \text{ lb}} \times \dfrac{0.1 \text{ unit}}{\text{kg} \times \text{h}} \times \dfrac{100 \text{ mL}}{100 \text{ units}} = 2.25 \text{ mL/h}$

11. $21 \text{ lb} \times \dfrac{0.45 \text{ kg}}{1 \text{ lb}} \times \dfrac{\overset{3}{30} \text{ mg}}{\text{kg}} \times \dfrac{5 \text{ mL}}{\underset{10}{100 \text{ mg}}} = 14.175$ or   14.2   mL   of Lorabid in divided doses (7.1 mL q12h)

12. $0.68 \text{ m}^2 \times \dfrac{\overset{12}{300} \text{ mg}}{\text{m}^2} \times \dfrac{5 \text{ mL}}{\underset{5}{125 \text{ mg}}} = 8.16$ or   8.2 mL of Biaxin

13. $4 \text{ mL} \times \dfrac{0.025 \text{ g}}{100 \text{ mL}} \times \dfrac{1000 \text{ mg}}{1 \text{ g}} = 1 \text{ mg of vitamin A in 4 mL of solution}$

14. $0.5 \text{ m}^2 \times \dfrac{\overset{8}{400} \text{ mg}}{\text{m}^2} \times \dfrac{\overset{}{5} \text{ mL}}{\underset{5}{250 \text{ mg}}} = 4 \text{ mL of Augmentin}$

15. $30 \text{ kg} \times \dfrac{30 \text{ mg}}{\text{kg}} = 900 \text{ mg/day in divided dose}$

$30 \text{ kg} \times \dfrac{50 \text{ mg}}{\text{kg}} = 1500 \text{ mg/day in divided dose}$

$\dfrac{250 \text{ mg}}{\underset{1}{6 \text{ h}}} \times \dfrac{\overset{4}{24} \text{ h}}{\text{day}} = 1000 \text{ mg is a safe dose for this child}$

16. $35 \text{ kg} \times \dfrac{35 \text{ mg}}{\text{kg}} \times \dfrac{1 \text{ g}}{1000 \text{ mg}} = 1.225 \text{ g of Mefoxin pre operative}$

$1.225 \text{ g} \times \dfrac{\overset{4}{24} \text{ h}}{\underset{1}{6 \text{ h}}} = 4.9 \text{ g of Mefoxin post operative}$

The total amount of Mefoxin is 6.125 g, pre and post operative

17. $\overset{3}{150} \text{ mg} \times \dfrac{5 \text{ mL}}{\underset{1}{50 \text{ mg}}} = 15 \text{ mL of Vantin}$

18. $\dfrac{100 \text{ mL}}{\underset{1}{30 \text{ min}}} \times \dfrac{\overset{2}{60} \, \mu\text{gtt}}{\text{mL}} = 200 \, \mu\text{gtt per minute of Rocephin}$

19. $\overset{4}{200} \text{ mg} \times \dfrac{5 \text{ mL}}{\underset{5}{250 \text{ mg}}} = 4 \text{ mL of Vancocin}$

20. $42 \text{ lb} \times \dfrac{0.45 \text{ kg}}{1 \text{ lb}} \times \dfrac{\overset{1}{25} \text{ mg}}{\text{kg}} \times \dfrac{5 \text{ mL}}{\underset{1}{30 \text{ mg}}} = 9.45$ or   9.5 mL of Ampicillin

Cumulative Review Exercises

1. 525 mg

2. 30 units

3. a. 200 mg

b. 1 tab

4. 0.5 mL

5. 20 mL

6. 2 cap

7. 60.75 mg

8. 60 gtt/min

9. 2.5 mL/min

10. 14.7 h; infusion will finish at 11:42 A.M. the following morning

11. gr $\dfrac{3}{100}$

12. 2 tab

13. Take 66.7 mL of the $\dfrac{1}{2}$ strength solution and add water to the level of 100 mL.

14. 1 tab

15. 5.25 mL

Answers to Comprehensive Self-Tests

Comprehensive Self-Test 1

1. $\overset{1}{\cancel{500}} \text{ tab} \times \dfrac{40 \text{ mg}}{\text{tab}} \times \dfrac{1 \text{ g}}{\underset{2}{\cancel{1000} \text{ mg}}} = 20$ g of Prozac

2. $375 \text{ mg} \times \dfrac{1 \text{ g}}{1000 \text{ mg}} = 0.375$ g of Naproxen in 1 tab

3. $1 \text{ mL} \times \dfrac{\overset{50}{\cancel{2500}} \text{ mcg}}{\underset{1}{\cancel{50} \text{ mL}}} = 50$ micrograms of fentanyl

4. $\dfrac{0.8 \text{ g}}{\text{dose}} \times \dfrac{1000 \text{ mg}}{\text{g}} \times \dfrac{2 \text{ dose}}{\text{day}} = 1600$ mg/day of Cimetidine

5. $0.15 \text{ g} \times \dfrac{\overset{20}{\cancel{1000}} \text{ mg}}{1 \text{ g}} \times \dfrac{1 \text{ tab}}{\underset{3}{\cancel{150} \text{ mg}}} = 1$ tab of desipramine

6. $600 \text{ mg} \times \dfrac{1 \text{ tab}}{200 \text{ mg}} = 3$ tab of Trovan

7. $1.5 \text{ mg} \times \dfrac{5 \text{ mL}}{0.5 \text{ mg}} = 15$ mL of dexamethasone

8. a. $90 \text{ kg} \times \dfrac{0.3 \text{ mcg}}{\text{kg}} \times \dfrac{1 \text{ mL}}{4 \text{ mcg}} = 6.75$ mL of Stimate

   b. $\dfrac{56.75 \text{ mL}}{30 \text{ min}} = 1.89$ or 1.9 milliters per minute

9. a. $1 \text{ mL} \times \dfrac{50 \text{ mg}}{250 \text{ mL}} = 0.2$ mg/mL is the concentration of Nipride in 1 mL

   b. $\overset{9}{\cancel{90}} \text{ kg} \times \dfrac{4 \text{ mcg}}{\text{kg} \times \text{min}} \times \dfrac{1 \text{ mg}}{\underset{4}{\cancel{1000} \text{ mcg}}} \times \dfrac{\overset{1}{\cancel{250}} \text{ mL}}{\underset{5}{\cancel{50} \text{ mg}}} \times \dfrac{60 \text{ min}}{1 \text{ h}} =$

   108 mL/h of the Nipride solution

10. $\overset{4}{\cancel{400}}\ \cancel{mL} \times \dfrac{0.5\ g}{\underset{1}{\cancel{100}\ \cancel{mL}}} = 2\ g$ of boric acid crystals; add H_2O to level of 400 mL

11. $0.01\ \cancel{g} \times \dfrac{\overset{200}{\cancel{1000}\ \cancel{mg}}}{1\ \cancel{g}} \times \dfrac{1\ tab}{\underset{1}{\cancel{5}\ \cancel{mg}}} = 2$ tab of glipizide

12. a. $130\ \cancel{lb} \times \dfrac{0.45\ \cancel{kg}}{1\ \cancel{lb}} \times \dfrac{0.01\ \cancel{mg}}{\cancel{kg}} \times \dfrac{10\ mL}{1\ \cancel{mg}} = 5.85$ or 5.9 mL of Corvert

  b. $\dfrac{55.9\ mL}{10\ min} = 5.6\ mL/min$

13. a. Cardura 6 mg; Bumex 2 mg; K-Tab 20 mEq; Norvasc 10 mg; Digoxin 0.125 mg; Glucotrol XL 5 mg; Feldene 40 mg.

  b. Trovan 400 mg; on 5/9/03 give Zithromax 600 mg.

14. a. Zithromax, 600 mg

  b. $\overset{3}{\cancel{600}}\ \cancel{mg} \times \dfrac{5\ mL}{\underset{1}{\cancel{200}\ \cancel{mg}}} = 15\ mL$ of Zithromax

15. $\overset{2}{\cancel{20}}\ \cancel{mEq} \times \dfrac{750\ mg}{\underset{1}{\cancel{10}\ \cancel{mEq}}} = 1500\ mg$ of potassium chloride

16. $5\ \cancel{mg} \times \dfrac{1000\ mcg}{1\ \cancel{mg}} = 5000\ mcg$ of Glucotrol XL

17. $\overset{2}{\cancel{400}}\ \cancel{mg} \times \dfrac{1\ tab}{\underset{1}{\cancel{200}\ \cancel{mg}}} = 2$ tab of Trovan

18. 1 capsule of Feldene

19. $0.125\ \cancel{mg} \times \dfrac{1000\ mcg}{1\ \cancel{mg}} = 125\ mcg$ of Digoxin

20. Elavil, 50 mg

21. $\dfrac{2\ mg}{1\ \cancel{day}} \times \dfrac{1\ g}{1000\ \cancel{mg}} \times \dfrac{7\ \cancel{days}}{1} = 0.014\ g$ of Bumex in 7 days

22. Either 3 (2 mg) tablets or 1 (2 mg) and 1 (4 mg) tablet of Cardura

23. a. $95\ \cancel{lb} \times \dfrac{0.45\ \cancel{kg}}{\cancel{lb}} \times \dfrac{0.15\ \cancel{mg}}{\cancel{kg}} \times \dfrac{1\ mL}{1\ \cancel{mg}} = 6.4\ mL$ of Platinol

  $6.4\ mL = 6.4\ mg\ (1\ mL = 1\ mg)$, so $6.4\ \cancel{mg} \times \dfrac{1\ g}{1000\ \cancel{mg}} = 0.0064\ g$ of Platinol

  b. $\dfrac{506.4\ mL}{6\ h} = 84.4\ mL/h.$

24. a. $74\ \cancel{kg} \times \dfrac{0.3\ \cancel{mg}}{\cancel{kg}} \times \dfrac{\overset{1}{\cancel{10}}\ mL}{\underset{5}{\cancel{50}\ \cancel{mg}}} = 4.44$ or 4.4 mL of amphotericin B

  b. $\dfrac{254.4\ mL}{6\ h} = 42.4\ mL/h$ is the setting on the infusion pump

25. $220\ \cancel{lb} \times \dfrac{0.45\ \cancel{kg}}{\cancel{lb}} \times \dfrac{0.08\ \cancel{mg}}{\cancel{kg}} \times \dfrac{1\ mL}{5\ \cancel{mg}} = 1.6\ mL$ of Versed

Comprehensive Self-Test 2

1. $0.01 \cancel{g} \times \dfrac{1000 \cancel{mg}}{1 \cancel{g}} \times \dfrac{1 mL}{1 \cancel{mg}} = 10$ mL of Claritin

2. $0.04 \cancel{g} \times \dfrac{\overset{50}{\cancel{1000}} \cancel{mg}}{1 \cancel{g}} \times \dfrac{1 cap}{\underset{1}{\cancel{20}} \cancel{mg}} = 2$ cap of Nexium

3. $\overset{1}{\cancel{250}} \cancel{mcg} \times \dfrac{1 \cancel{mg}}{\underset{4}{\cancel{1000}} \cancel{mcg}} \times \dfrac{1 tab}{0.125 \cancel{mg}} = \dfrac{1 tab}{0.5} = 2$ tab of digoxin

4. a. $0.3 \cancel{g} \times \dfrac{\cancel{1000} \cancel{mg}}{1 \cancel{g}} \times \dfrac{1 cap}{\cancel{100} \cancel{mg}} = 3$ cap of Retrovir q6h

   b. $\dfrac{3\, cap}{\underset{1}{\cancel{6}}\, \cancel{h}} \times \dfrac{\overset{4}{\cancel{24}}\, \cancel{h}}{\cancel{day}} \times 30\, \cancel{days} = 360$ cap of Retrovir are required for 30 days

5. $\dfrac{0.09 \cancel{g}}{week} \times \dfrac{1000\, mg}{1 \cancel{g}} = 90$ mg of Prozac each week

6. $\overset{1000}{\cancel{60,000}} \cancel{mcg} \times \dfrac{1 \cancel{mg}}{1000 \cancel{mcg}} \times \dfrac{1 tab}{\underset{1}{\cancel{60}} \cancel{mg}} = 1$ tab of Evista

7. $0.8 \cancel{g} \times \dfrac{\overset{5}{\cancel{1000}} \cancel{mg}}{\cancel{g}} \times \dfrac{1 tab}{\underset{2}{\cancel{400}} \cancel{mg}} = 2$ tab of Cimetidine

8. $\dfrac{1010\, mL}{2\, h} = 42.1$ mL/h of Mefoxin is the rate set on the infusion pump

9. $\dfrac{110\, mL}{24\, h} = 4.6$ mL/h of Aredia

10. $3 \cancel{mL} \times \dfrac{0.03 \cancel{g}}{\cancel{100} \cancel{mL}} \times \dfrac{\cancel{1000}\, mg}{1 \cancel{g}} = 0.9$ mg of Phospholine iodide

11. $\overset{5}{\cancel{50}} \cancel{mcg} \times \dfrac{1\, mL}{\underset{2}{\cancel{20}} \cancel{mcg}} = 2.5$ mL of zinc sulfate

12. $\dfrac{\overset{10}{\cancel{500}}\, mL}{\underset{3}{\cancel{150}} \cancel{mg}} \times \dfrac{0.05 \cancel{mg}}{1\, min} = 0.17$ mL/min of Yutopar

13. $\dfrac{202 \cancel{mL}}{\underset{3}{\cancel{60}}\, min} \times \dfrac{\overset{1}{\cancel{20}}\, gtt}{1 \cancel{mL}} = 67$ drops per minute of Erythrocin

14. $110 \cancel{lb} \times \dfrac{0.45 \cancel{kg}}{1 \cancel{lb}} \times \dfrac{20\, mg}{\cancel{kg}} = 990$ mg of Erythromycin

15. $94 \cancel{lb} \times \dfrac{0.45 \cancel{kg}}{1 \cancel{lb}} \times \dfrac{12 \cancel{mg}}{\cancel{kg}} \times \dfrac{1 \cancel{g}}{1000 \cancel{mg}} \times \dfrac{2.5\, mL}{1 \cancel{g}} = 1.27$ or 1.3 mL of Streptomycin

16. $\dfrac{100\,\text{mL}}{15\,\text{min}} = 6.7\,\text{mL/min of Monocid}$

17. $\dfrac{200\,\text{mL}}{60\,\text{min}} = 3.3\,\text{mL/min of Ciprofloxacin}$

18. $\overset{10}{\cancel{500}}\,\cancel{\text{mg}} \times \dfrac{1\,\text{mL}}{\underset{1}{\cancel{50}\,\cancel{\text{mg}}}} = 10\,\text{mL will contain 500 mg acyclovir}$

19. a. 60 mL contain 300 mg of Trovan

    b. $\dfrac{260\,\text{mL}}{2\,\text{h}} = 130\,\text{mL/h}$

20. 2 tab of Glucotrol

21. a. $25,\cancel{000}\,\cancel{\text{units}} \times \dfrac{1\,\text{mL}}{10,\cancel{000}\,\cancel{\text{units}}} = 2.5\,\text{mL of heparin}$

    b. $\dfrac{\overset{1}{\cancel{1250}\,\cancel{\text{units}}}}{\text{h}} \times \dfrac{252.5\,\text{mL}}{\underset{20}{\cancel{25,000}\,\cancel{\text{units}}}} = 12.6\,\text{mL/h}$

22. $\overset{2}{\cancel{25}}\,\cancel{\text{mg}} \times \dfrac{1\,\text{tab}}{\underset{1}{\cancel{12.5}\,\cancel{\text{mg}}}} = 2\,\text{tab of Meclizine}$

23. a. $\dfrac{2\,\text{tab}}{\cancel{\text{day}}} \times 7\,\cancel{\text{days}} = 14\,\text{tab of ferrous gluconate}$

24. $6\,\cancel{\text{mg}} \times \dfrac{1\,\cancel{\text{g}}}{1000\,\cancel{\text{mg}}} \times \dfrac{1\,\text{tab}}{0.002\,\cancel{\text{g}}} = 3\,\text{tab of Cardura}$

25. 9 P.M.

Comprehensive Self-Test 3

1. $\overset{3}{\cancel{15}}\,\cancel{\text{mg}} \times \dfrac{5\,\text{mL}}{\underset{2}{\cancel{10}\,\cancel{\text{mg}}}} = 7.5\,\text{mL of Atarax}$

2. $60\,\cancel{\text{mg}} \times \dfrac{1\,\text{mL}}{25\,\cancel{\text{mg}}} = 2.4\,\text{mL of Zantac}$

3. $70\,\cancel{\text{kg}} \times \dfrac{0.28\,\cancel{\text{mg}}}{\cancel{\text{kg}} \times \text{min}} \times \dfrac{250\,\text{mL}}{\cancel{2000}\,\cancel{\text{mg}}} \times \dfrac{60\,\mu\text{gtt}}{\cancel{\text{mL}}} = 147$ microdrops per minute of oxacillin

4. $\dfrac{\overset{1}{\cancel{250}\,\text{mL}}}{\underset{2}{\cancel{500}\,\cancel{\text{mg}}}} \times \dfrac{50\,\cancel{\text{mg}}}{\text{h}} = 25\,\text{mL/h of theophylline}$

5. $\dfrac{750\,\text{mL}}{\cancel{20,000,000}\,\cancel{\text{units}}} \times \dfrac{\cancel{2,000,000}\,\cancel{\text{units}}}{\text{h}} = 75\,\text{mL/h of penicillin}$

6. $\dfrac{500\,\text{mL}}{\underset{2}{\cancel{120}\,\text{min}}} \times \dfrac{\overset{1}{\cancel{60}}\,\mu\text{gtt}}{1\,\cancel{\text{mL}}} = 250\,\mu\text{gtt/min}$

7. $\dfrac{100 \text{ mL}}{30 \text{ min}} = 3.3 \text{ mL/min}$

8. $\overset{4}{200} \text{ mL} \times \dfrac{10 \text{ mL}}{100 \text{ mL}} \times \dfrac{\overset{1}{100} \text{ mL}}{\underset{1}{50} \text{ mL}} = 40$ mL of the 50% solution (boric acid) and add H_2O to the level of 200 mL

9. $2000 \text{ mL} \times \dfrac{0.45 \text{ g}}{100 \text{ mL}} = 9$ g of sodium chloride

10. a. 10 mL of Floxcin

    b. $\dfrac{110 \text{ mL}}{\underset{3}{90} \text{ min}} \times \dfrac{\overset{2}{60} \,\mu\text{gtt}}{\text{mL}} = 73 \,\mu\text{gtt/min of Floxin}$

11. $\overset{12}{300} \text{ mg} \times \dfrac{5 \text{ mL}}{\underset{5}{125} \text{ mg}} = 12$ mL of amoxicillin

12. $60 \text{ kg} \times \dfrac{15 \text{ mg}}{\text{kg}} \times \dfrac{\overset{1}{5} \text{ mL}}{\underset{4}{200} \text{ mg}} = 22.5$ mL of Depakene

13. $\dfrac{0.04 \text{ g}}{\text{dose}} \times \dfrac{1000 \text{ mg}}{\text{g}} \times \dfrac{1 \text{ mL}}{\underset{5}{10} \text{ mg}} \times \dfrac{\overset{1}{2} \text{ doses}}{\text{day}} = 8$ mL of Furosemide in one day

14. $0.02 \text{ g} \times \dfrac{1000 \text{ mg}}{\text{g}} \times \dfrac{1 \text{ mL}}{30 \text{ mg}} = 0.66$ or 0.7 mL of Talwin

15. $\overset{4}{60} \text{ mg} \times \dfrac{1 \text{ tab}}{\underset{1}{15} \text{ mg}} = 4$ tab of Nardil in one day

16. $44 \text{ lb} \times \dfrac{0.45 \text{ kg}}{\text{lb}} \times \dfrac{5 \text{ mg}}{\text{kg}} \times \dfrac{\overset{1}{5} \text{ mL}}{\underset{20}{100} \text{ mg}} = 4.95$ or 5 mL of Motrin

17. a. $\dfrac{17 \text{ gtt}}{\text{min}} \times \dfrac{1 \text{ mL}}{\underset{1}{10} \text{ gtt}} \times \dfrac{\overset{6}{60} \text{ min}}{1 \text{ h}} = 102 \text{ mL/h}$

    b. $\dfrac{102 \text{ mL}}{\text{h}} \times 9.5 \text{ h} = 969$ mL in 9.5 h

18. $121 \text{ lb} \times \dfrac{0.45 \text{ kg}}{\text{lb}} \times \dfrac{0.5 \text{ mcg}}{\text{kg}} \times \dfrac{1 \text{ mL}}{50 \text{ mcg}} = 0.5$ mL of Sublimaze

19. $120 \text{ mg} \times \dfrac{1 \text{ g}}{1000 \text{ mg}} \times \dfrac{1 \text{ cap}}{0.12 \text{ g}} = 1$ cap of Inderal

20. a. $\dfrac{2000 \text{ mg}}{500 \text{ mL}} = 4$ mg of lidocaine per mL

    b. $\dfrac{20 \text{ mL}}{\text{h}} \times \dfrac{4 \text{ mg}}{1 \text{ mL}} = 80$ mg of lidocaine per hour

    c. $\dfrac{80 \text{ mg}}{60 \text{ min}} = 1.3$ mg of lidocaine per minute

21. $200\text{0 mL} \times \dfrac{1 \text{ g}}{10\text{0 mL}} \times \dfrac{1 \text{ tab}}{5 \text{ g}} = 4$ tab of Neosporin; add H_2O to the level of 2000 mL

22. $\overset{1}{2\text{0 mg}} \times \dfrac{\text{gr } 1}{\underset{3}{6\text{0 mg}}} \times \dfrac{1 \text{ tab}}{\text{gr } \dfrac{1}{6}} = \dfrac{1 \text{ tab}}{0.5}$ or 2 tab of Tamoxifen

23. $\dfrac{50 \text{ mL}}{\underset{1}{2\text{0 min}}} \times \dfrac{\overset{1}{2\text{0 gtt}}}{1 \text{ mL}} = 50$ gtt/min of Kefurox

24. $\text{gr } \dfrac{1}{\underset{10}{60\text{0}}} \times \dfrac{\overset{1}{6\text{0 mg}}}{\text{gr } 1} = 0.1$ mg

25. $0.32 \text{ mg} \times \dfrac{1.25 \text{ mL}}{0.5 \text{ mg}} = 0.8$ mL of atropine sulfate

Comprehensive Self-Test 4

1. $1.9 \text{ m}^2 \times \dfrac{\overset{1}{27\text{5 mg}}}{\text{m}^2} \times \dfrac{1 \text{ tab}}{\underset{1}{27\text{5 mg}}} = 1.9$ tab   or   2 tab of Naproxen

2. $1 \text{ mg} \times \dfrac{1 \text{ cap}}{0.5 \text{ mg}} = \dfrac{1 \text{ cap}}{0.5}$ or   2 cap of Tikosyn

3. $\dfrac{0.5 \text{ mg}}{\underset{1}{8 \text{ h}}} \times \dfrac{1 \text{ tab}}{0.25 \text{ mg}} \times \overset{3}{24 \text{ h}} = 6$ tab of alprazolam in 24 hour

4. $0.01 \text{ g} \times \dfrac{1000 \text{ mg}}{1 \text{ g}} \times \dfrac{1 \text{ tab}}{5 \text{ mg}} = 2$ tab of glipizide

5. $0.8 \text{ g} \times \dfrac{\overset{5}{100\text{0 mg}}}{1 \text{ g}} \times \dfrac{1 \text{ tab}}{\underset{1}{20\text{0 mg}}} = 4$ tab of amiodarone

6. a. 10 mg of furosemide

    b. 60 mL of furosemide in bottle

7. $\dfrac{40\text{0 mL} \times \dfrac{10 \text{ mL}}{10\text{0 mL}}}{\dfrac{10\text{0 mL}}{10\text{0 mL}}} = 40$ mL of the 100% solution of Chlorox and add H_2O to the level of 400 mL

8. $2 \text{ mL} \times \dfrac{\overset{1}{100\text{0 mg}}}{\underset{1}{100\text{0 mL}}} = 2$ mg of epinephrine 1:1000 are contained in 2 mL of 1% epinephrine solution

9. a. $2 \text{ mL} \times \dfrac{15 \text{ gtt}}{1 \text{ mL}} = 30$ drops in a 2-mL vial of scopolamine 0.25%

  b. $30 \text{ drops} \times \dfrac{1 \text{ day}}{2 \text{ drops}} = 15$ days

  c. $2 \text{ mL} \times \dfrac{0.25 \text{ g}}{100 \text{ mL}} = 0.005$ g in the vial

10. $0.1 \text{ g} \times \dfrac{1000 \text{ mg}}{1 \text{ g}} \times \dfrac{1 \text{ mL}}{100 \text{ mg}} = 1$ mL of Kineret

11. $1.5 \text{ g} \times \dfrac{1000 \text{ mg}}{\text{g}} \times \dfrac{1 \text{ cap}}{500 \text{ mg}} = 3$ cap of Tylenol

12. $\dfrac{800 \text{ mg}}{12 \text{ h}} \times \dfrac{1 \text{ g}}{1000 \text{ mg}} \times \dfrac{1 \text{ tab}}{0.8 \text{ g}} \times \dfrac{24 \text{ h}}{\text{day}} \times \dfrac{5 \text{ day}}{1} = 10$ tab of Motrin

13. $1000 \text{ mL} \times \dfrac{20 \text{ gtt}}{\text{mL}} \times \dfrac{1 \text{ min}}{40 \text{ gtt}} \times \dfrac{1 \text{ h}}{60 \text{ min}} = 8.33 \text{ h}$ or 8 h and 20 min

14. a. $2.2 \text{ m}^2 \times \dfrac{1800 \text{ mg}}{\text{m}^2} = 3960$ mg of Cefobid

  b. $\dfrac{240 \text{ mL}}{3 \text{ h}} = 80$ mL/h of Cefobid infusion

15. a. $80 \text{ lb} \times \dfrac{0.45 \text{ kg}}{1 \text{ lb}} \times \dfrac{4.4 \text{ mg}}{\text{kg}} = 158.4$ mg of Vibramycin

  b. $158.4 \text{ mg} \times \dfrac{250 \text{ mL}}{200 \text{ mg}} = 198$ mL of premixed Vibramycin solution

  c. $\dfrac{198 \text{ mL}}{4 \text{ h}} \times \dfrac{1 \text{ h}}{60 \text{ min}} = 0.83$ mL per minute of the Vibramycin infusion

16. $\dfrac{100 \text{ mL}}{60 \text{ min}} \times \dfrac{15 \text{ gtt}}{\text{mL}} = 25$ gtt/min of the Levaquin infusion

17. a. $75 \text{ kg} \times \dfrac{0.5 \text{ mg}}{\text{kg}} = 37.5$ mg of abciximab

  b. $37.5 \text{ mg} \times \dfrac{1 \text{ mL}}{2 \text{ mg}} = 18.75$ mL of the drug; add to 250 mL of normal saline

  c. $\dfrac{268.75 \text{ mL}}{12 \text{ h}} = 22.4$ mL/h of the abciximab infusion

18. $8 \text{ tsp} \times \dfrac{5 \text{ mL}}{1 \text{ tsp}} \times \dfrac{\text{oz } 1}{30 \text{ mL}} = 1\dfrac{1}{3}$ oz

19. $\text{gr}\,\dfrac{1}{5} \times \dfrac{\overset{4}{\cancel{60}}\,\text{mg}}{\cancel{\text{gr}}} \times \dfrac{1\,\text{mL}}{\underset{1}{\cancel{15}\,\cancel{\text{mg}}}} = 0.8\,\text{mL of morphine sulfate}$

20. $\overset{4}{\cancel{100}}\,\text{mg} \times \dfrac{1\,\text{tab}}{\underset{1}{\cancel{25}\,\cancel{\text{mg}}}} = 4\,\text{tab of atenolol}$

21. $0.025\,\cancel{\text{g}} \times \dfrac{\overset{40}{\cancel{1000}}\,\text{mg}}{1\,\cancel{\text{g}}} \times \dfrac{1\,\text{tab}}{\underset{1}{\cancel{25}\,\cancel{\text{mg}}}} = 1\,\text{tab of amitriptyline}$

22. $\dfrac{0.6\,\cancel{\text{g}}}{\cancel{\text{dose}}} \times \dfrac{1000\,\text{mg}}{\cancel{\text{g}}} \times \dfrac{2\,\cancel{\text{doses}}}{\cancel{\text{day}}} \times 21\,\cancel{\text{days}} = 25{,}200\,\text{mg of ranitidine}$

23. $0.0075\,\cancel{\text{g}} \times \dfrac{1000\,\cancel{\text{mg}}}{1\,\cancel{\text{g}}} \times \dfrac{1000\,\cancel{\text{mcg}}}{1\,\cancel{\text{mg}}} \times \dfrac{1\,\text{tab}}{7500\,\cancel{\text{mcg}}} = 1\,\text{tab of Coumadin}$

24. $\dfrac{44\,\cancel{\text{mcg}}}{\cancel{\text{dose}}} \times \dfrac{1\,\text{mg}}{1000\,\cancel{\text{mcg}}} \times \dfrac{3\,\cancel{\text{doses}}}{\text{week}} = 0.132\,\text{mg in 3 days (TIW) of the drug Interferon beta–1A}$

25. $200\,\text{mL} \times \dfrac{1\,\cancel{\text{mL}}}{3\,\cancel{\text{mL}}} \times \dfrac{2\,\cancel{\text{mL}}}{1\,\cancel{\text{mL}}} = 133\,\text{mL of the}\ \dfrac{1}{2}\ \text{strength Isocal; add}\ H_2O$ to the level of 200 mL

Comprehensive Self-Test 5

1. $\dfrac{20\,\cancel{\text{mL}}}{1\,\text{h}} \times \dfrac{\overset{100}{\cancel{25{,}000}}\,\text{units}}{\underset{1}{\cancel{250}\,\cancel{\text{mL}}}} = 2000\,\text{units of heparin per hour}$

2. $\dfrac{\cancel{1400}\,\cancel{\text{units}}}{\text{h}} \times \dfrac{500\,\text{mL}}{\cancel{50{,}000}\,\cancel{\text{units}}} = 14\,\text{mL per hour of heparin solution}$

3. a. Add 10 mL of sterile diluent to the 50-mg vial of Alkeran

   b. $1.2\,\cancel{\text{m}^2} \times \dfrac{16\,\cancel{\text{mg}}}{\cancel{\text{m}^2}} \times \dfrac{\overset{1}{\cancel{10}}\,\text{mL}}{\underset{5}{\cancel{50}\,\cancel{\text{mg}}}} = 3.84$ or 3.8 mL of Alkeran must be added to 100 mL 0.9% normal saline

   c. $\dfrac{103.8\,\text{mL}}{20\,\text{min}} = 5.2\,\text{mL/min}$

4. a. $22\,\cancel{\text{mg}} \times \dfrac{1\,\text{mL}}{10\,\cancel{\text{mg}}} = 2.2\,\text{mL of protamine sulfate}$

   b. $\dfrac{27.2\,\text{mL}}{10\,\text{min}} = 2.7\,\text{mL/min}$

5. $\dfrac{\overset{2}{\cancel{100}}\,\text{mL}}{\underset{1}{\cancel{50}\,\cancel{\text{mg}}}} \times \dfrac{6.25\,\cancel{\text{mg}}}{\text{h}} = 12.5\,\text{mL/h of Zantac infusion}$

6. $\dfrac{0.75 \text{ g}}{\text{dose}} \times \dfrac{\overset{4}{1000} \text{ mg}}{\text{g}} \times \dfrac{1 \text{ tab}}{\underset{1}{250} \text{ mg}} \times \dfrac{2 \text{ doses}}{\text{day}} = 6 \text{ tab/day of Cipro}$

7. $0.4 \text{ g} \times \dfrac{1000 \text{ mg}}{\text{g}} \times \dfrac{1 \text{ tab}}{400 \text{ mg}} = 1 \text{ tab of Maxaquin}$

8. a. $600 \text{ mg} \times \dfrac{1 \text{ g}}{1000 \text{ mg}} = 0.6 \text{ gram of Floxin}$

   b. $\dfrac{100 \text{ mL}}{\underset{9}{90} \text{ min}} \times \dfrac{\overset{1}{10} \text{ gtt}}{\text{mL}} = 11 \text{ gtt/min of Floxin solution}$

9. a. $\dfrac{\overset{4}{2000} \text{ mg}}{\underset{1}{500} \text{ mL}} = 4 \text{ mg/milliliter is the concentration of lidocaine}$

   b. $\dfrac{\overset{4}{24} \text{ mL}}{\text{h}} \times \dfrac{4 \text{ mg}}{\text{mL}} \times \dfrac{1 \text{ h}}{\underset{10}{60} \text{ min}} = 1.6 \text{ mg/min}$

   c. $\dfrac{1.6 \text{ mg}}{\text{min}} \times \dfrac{60 \text{ min}}{1 \text{ h}} = 96 \text{ mg/h of lidocaine}$

10. $\overset{20}{1000} \text{ mL} \times \dfrac{1 \text{ h}}{\underset{1}{50} \text{ mL}} = 20 \text{ h}$, so the infusion will be completed at 9 A.M. on the following day

11. $\dfrac{\overset{1}{500} \text{ mL}}{\underset{100}{50{,}000} \text{ units}} \times \dfrac{1500 \text{ units}}{\underset{1}{60} \text{ min}} \times \dfrac{\overset{1}{60} \mu\text{gtt}}{\text{mL}} = 15 \ \mu\text{gtt/min}$

12. $\overset{4}{400} \text{ mg} \times \dfrac{5 \text{ mL}}{\underset{1}{100} \text{ mg}} = 20 \text{ mL of Lorabid}$

13. $1.2 \text{ m}^2 \times \dfrac{\overset{6}{240} \text{ mg}}{\text{m}^2} \times \dfrac{\overset{}{5} \text{ mL}}{\underset{5}{200} \text{ mg}} = 7.2 \text{ mL of Lorabid}$

14. $\dfrac{250 \text{ mL}}{288 \text{ unit}} \times \dfrac{12 \text{ unit}}{\text{h}} = 10.4 \text{ mL/h of the insulin infusion}$

15. $90 \text{ kg} \times \dfrac{0.05 \text{ mg}}{\text{kg}} \times \dfrac{1 \text{ mL}}{1 \text{ mg}} = 4.5 \text{ mL of doxacurium}$

16. $40 \text{ lb} \times \dfrac{0.45 \text{ kg}}{1 \text{ lb}} \times \dfrac{0.5 \text{ mg}}{\text{kg}} \times \dfrac{1 \text{ mL}}{10 \text{ mg}} = 0.9 \text{ mL of Tracrium}$

17. a. 45 mL must be added to the vial of Kefzol

    b. $\dfrac{55 \text{ mL}}{20 \text{ min}} = 2.75 \text{ mL/min of the Kefzol solution}$

18. $\dfrac{\overset{1}{150} \text{ mg}}{\text{dose}} \times \dfrac{1 \text{ tab}}{\underset{1}{150} \text{ mg}} \times \dfrac{2 \text{ doses}}{\text{day}} = 2 \text{ tab per day of Zantac}$

19. $0.45 \text{ g} \times \dfrac{1000 \text{ mg}}{\text{g}} \times \dfrac{1 \text{ tab}}{150 \text{ mg}} = 3$ tab of Zantac

20. $3 \text{ mg} \times \dfrac{5 \text{ mL}}{2 \text{ mg}} = 7.5$ mL of Artane

21. $7 \text{ mg} \times \dfrac{1 \text{ mL}}{10 \text{ mg}} = 0.7$ mL of dexamethasone

22. a. $1.2 \text{ m}^2 \times \dfrac{12 \text{ mg}}{\text{m}^2} \times \dfrac{1 \text{ mL}}{1 \text{ mg}} = 14.4$ mL of Idamycin

    b. $\dfrac{14.4 \text{ mL}}{15 \text{ min}} = 0.96$ mL/min

23. $0.1 \text{ mg} \times \dfrac{1 \text{ cap}}{0.05 \text{ mg}} = 2$ cap of Lanoxin

24. $3 \text{ tab} \times \dfrac{1 \text{ g}}{1000 \text{ mg}} \times \dfrac{75 \text{ mg}}{\text{tab}} = 0.225$ g of Wellbutrin

25. $\overset{2}{8} \text{ mg} \times \dfrac{1 \text{ tab}}{\underset{1}{4} \text{ mg}} = 2$ tab of Avandia

Comprehensive Self-Test 6

1. $1.8 \text{ m}^2 \times \dfrac{300 \text{ mg}}{\text{m}^2} \times \dfrac{5 \text{ mL}}{200 \text{ mg}} = 13.5$ mL of Zithromax

2. $1.7 \text{ m}^2 \times \dfrac{1000 \text{ mcg}}{\text{m}^2} \times \dfrac{1 \text{ mg}}{1000 \text{ mcg}} \times \dfrac{1 \text{ mL}}{1 \text{ mg}} = 1.7$ mL of glucagon

3. $0.3 \text{ m}^2 \times \dfrac{0.2 \text{ mg}}{\text{m}^2} \times \dfrac{1000 \text{ mcg}}{1 \text{ mg}} \times \dfrac{1 \text{ mL}}{50 \text{ mcg}} = 1.2$ mL of digoxin

4. a. $1.6 \text{ m}^2 \times \dfrac{160 \text{ mg}}{\text{m}^2} = 256$ mg of Keflex

    b. $256 \text{ mg} \times \dfrac{1 \text{ mL}}{125 \text{ mg}} = 2$ mL of Keflex

5. a. $125 \text{ lb} \times \dfrac{0.45 \text{ kg}}{\text{lb}} \times \dfrac{10 \text{ mg}}{\text{kg}} = 562.5$ mg of Rocephin

    b. $562.5 \text{ mg} \times \dfrac{1 \text{ g}}{1000 \text{ mg}} \times \dfrac{50 \text{ mL}}{2 \text{ g}} = 14.1$ mL of Rocephin

6. $\dfrac{40 \text{ mL}}{30 \text{ min}} = 1.33$ mL/min of digoxin immune Fab

7. $\dfrac{250 \text{ mL}}{300 \text{ min}} \times \dfrac{60 \, \mu\text{gtt}}{1 \text{ mL}} = 50 \, \mu\text{gtt/min of Amicar}$

8. $\overset{8}{\cancel{1200}} \text{ mg} \times \dfrac{1 \text{ cap}}{\underset{1}{\cancel{150} \text{ mg}}} = 8 \text{ cap of Agenerase}$

9. a. $200 \cancel{\text{ lb}} \times \dfrac{0.45 \cancel{\text{ kg}}}{\cancel{\text{lb}}} \times \dfrac{\overset{3}{\cancel{150} \cancel{\text{ mg}}}}{\cancel{\text{kg}}} \times \dfrac{1 \text{ mL}}{\underset{4}{\cancel{200} \cancel{\text{ mg}}}} = 67.5 \text{ mL of acetylcystine}$

   b. $\dfrac{267.5 \text{ mL}}{15 \text{ min}} = 17.8 \text{ mL of acetylcystine solution per minute}$

10. $\dfrac{250 \cancel{\text{ mL}}}{\underset{3}{\cancel{90} \text{ min}}} \times \dfrac{\overset{2}{\cancel{60}} \mu\text{gtt}}{\cancel{\text{mL}}} = 166.6 \quad \text{or} \quad 167 \, \mu\text{gtt/min}$

11. $\dfrac{250 \text{ mL}}{60 \text{ min}} = 4.2 \text{ mL/min}$

12. a. $60 \cancel{\text{ kg}} \times \dfrac{50 \cancel{\text{ mcg}}}{\cancel{\text{kg}}} \times \dfrac{1 \text{ mL}}{200 \cancel{\text{ mcg}}} = 15 \text{ mL of Primacor}$

   b. $\dfrac{15 \text{ mL}}{10 \text{ min}} = 1.5 \text{ mL/min}$

13. $120 \cancel{\text{ mg}} \times \dfrac{1 \text{ g}}{1000 \cancel{\text{ mg}}} = 0.12 \text{ g in 1 tablet of verapamil}$

14. $136 \cancel{\text{ lb}} \times \dfrac{0.45 \cancel{\text{ kg}}}{\cancel{\text{lb}}} \times \dfrac{8.2 \cancel{\text{ mg}}}{\cancel{\text{kg}}} \times \dfrac{1 \text{ tab}}{500 \cancel{\text{ mg}}} = 1 \text{ tab of Amoxil}$

15. $\overset{2}{\cancel{20} \cancel{\text{ mg}}} \times \dfrac{1 \text{ tab}}{\underset{1}{\cancel{10} \cancel{\text{ mg}}}} = 2 \text{ tab of enalapril}$

16. $\dfrac{\overset{1}{\cancel{20} \cancel{\text{ mg}}}}{\cancel{\text{tab}}} \times \dfrac{\text{gr } 1}{\underset{3}{\cancel{60} \cancel{\text{ mg}}}} \times \dfrac{2 \text{ tab}}{1} = \text{grain } \dfrac{2}{3} \text{ of Prozac in 2 tab}$

17. a. D. O'Donavan, M.D.

   b. Imitrex and Regular insulin

   c. Sinemet; Entacapone

18. a. Imitrex administered at 10 A.M. and 6 P.M. 12/4/03

   b. RN Lou Rase

   c. Zantac, Sinemet, and Entacapone

   d. 8 doses of Entacapone 200 mg

19. a. 2 mL of Zantac

   b. $\dfrac{52 \text{ mL}}{20 \text{ min}} = 2.6 \text{ mL/min}$

20. $\dfrac{20 \cancel{\text{ mL}}}{20 \text{ min}} \times \dfrac{60 \, \mu\text{gtt}}{\cancel{\text{mL}}} = 60 \, \mu\text{gtt/min}$

21. $800 \text{ mL} \times \dfrac{\overset{1}{\cancel{15}} \text{ gtt}}{\text{mL}} \times \dfrac{1 \text{ min}}{31 \text{ gtt}} \times \dfrac{1 \text{ h}}{\underset{4}{\cancel{60} \text{ min}}} = 6.45 \text{ h}$ or   6 h and 27 min

22. $\dfrac{\overset{1}{\cancel{250}} \text{ mL}}{\underset{2}{\cancel{500} \text{ mg}}} \times \dfrac{2 \text{ mg}}{\text{min}} \times \dfrac{60 \text{ min}}{1 \text{ h}} = 60 \text{ mL/h}$

23. $\overset{5}{\cancel{25}} \text{ mg} \times \dfrac{1 \text{ mL}}{\underset{1}{\cancel{5} \text{ mg}}} = 5 \text{ mL of labetalol}$

24. $\dfrac{5\cancel{1}0 \text{ mL}}{100 \text{ mg}} \times \dfrac{0.05 \text{ mg}}{\text{min}} \times \dfrac{60 \text{ min}}{\text{h}} = 15.3 \text{ mL/h of Bretylate}$

25. a. $\dfrac{70 \text{ mL}}{500 \text{ mg}} \times \dfrac{0.1 \text{ mg}}{\text{kg} \times \text{min}} \times \dfrac{0.45 \text{ kg}}{\text{lb}} \times \dfrac{220 \text{ lb}}{1} \times \dfrac{15 \text{ gtt}}{\text{mL}}$

$= 20.19$ or   21 gtt/min

b. $\dfrac{21 \text{ gtt}}{\text{min}} \times \dfrac{1 \text{ mL}}{\underset{1}{\cancel{15} \text{ gtt}}} \times \dfrac{\overset{4}{\cancel{60} \text{ min}}}{\text{h}} = 84 \text{ mL/h}$

Comprehensive Self-Test 7

1. $8 \text{ lb} \times \dfrac{0.45 \text{ kg}}{1 \text{ lb}} \times \dfrac{\overset{1}{\cancel{25}} \text{ mg}}{\text{kg}} \times \dfrac{5 \text{ mL}}{\underset{5}{\cancel{125} \text{ mg}}} = 3.6 \text{ mL of neomycin sulfate}$

2. $44 \text{ lb} \times \dfrac{0.45 \text{ kg}}{1 \text{ lb}} \times \dfrac{10 \text{ mg}}{\text{kg}} \times \dfrac{\overset{1}{\cancel{5}} \text{ mL}}{\underset{25}{\cancel{125} \text{ mg}}} = 7.9 \text{ mL of Amoxicillin}$

3. $\dfrac{100 \text{ mL}}{\underset{4}{\cancel{60} \text{ min}}} \times \dfrac{\overset{1}{\cancel{15}} \text{ gtt}}{\text{mL}} = 25 \text{ gtt/min}$

4. $3000 \text{ mL} \times \dfrac{1 \text{ mL}}{\underset{1}{\cancel{100} \text{ mL}}} \times \dfrac{\overset{1}{\cancel{100}} \text{ mL}}{5 \text{ mL}} = 600 \text{ mL of the 5\% neosporin solution; add } H_2O \text{ up to the level of } 3000 \text{ mL}$

5. $0.5 \text{ mL} \times \dfrac{\overset{1}{\cancel{1000}} \text{ mg}}{\underset{1}{\cancel{1000} \text{ mL}}} = 0.5 \text{ mg of Epinephrine}$

6. $250 \text{ mg} \times \dfrac{5 \text{ mL}}{62.5 \text{ mg}} = 20 \text{ mL of Dynapen}$

7. a. $90 \text{ kg} \times \dfrac{2.5 \text{ mg}}{\text{kg}} = 225 \text{ mg of gentamycin}$

b. $\dfrac{210\,\text{mL}}{1.5\,\text{h}} = 140\,\text{mL/h}$

8. $0.3\,\text{g} \times \dfrac{1000\,\text{mg}}{1\,\text{g}} \times \dfrac{1\,\text{tab}}{300\,\text{mg}} = \dfrac{3\,\text{tab}}{3}$ or 1 tab of tenofovir

9. $1200\,\text{mg} \times \dfrac{1\,\text{g}}{1000\,\text{mg}} \times \dfrac{1\,\text{cap}}{0.2\,\text{g}} = \dfrac{12\,\text{cap}}{2} = 6\,\text{cap of saquinavir}$

10. $\overset{3}{750}\,\text{mg} \times \dfrac{1\,\text{g}}{\underset{4}{1000}\,\text{mg}} \times \dfrac{1\,\text{tab}}{0.25\,\text{g}} = \dfrac{3\,\text{tab}}{1} = 3\,\text{tab of relfinavir}$

11. $\dfrac{0.075\,\text{g}}{12\,\text{h}} \times \dfrac{1000\,\text{mg}}{1\,\text{g}} \times \dfrac{1\,\text{cap}}{75\,\text{mg}} \times \dfrac{24\,\text{h}}{\text{day}} \times 5\,\text{days} = 10\,\text{cap of Tamiflu in 5 days}$

12. $30\,\text{mg} \times \dfrac{1\,\text{g}}{1000\,\text{mg}} \times \dfrac{1\,\text{tab}}{0.015\,\text{g}} = 2\,\text{tab of Actos}$

13. $0.008\,\text{g} \times \dfrac{1000\,\text{mg}}{1\,\text{g}} \times \dfrac{1\,\text{tab}}{8\,\text{mg}} = 1\,\text{tab of Aceon}$

14. a. $174\,\text{lb} \times \dfrac{0.45\,\text{kg}}{1\,\text{lb}} \times \dfrac{10\,\text{mg}}{\text{kg}} \times \dfrac{1\,\text{mL}}{50\,\text{mg}} = 15.7\,\text{mL of amiodarone}$

b. $\dfrac{265.7\,\text{mL}}{24\,\text{h}} = 11.1\,\text{mL/h}$

15. $90\,\text{kg} \times \dfrac{0.05\,\text{mg}}{\text{kg}} \times \dfrac{\overset{1}{1000}\,\text{mL}}{\underset{1}{1000}\,\text{mg}} = 4.5\,\text{cubic centimeter of 1\% lidocaine}$

16. $\dfrac{100\,\text{mg}}{2\,\text{mL}}$ so you will give 2 mL of phenytoin IM to patient

17. $0.5\,\text{mg} \times \dfrac{1\,\text{mL}}{1\,\text{mg}} = 0.5\,\text{mL of Glucagon}$

18. $\overset{2}{6}\,\text{mg} \times \dfrac{1\,\text{mL}}{\underset{1}{3}\,\text{mg}} = 2\,\text{mL of adenosine}$

19. $\overset{1}{25}\,\text{g} \times \dfrac{\overset{2}{100}\,\text{mL}}{\underset{1}{25}\,\text{g}} \times \dfrac{1\,\text{bottle}}{\underset{1}{50}\,\text{mL}} = 2\,\text{bottles of albumin}$

20. a. 2000 mg of Cafadyl in 100 mL

b. $\dfrac{100\,\text{mL}}{120\,\text{min}} \times \dfrac{60\,\mu\text{gtt}}{\text{mL}} = 50\,\mu\text{gtt/min}$

21. $\overset{2}{\cancel{320}} \text{ mg} \times \dfrac{1 \text{ tab}}{\underset{1}{\cancel{160} \text{ mg}}} = 2 \text{ tab of Betapace}$

22. a. $34 \cancel{\text{ kg}} \times \dfrac{0.06 \text{ mg}}{\cancel{\text{kg}}} = 2.04 \text{ mg of Somatropin}$

    b. $2.04 \cancel{\text{ mg}} \times \dfrac{5 \text{ mL}}{5 \cancel{\text{ mg}}} = 2.04 \text{ mL of Somatropin}$

23. a. $\overset{1}{\cancel{400}} \cancel{\text{ mg}} \times \dfrac{200 \text{ mL}}{\underset{1}{\cancel{400}} \cancel{\text{ mg}}} = 200 \text{ mL contain 200 mg of Cipro}$

    b. 200 mL in 1 h

24. $\overset{3}{\cancel{1875}} \cancel{\text{ mg}} \times \dfrac{5 \text{ mL}}{\underset{2}{\cancel{1250}} \cancel{\text{ mg}}} = 7.5 \text{ mL of calcium carbonate}$

25. $\cancel{\text{gr}} \dfrac{1}{\cancel{1000}} \times \dfrac{\cancel{60} \text{ mg}}{\cancel{\text{gr}} 1} = 0.06 \text{ mg}$

APPENDIX B

Common Abbreviations on Medication Orders

To someone unfamiliar with prescriptive abbreviations, medication orders may look like a foreign language. To interpret prescriptive orders accurately and to administer drugs safely, a qualified person must have a thorough knowledge of common abbreviations. For instance, when the prescriber writes, "**Hydromorphone 1.5 mL IM q4h pc & hs**," the administrator knows how to interpret it as "Hydromorphone, 1.5 milliliters, intramuscular, every four hours, after meals and at hour of sleep." Study the following list of common abbreviations for smooth navigation through the medication orders in this book. For measurement abbreviations, refer to Appendix C.

Abbreviation	Meaning	Abbreviation	Meaning
$\overline{a}$	before (abante)	elix	elixir
$\overline{aa}$	of each	F	Fahrenheit
ac	before meals (ante cibum)	g	gram
		gr	grain
ad	up to (ad)	gtt	drop
ad lib	as desired (ad libitum)	h, hr, H	hour
A.M., am	morning	hs, HS	hour of sleep; bedtime (hora somni)
amp	ampule		
aq	aqueous water	IC	intracardia
bi	two	ID	intradermal
bid, BID	two times a day	IM	intramuscular
$\overline{c}$	with	IV	intravenous
C	Celsius; centigrade	IVP	intravenous push
cap	capsule	IVPB	intravenous piggyback
cc	cubic centimeter	kg	kilogram
CVP	central venous pressure	KVO	keep vein open
d	day	L	liter
DC, dc	discontinue	LA	long acting
dr or ℨ	dram	lb	pound
D/W	dextrose in water	LIB	left in bag, left in bottle
D5W or D/5/W or D_5W	5% dextrose in water	ℳ	minim
Dx	diagnosis	mcg or μg	microgram

Abbreviation	Meaning	Abbreviation	Meaning
mEq	milliequivalent	q2h	every two hours
mg	milligram	q3h	every three hours
min	minute	q4h	every four hours
mL	milliliter	q6h	every six hours
mU	milliunit	q8h	every eight hours
n	night	q12h	every 12 hours
NKA	no known allergies	qid, QID	four times a day *(quarter in die)*
NPO	nothing by mouth *(per ora)*		
NS	normal saline	qod	every other day
NSAID	nonsteroidal anti-inflammatory drug	qn	every night *(quaque noct)*
		qs	quantity sufficient or sufficient amount *(quantitas sufficiens)*
od	every day *(omni die)*		
OD	right eye *(oculus dexter)*		
OS	left eye *(oculus sinister)*	R/O	rule out
OU	both eyes	R	respiration
℥ or oz	ounce	s̄	without *(sine)*
p̄	after	sc, SC, SQ	subcutaneous
PEG	percutaneous endoscopic gastrostony tube	sl, sL	under the tongue (sublingual)
		SR	sustained release
		s̄s̄ ss	one-half
P	pulse	sos	if necessary
pc	after meals *(post cibum)*	stat	immediately *(statum)*
PICC	peripherally inserted central catheter	supp	suppository
		susp	suspension
P.M., pm	afternoon, evening	T	temperature
po, PO	by mouth *(per os)*	t or tsp	teaspoon
postop	after surgery	T or tbs	tablespoon
preop	before surgery	tab	tablet
prn	when required or whenever necessary	tid, TID	three times a day *(ter in die)*
		TPN	total parenteral nutrition
pt	pint	u	unit
Pt	patient	wt	weight
q	every *(quaque)*	>	greater than
qd	every day *(quaque die)*	<	less than
qh	every hour *(quaque hora)*		

APPENDIX C

Units of Measurement in Metric, Household, and Apothecary Systems

Abbreviations

Volume	Metric		Household
milliliter	mL	microdrop	μgtt or mcgtt
liter	L	drop	gtt
cubic centimeter	cc	teaspoon	t or tsp
		tablespoon	T or tbs
Apothecary		fluid ounce	℥
minim	ℳ	pint	pt
fluid dram	ʒ	quart	qt
		gallon	gal

Weight	Metric		Household
microgram	μg or mcg	ounces	℥ or oz
milligram	mg	pound	lb
gram	g		
kilogram	kg		
Apothecary			
grain	gr		
dram	ʒ		

Length	Metric		Household
centimeter	cm	inch	in
meter	m	foot	ft
		yard	yd

Area	Metric
square meter	m^2

Numeric	Apothecary		Other
$\frac{1}{2}$	ss	milliunit	mU
		unit	u or U
$1\frac{1}{2}$	iss	milliequivalent	mEq
$2\frac{1}{2}$	iiss		
		Roman	
$7\frac{1}{2}$	viiss	1 I	7 VII
		2 II	10 X
		3 III	15 XV
		4 IV	20 XX
		5 V	25 XXV
		6 VI	30 XXX

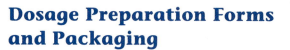

Dosage Preparation Forms and Packaging

Preparation Forms

Medications are manufactured in many preparation forms. Each form serves a distinct purpose. One form might release medication into the body at a slower rate than another. One form might be manufactured to facilitate swallowing. Use the following definitions of preparation forms as a reference for understanding medication orders.

Aqueous solution   One or more medications completely dissolved in water.

Capsule   Gelatinous container enclosing a powder, a liquid, or time-release granules of medication.

Elixir   Medication dissolved in a mixture of water, alcohol, sweeteners, and flavoring.

Metered-dose inhaler   Aerosol device containing multiple doses of medication for inhalation.

Ointment   Semisolid preparation of medication to be applied to the skin.

Suppository   Mixture of medication with a firm base that melts at body temperature and is molded into a shape suitable for insertion into body cavities.

Suspension   Finely divided particles of medication undissolved in water.

Syrup   Medication in water and sugar solution.

Tablet   Powdered medication compressed or molded into a small disk.

Transdermal patch   Adhesive disk that attaches to the skin with a center reservoir containing medication to be slowly absorbed through the skin.

Parenteral Packaging

There are three common types of parenteral medication containers for sterile solutions.

Ampule   Sealed glass container with only one dose of powdered or liquid medication.

Prefilled cartridge   Single-dose syringe with an attached needle. A metal or plastic holder is used to inject the medication.

Vial   Sealed glass container of a liquid or powdered medication with a rubber stopper, allowing multiple-dose use.

APPENDIX E

Celsius and Fahrenheit Temperature Conversions

Reading and recording a temperature is a crucial step in assessing a patient's health. Temperatures can be measured using either the Fahrenheit (F) scale or the Celsius or centigrade (C) scale. Most health-care settings use Fahrenheit, but some are switching to Celsius. Celsius/Fahrenheit equivalency tables make it easy to convert Celsius to Fahrenheit, or vice versa. Still, it is useful to be able to make this conversion yourself.

You can use the following rules to convert from one temperature scale to the other

---
NOTE

$$F = \frac{9}{5}C + 32 \quad \text{or} \quad C = \frac{5}{9}(F - 32)$$

For those unfamiliar with algebra, the following rules are equivalent to the algebraic formulas.

First rule: To convert to Celsius. Subtract 32 and then divide by 1.8.

Second rule: To convert to Fahrenheit. Multiply by 1.8 and then add 32.

NOTE

Temperatures are rounded to the nearest tenth.

Example E.1

Convert 102.5° F to Celsius.

Using the first rule, we subtract 32.

$$\begin{array}{r} 102.5 \\ -32.0 \\ \hline 70.5 \end{array}$$

Then we divide by 1.8.

$$1.8 \overline{)70.5\,000} \quad 39.17$$

So, 102.5° F equals 39.2° C.

Example E.2

Convert 3° C to Fahrenheit.

Using the second rule, we first multiply by 1.8.

$$
\begin{array}{r}
1.8 \\
\times 3 \\
\hline
5.4
\end{array}
$$

Then we add 32.

$$
\begin{array}{r}
5.4 \\
+32.0 \\
\hline
37.4
\end{array}
$$

So, 3° C equals 37.4° F.

APPENDIX F

Tables of Weight Conversions

Use the following tables to convert between the metric kilogram and the household pound.

Table F.1

Pounds to Kilograms					
lb	**kg**	**lb**	**kg**	**lb**	**kg**
2.2	1.0	120	54.5	240	109.1
5	2.3	125	56.8	245	111.4
10	4.5	130	59.1	250	113.6
15	6.8	135	61.4	255	115.9
20	9.1	140	63.6	260	118.2
25	11.4	145	65.9	265	120.5
30	13.6	150	68.2	270	122.7
35	15.9	155	70.5	275	125
40	18.2	160	72.7	280	127.3
45	20.5	165	75	285	129.5
50	22.7	170	77.3	290	131.8
55	25	175	79.5	295	134.1
60	27.3	180	81.8	300	136.4
65	29.5	185	84.1	305	138.6
70	31.8	190	86.4	310	140.9
75	34.1	195	88.6	315	143.2
80	36.4	200	90.9	320	145.5
85	38.6	205	93.2	325	147.7
90	40.9	210	95.5	330	150
95	43.2	215	97.7	335	152.3
100	45.5	220	100	340	154.5
105	47.7	225	102.3	345	156.8
110	50	230	104.5	350	159.1
115	52.3	235	106.8	355	161.4

Table F.2

Kilograms to Pounds

kg	lb	kg	lb	kg	lb
2	4.4	56	123.2	110	242
4	8.8	58	127.6	112	246.4
6	13.2	60	132	114	250.8
8	17.6	62	136.4	116	255.2
10	22	64	140.8	118	259.6
12	26.4	66	145.2	120	264
14	30.8	68	149.6	122	268.4
16	35.2	70	154	124	272.8
18	39.6	72	158.4	126	277.2
20	44	74	162.8	128	281.6
22	48.4	76	167.2	130	286
24	52.8	78	171.6	132	290.4
26	57.2	80	176	134	294.8
28	61.6	82	180.4	136	299.2
30	66	84	184.8	138	303.6
32	70.4	86	189.2	140	308
34	74.8	88	193.6	142	312.4
36	79.2	90	198	144	316.8
38	83.6	92	202.4	146	321.2
40	88	94	206.8	148	325.6
42	92.4	96	211.2	150	330
44	96.8	98	215.6	152	334.4
46	101.2	100	220	154	338.8
48	105.6	102	224.4	156	343.2
50	110	104	228.8	158	347.6
52	114.4	106	233.2	160	352
54	118.8	108	237.6	162	356.4

APPENDIX G

Nomograms

Dosages are sometimes based on a patient's body surface area (BSA), and nomograms are the equivalency charts used to determine the patient's BSA.

Pediatric Nomogram

The boxed column listing weight on the left and surface in square meters on the right can be used when a child is of normal height for his or her weight.

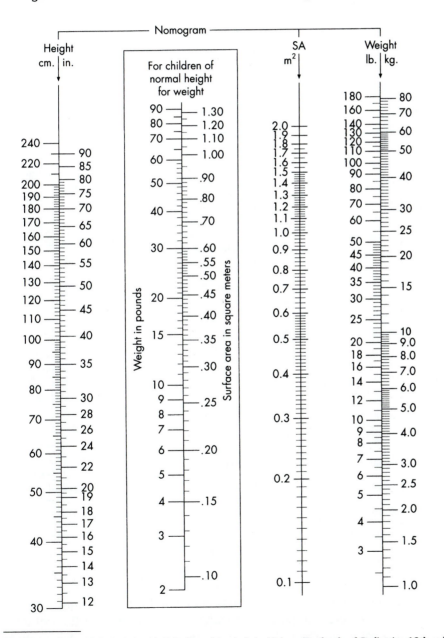

Courtesy of R.E. Behrman and V.C. Vaughn, (eds.), *Nelson Textbook of Pediatrics* 13th ed., Philadelphia: W.B. Saunders Co., 1987. Reprinted with permission

Adult Nomogram

HEIGHT	BODY SURFACE AREA	WEIGHT

To use the nomogram, you need the patient's weight and height. Draw a straight line between the patient's height (first column) and the patient's weight (last column). The point at which the line crosses the SA column is the estimated **BSA in square meters**.

APPENDIX H

Ratio and Proportion Method for Dosage Calculation

There are methods other than Dimensional Analysis that can be used to calculate drug dosages.

Memorized formulas like

$$\text{Amount to administer} = \frac{\text{Desired dose}}{\text{Dose on hand}} \times \text{Quantity on hand}$$

were once popular.

Another technique uses a ratio and proportion approach and is illustrated in the following examples.

Example H.1

If each tablet contains 5 mg, how many tablets contain 15 mg?
The information in the example is summarized in the following table:

Known equivalent	1 tablet = 5 mg
Unknown equivalent	x tablets = 15 mg

The equivalents in the table are written as fractions (ratios) and are equated to form the following proportion:

$$\frac{1 \text{ tab}}{5 \text{ mg}} = \frac{x \text{ tab}}{15 \text{ mg}}$$

x is found by algebraically solving the proportion

$$\frac{1}{5} = \frac{x}{15}$$

Now, cross-multiply

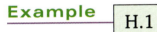

$$5x = 15$$

Now, divide both sides by 5

$$\frac{5x}{5} = \frac{15}{5}$$

Cancel

$$\frac{\cancel{5}x}{\cancel{5}} = \frac{\overset{3}{\cancel{15}}}{\cancel{5}}$$

$$x = 3$$

So, 3 tablets contain 15 mg.

Example H.2

A vial label states: $\dfrac{75\,\text{mg}}{5\,\text{mL}}$. How many milliliters of this solution contains 10 milligrams of the drug?

The information in the example is summarized in the following table:

Known equivalent	75 mg = 5 mL
Unknown equivalent	10 mg = x mL

The equivalents in the table are written as fractions (ratios) and are equated to form the following proportion:

$$\frac{75\,\text{mg}}{5\,\text{mL}} = \frac{10\,\text{mg}}{x\,\text{mL}}$$

x is found by algebraically solving the proportion

$$\frac{75}{5} = \frac{10}{x}$$

Now, cross-multiply

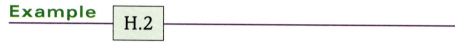

$$50 = 75x$$

Now, divide both sides by 75

$$\frac{50}{75} = \frac{75x}{75}$$

Cancel

$$\frac{\overset{2}{\cancel{50}}}{\underset{3}{\cancel{75}}} = \frac{\cancel{75}x}{\cancel{75}}$$

$$x = \frac{2}{3} \quad \text{or} \quad 0.67$$

So, 0.67 mL contains 10 mg of the drug.

Example   H.3

If an IV containing 880 mL is to infuse in 8 hours, then how long will it take for 350 mL of this IV to infuse?

The information in the example is summarized in the following table:

Known equivalent	880 mL = 8 h
Unknown equivalent	350 mL = x h

The equivalents in the table are written as fractions (ratios) and are equated to form the proportion below:

$$\frac{880 \text{ mL}}{8 \text{ h}} = \frac{350 \text{ mL}}{x \text{ h}}$$

x is found by algebraically solving the proportion

$$\frac{880}{8} = \frac{350}{x}$$

Now, cross-multiply

$$\frac{880}{8} \diagdown \frac{350}{x}$$

$$880x = 2800$$

Now, divide both sides by 880

$$\frac{880x}{880} = \frac{2800}{880}$$

Cancel

$$\frac{\cancel{880}x}{\cancel{880}} = \frac{2800}{880}$$

$$x = \frac{2800}{880} \quad \text{or} \quad 3.18$$

So, it will take about 3.18 hours for 350 mL to infuse.

To change 0.18 h to minutes, ratio and proportion could also be used.

Known equivalent	1 h = 60 min
Unknown equivalent	0.18 h = x min

The equivalents in the table are written as fractions (ratios) and are equated to form the proportion below:

$$\frac{1\,h}{60\,min} = \frac{0.18\,h}{x\,min}$$

x is found by algebraically solving the proportion

$$\frac{1}{60} = \frac{0.18}{x}$$

Now, cross-multiply

$$\frac{1}{60} \underset{\diagdown}{\times} \frac{0.18}{x}$$

$$10.8 = x$$

So, it will take about 3 hours and 11 minutes for 350 mL to infuse.

INDEX